AF615771

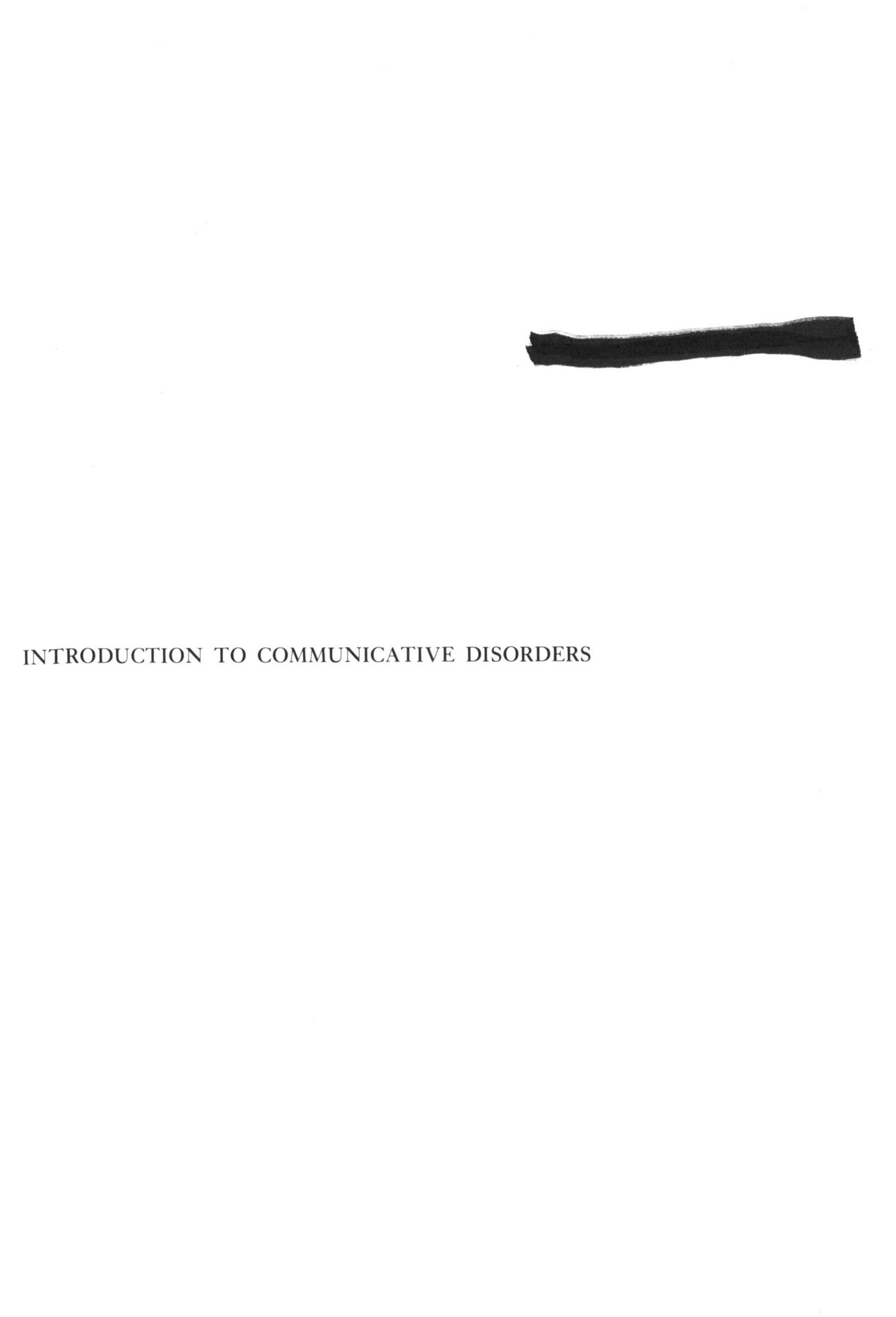

INTRODUCTION TO COMMUNICATIVE DISORDERS

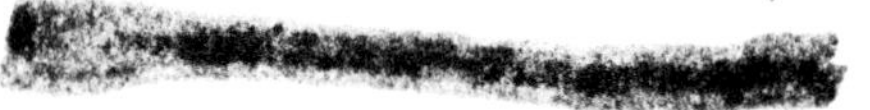

INTRODUCTION TO COMMUNICATIVE DISORDERS

Margaret C. Byrne
University of Kansas

Chris C. Shervanian
Northeastern Illinois University

HARPER & ROW, PUBLISHERS
New York, Hagerstown, San Francisco, London

Sponsoring Editor: Larry Sifford
Project Editor: David Nickol
Designer: T. R. Funderburk
Production Supervisor: Kewal K. Sharma
Compositor: Bi-Comp, Incorporated
Printer and binder: Halliday Lithograph Corporation
Art Studio: Danmark & Michaels Inc.
Photographs: Richard Gwin
Cover design: Donya Melanson Associates/Illustration: Dorothy Kegel

INTRODUCTION TO COMMUNICATIVE DISORDERS

Library of Congress Cataloging in Publication Data

Byrne, Margaret C
Introduction to communicative disorders.

Includes index.
1. Communicative disorders. 2. Communicative disorders in children. I. Shervanian, Chris C., Date– joint author. II. Title. [DNLM: 1. Language disorders. 2. Speech disorders. 3. Speech therapy. WM475 B995i]
RC423.B95 616.8'55 76-46409
ISBN 0-06-041116-3

CONTENTS

PREFACE

This text deals with the processes of oral communication and the deficits that can occur during and following their normal development. We have written it primarily for two groups of readers—those who are exploring various aspects of communicative disorders as a potential professional field and those teachers and teachers-in-training who expect to be working with children. The former group may eventually become speech and language clinicians, teachers of the hearing impaired, audiologists, speech pathologists, or speech and hearing scientists. The latter group may be the elementary classroom teachers, resource-room specialists who provide a wide variety of services for exceptional children, itinerant teachers who plan educational intervention for many pupils in different school buildings, and teachers and supervisors in special education programs.

In preparing this book we were guided by several purposes. Our first purpose is to provide a system for studying an individual's language and communications skills. Therefore, we have described the normal aspects of the structure of language—the sounds that make up the words, the grammar of language, and its semantics—and the functions. We then discuss the acquisition of each of these aspects and, with what is normal as a guide, the types of deficits that occur.

Our second purpose is to review the factors that contribute to normal and abnormal communication. We refer to these as the determinants—physical, psychological, and social. Here again we consider the normal and the pathological aspects of each, using the themes of structure, function, and deficit. We show the interrelationships among the determinants and our resultant difficulty in determining why a deficit has developed.

Our third purpose is to help the student to understand the contributions that many people make to the development of a child's communication and the maintenance of the adult's system and to provide general principles for programs of intervention or remediation. We describe current representative programs so that teachers and clinicians can begin to evaluate the many approaches that are available.

Our final and overriding purpose is to encourage students and parents to develop a positive philosophy about our relations and responsibilities to those with delays and deficits in language and communication. Our laws mandate that every person must be provided with an educational program that fits his or her needs. Our social obligation is to support and participate in planning for the integration of all those with special problems in our society. Many of them cannot speak for themselves.

We have organized our book to cover topics in the following sequence. Chapter 1 presents a description of communicative disorders, an overview of their magnitude, the responsibilities of the profession of speech pathology and audiology, which deals with these disorders, the forces that are shaping the profession, and our theoretical frame of reference of the multiple determinants of language and communication. Chapter 2 is concerned with the structure and functions of language, Chapter 3 with its acquisition and deficits. In Chapters 4, 5, and 6 we present the three major categories of normal and pathological determinants—the physical, which deal with the anatomical and physiological structures; the psychological, which present the structures of cognition, learning, and personality; and the social, which cover the structures of class, role, and social institutions. In Chapter 7 we discuss the roles of the parent, clinician, and teacher in child language development and offer some general guidelines for program planning for the clinician and the teacher. In that chapter some existing programs are described and ideas for developing new ones are suggested. Since students are most accessible for programs designed to develop their optimal skills in language and communication in the school, Chapter 8 deals in greater detail with the role of the clinician in school programming. The epilogue provides a brief summary.

We would like to thank our students and our friends who have contributed in many ways to the completion of this book.

Margaret C. Byrne
Chris C. Shervanian

INTRODUCTION TO COMMUNICATIVE DISORDERS

INTRODUCTION TO COMMUNICATION AND ITS DISORDERS
Chapter 1

This chapter provides an overview of the field of communication disorders. It begins with a description of communication and its many processes. The disorders are identified and data on incidence are reviewed. The profession of speech pathology and audiology and the responsibilities of its members are discussed. The value of studying why children and adults talk as they do is considered. The social changes that are influencing the work of the speech specialist are discussed briefly. And, finally, a frame of reference for thinking about normal and abnormal communication is presented.

DESCRIPTION

Although we have many modes for conveying our ideas, most of us are concerned primarily with three: we talk, we write, and we use gestures. The person with whom we are communicating can listen to our words, read the message we write, and observe our signs and gestures. The sender of a message selects an appropriate set of symbols or signs to convey an idea; and the receiver has the task of understanding the message, and making an appropriate response.

The word *communication* conveys different meanings to various professional groups. The speech pathologists and audiologists are concerned with several components: (1) the expressive aspects that include its formulation into meaningful words and sentences; (2) its transmission; (3) its reception, including hearing and comprehension; and (4) its social psychological or its interpersonal aspects. Since it is a social act, it involves individuals and groups of people. The greatest concern of speech pathologists and audiologists is with speaking and listening rather than the writing and reading, although we recognize the interrelationship among the four.

The study of the disorders of communication involves all the processes that contribute to communication that may have gone awry. These include language, paralanguage, speech production, audition, cognition, and the interpersonal relations that underly communication.

Those who are concerned with communication disorders draw upon the research of fellow speech pathologists, audiologists, and speech and hearing scientists on the normal and abnormal aspects of communication. They also utilize information from other fields—linguistics, psychology, sociology, physiology, physics, neurology, child development, and education. They reintegrate the data and formulate new principles to guide their work.

In order to obtain an understanding of the complex nature of communication disorders, it seems appropriate first to describe or define the processes involved.

LANGUAGE

In order to communicate with one another, people use a code, that is, a system of symbols or signs to stand for "real" things. The assigned meanings of the symbols are agreed upon by the members of a society. To serve the purpose of conveying a message the symbols are strung together in accordance with rules and forms also agreed upon by the society. The symbols and the rules constitute language. We shall be studying four major components of language—its phonology, morphology, syntax, and semantics.

PARALANGUAGE

There are other ways to convey meaning—gestures, facial expressions, body movements, and other aspects of appearance, such as clothes. These nonverbal means of communication are called paralanguage.

Sometimes the meaning of words is contradicted by nonverbal cues. We tell a child he's been a naughty boy, but at the same time we smile at him. We can say *no*, but our eyes signal *yes*. We cannot always be sure to what we react in the communication exchange. When the mother says to her 12-month-old child, "No, no no. You mustn't eat the dirt," the child with a fistful of mud close to his mouth may hesitate because of his mother's words, her accompanying gestures, or a combination of these cues.

Paralanguage is also associated with oral language, but it is distinct from it. According to Trager (1958), it includes the pitch of the voice—its highness or lowness; the quality or timbre; the loudness or variations in loudness; the tempo or rate; and rhythm or fluency. In addition, it includes vocalizations such as giggling, crying, and utterances such as *uh-hu* that have meaning but are not the usual phonological pattern of English.

SPEECH PRODUCTION

The physical process of speech production utilizes structures located in the upper half of the human body. It involves coordinated movements of the mechanisms of breathing and voice and speech sound production. Impulses for speech originate in the brain and are carried out by the appropriate muscle groups.

The French use the word *la langue* to indicate the code and *la parole* to indicate the production of the code. In English these are referred to as language and speech production, respectively.

AUDITION

Most of us learn a language as a result of hearing others use it. The hearing mechanism, the sensory system which provides for the reception of audible signals, is an integral part of the processing of information by the brain. It also serves as a self-monitoring device in speech production.

COGNITION

Cognition is the act of knowing. It includes awareness, perception, conceptualization, differentiation, and thought. Some equate cognition with conceptualization and others describe it as thought, but however it is defined cognition enables the individual to learn about his world and hopefully to manage himself competently in his society as a result. In the communication system it is cognition that enables the individual to comprehend, interpret, and use the symbols.

INTERPERSONAL RELATIONS

Communication is concerned with people's reactions to one another. When two or more individuals greet one another, tell about an event, or ask opinions, they are engaged in a social act which involves transmission, reception, understanding, and response.

COMMUNICATION DISORDERS

An oral communication disorder is speaking or listening behavior that deviates from the standard or accepted patterns, as judged by the speaker himself or by the listener. Standards are set by the speakers and listeners who are recognized in our society as average communicators. Patterns for emulation are provided by social leaders, political figures, educators, and television personalities. Children are still developing their command of language until age 12, so their methods of expressing themselves are evaluated according to norms established for various age groups. An individual may judge his communication pattern inadequate, even though it is regarded as acceptable by his listeners. Or, an individual may consider his speech adequate, but become aware of his listeners' lack of acceptance of his speech production or language. For these individuals, their communication patterns trigger an internal negative evaluation and result in a downgrading of their personal esteem.

Deviations in the expressive portion of communication have been classified in different ways by speech pathologists. The two major categories are deviations in the code and in its production. *Language disorders* are deviations in any aspect of its structure or its functions. The structure of language consists of its phonologic, morphologic, syntactic, and semantic aspects. Its functions are the uses to which it is put. *Articulation disorders* are those associated with the inadequate production of speech sounds in words, phrases, and sentences. Examples of deviations are sound substitutions, omissions, and distortions. When there are many inconsistent errors, the speech may be unintelligible, that is, the message may be lost. Another form of disorder, called a *voice disorder*, is a marked difference from others of the same sex, age, and cultural background in the pitch, loudness, or quality of voice of an individual. *Stuttering, or dysfluency*, is a disturbance in the rhythm of speech, marked by intermittent blocking, repetition, or prolongation of the sounds, syllables, words, phrases, sentences, or postures of the speech production mechanism.

Deviations in reception include those of hearing and comprehension. Hearing losses may be conductive or sensorineural, or a combination of the two. Deficits in comprehension are those associated with understanding the message. One type is aphasia.

Deviations in interpersonal relations are those related to personality factors in neuroses and psychoses. In addition there are others that are associated with the somatopsychologic aspects of communication.

The communicative disorders may represent a failure in development, a failure to master the appropriate level of communication, a loss following normal development, or an inappropriate use of the communication system. The deficits may be classified as mild, moderate, or severe from the point of view of the speaker or the listener.

INCIDENCE

Although the statistics vary depending upon the definitions used in surveys, incidence figures are high. A national study based on a random demographic sample of about 40,000 school pupils provided information about overall speech performance, voice, fluency, articulation, and hearing (Hull, 1969). Language analyses were not undertaken. Samples of conversational speech elicited through questions and presentation of pictures were audiorecorded and then evaluated on a rating scale by speech pathologists for speech proficiency, articulation, voice, and fluency. The adult General American dialect was used as the standard for judging the tapes. Hearing was measured in a sound-treated booth, using pure-tone audiometry. Although a picture test was given to determine the accuracy of sound production, these data are not available. This carefully executed study provided the percentages of deviations shown in Figure 1–1.

There are some limitations we must consider when we interpret these data. We do not know how many of the sample were pupils from special classes—whether accelerated or special education classrooms. Since language analyses were not made, it is not possible to estimate the incidence of language deviations. However, the language used by the students contributes to their speech proficiency rating, because it is an important variable. The information on articulation is gross, because it is based on judgments about the taped conversational speech. Those with extreme hearing losses had been identified at younger ages for the most part and were already enrolled in schools for the deaf. We do not know how many of the students had multiple communication deficiencies.

In spite of the incompleteness of these data, they provide us with some important

Degree and Type of Deviation	Percent
Acceptable overall speech pattern	34.7
Mild overall speech deviation	53.1
Moderate overall speech deviations	10.6
Extreme overall speech deviation	*1.5*
Acceptable articulation	66.4
Moderate articulation deviations	31.6
Extreme articulation deviations	*2.0*
Acceptable voice	50.1
Moderate voice deviation	46.8
Extreme voice deviation	*3.1*
Acceptable fluency	99.2
Dysfluent	*.8*
Normal bilateral hearing	88.8
Reduced Hearing	*11.2*

Figure 1–1. National speech survey incidence of disorders, 1968–1969. (F. M. Hull et al. Based on data from *National speech and hearing survey interim report* (Project No. 50978). Washington, D.C.: Department of Health, Education, and Welfare, Office of Education, Bureau of Education for the Handicapped, 1969.)

clues about the communication disorders of a public school national sample. If we use only the percentages for extreme overall speech deviations, we have as a minimum 1.5 percent, or 3 out of every 200 pupils with very limited speech proficiency. If we include the group with moderate deviation, the percent rises to 12, or 12 out of 100 with problems. The latter figure is closer tò the percent currently enrolled for speech and hearing problems in some states.

In terms of the various disorders we note that 2 percent had extreme articulation deviations, 3.1 percent had extreme voice deviations, .8 percent were dysfluent, and 11.2 percent had reduced hearing (with reduced hearing defined as a loss of at least 20 dB in one ear).

The incidence of disorders by grade levels was also examined. There was an increase in the percentage of pupils in grades 1 through 12 who have acceptable overall speech patterns (Figure 1–2), acceptable articulation (Figure 1–3), and acceptable voice patterns (Figure 1–4). There was a decrease in the percent of students who stutter (Figure 1–5). Examination of the data on deviant hearing indicates that prevalence is highest in the first grade, declines until fourth grade, and stays relatively constant until twelfth grade when there is an increase.

In comparing the performances of first graders and twelfth graders, we find that at least 15 percent of the former but only about 50 percent of the latter have no speech deviations. We should ask ourselves: How did those first graders achieve adult speech patterns? Why haven't more of the twelfth graders developed acceptable proficiency? If some can, why not all or most? We will return to these questions later.

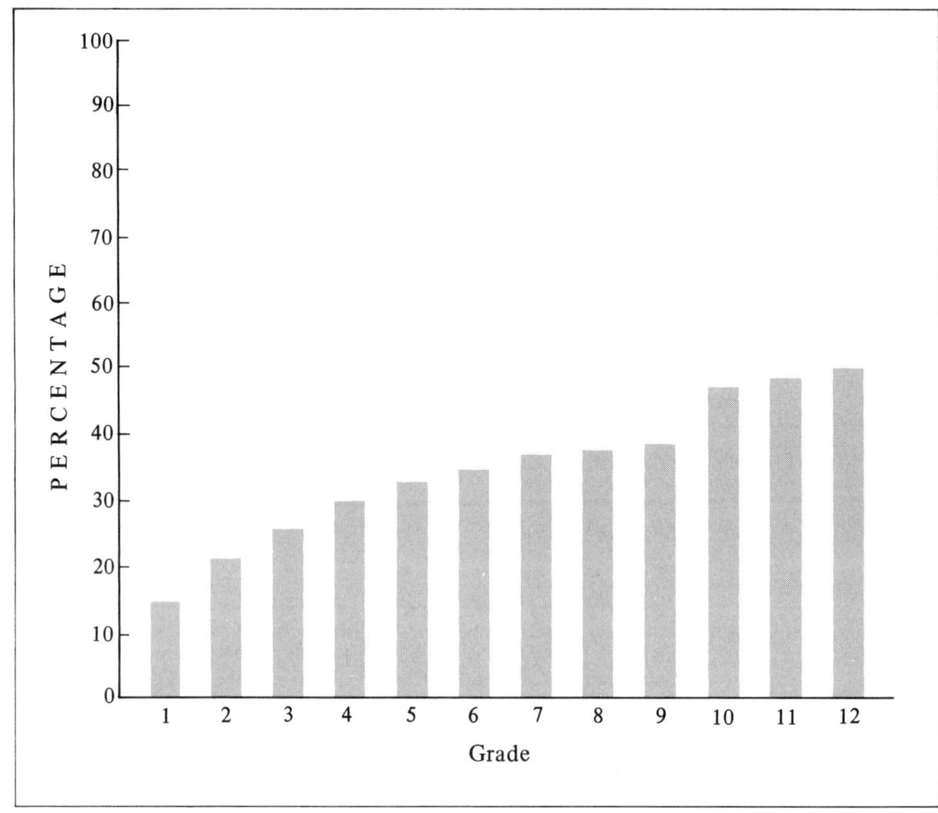

Figure 1–2. Acceptable overall speech patterns. (F. M. Hull et al. *National speech and hearing survey interim report* (Project No. 50978). Washington, D.C.: Department of Health, Education, and Welfare, Office of Education, Bureau of Education for the Handicapped, 1969.)

On the basis of information provided by state departments of education, the U.S. Bureau for the Education of the Handicapped estimated that for the academic year 1968–1969 there were more than two million students who needed speech, language, and hearing services. The estimate reflected both the excellent and inferior case-finding and reporting of the various states. Some states did not have a coordinator of speech and hearing services in their departments of education, to provide accurate data. In the intervening years, the number of school-age children has increased, and speech and language deficits have been redefined. Data from individual states seem more useful.

In 1974 the state of New Mexico published the results of its survey. It identified almost 8 percent of its school-age population as being speech impaired. The definition of speech impaired was "any deviation in speech or language which is outside the range of acceptable variation in a given environment." Bilingual children were not included in this total. If they had been, the percent would have been higher.

Since some conditions are identifiable at birth or shortly afterwards and since some states require that certain conditions be reported by the attending physician, we have some reliable data on their incidence. For example, 1 child in 800 live births will be born with a cleft palate; 1 in 700 will be identified as a child with cerebral palsy; 1 in

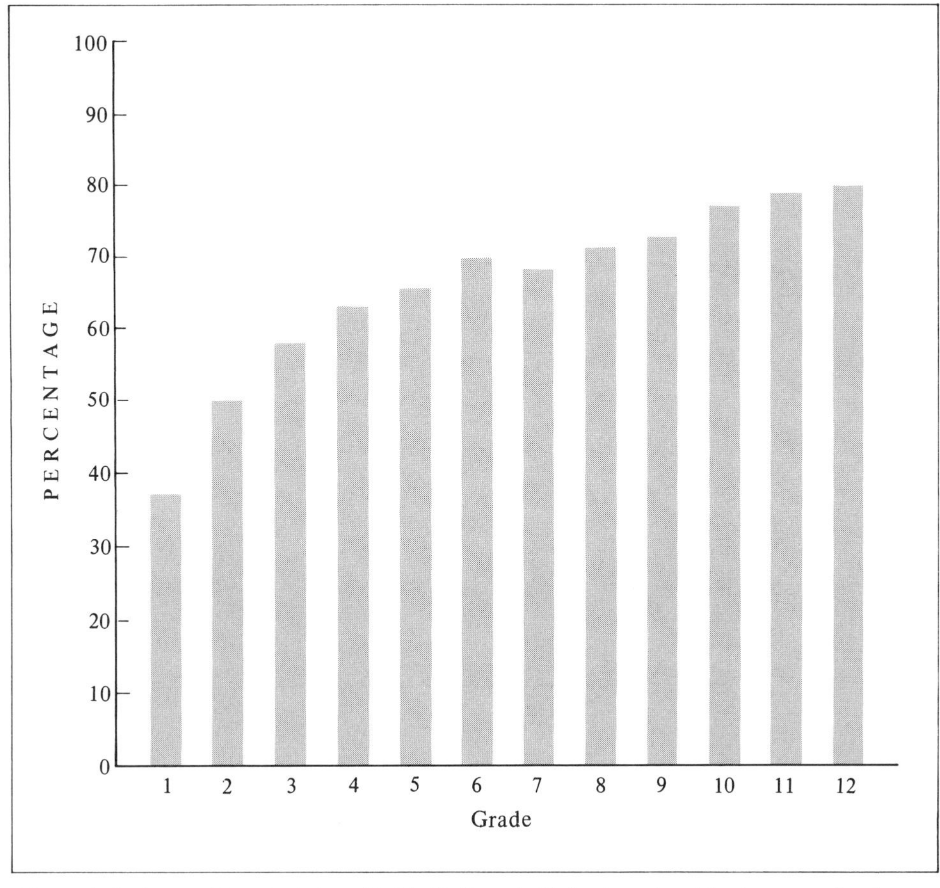

Figure 1–3. Acceptable articulation. (F. M. Hull et al. *National speech and hearing survey interim report* (Project No. 50978). Washington, D.C.: Department of Health, Education, and Welfare, Office of Education, Bureau of Education for the Handicapped, 1969.)

700 will have Down's syndrome (mongolism); 1 in 10,000 will have phenylketonuria (PKU), a metabolic disorder. All children with these conditions will require evaluation and many will need therapy.

There has been no decrease in the number of children with these various problems. In fact, it may be that there are more children being born today who have these and other deficits which require our evaluation and clinical intervention. The fact that many children who might have died at birth are being saved as a result of more effective medical care is an indicator that the incidence of communicative deficits will continue to increase rather than to decrease.

Our estimates about incidence for preschool and institutionalized individuals, school dropouts, and adults are quite gross or nonexistent. Marge (1972) indicated that 6.5 percent of those between 4 and 17 years had oral language disabilities. His figure includes appropriate percentages of mentally retarded, emotionally disturbed, learning disabled, deaf and hard-of-hearing, and those with articulation deficits.

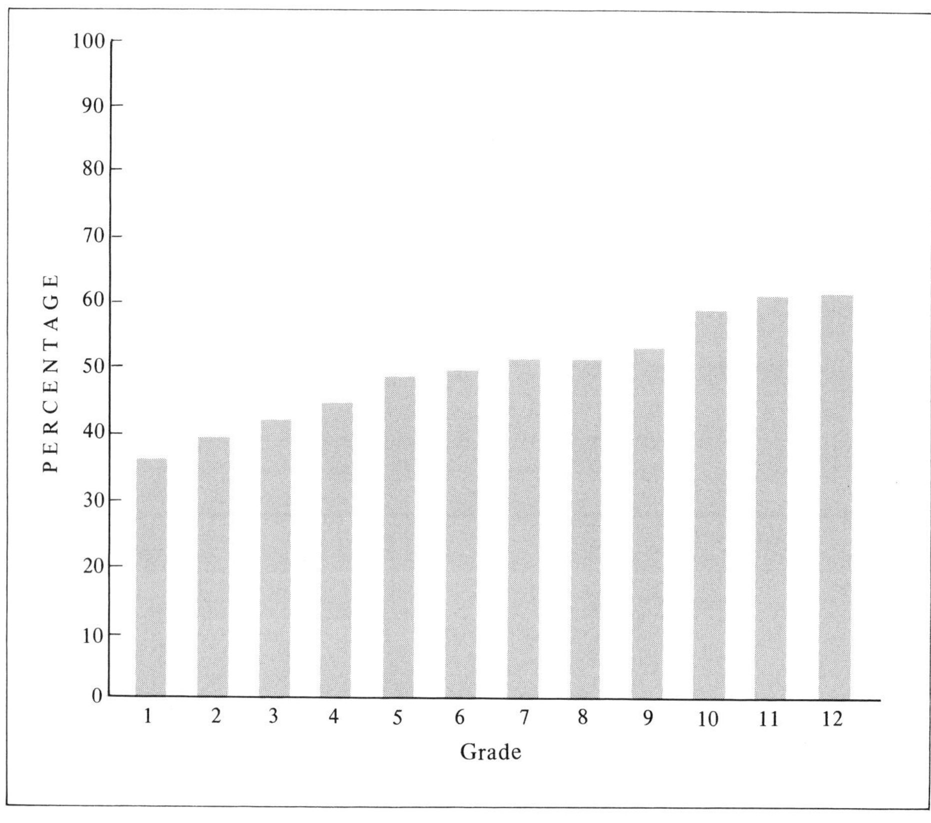

Figure 1–4. Acceptable voice patterns. (F. M. Hull et al. *National speech and hearing survey interim report* (Project No. 50978). Washington, D.C.: Department of Health, Education, and Welfare, Office of Education, Bureau of Education for the Handicapped, 1969.)

Programs for students who require special education have been increasing all over the country. There is a greater awareness of the need for different types of education for those who are learning disabled, physically handicapped, mentally retarded, and emotionally disturbed. There are no national incidence figures of communicative disorders among these groups. We would suspect that most of the retarded have either language code or production problems, that the severe emotionally disturbed will have communication and language breakdowns, that children with cerebral palsy or muscular dystrophy in the classes for physically handicapped will have speech production deficits, and a small proportion of those who are learning disabled will need help in achieving normal language usage. The deaf, of course, may have only a limited oral system when they get to school.

There are no national incidence figures that can be applied to the adult population. Insurance companies report that the population is living longer, thus increasing the likelihood of serious illness and cerebral accidents. Most individuals show some hearing loss as they approach 40 or 50 years of age. Various groups have estimated that there are at least 3 million persons over age 65 with hearing losses. Among residents of

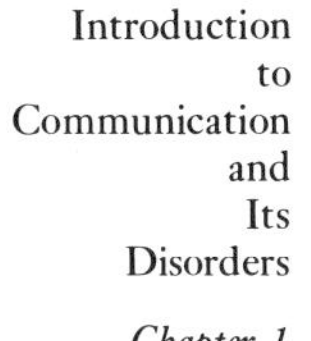

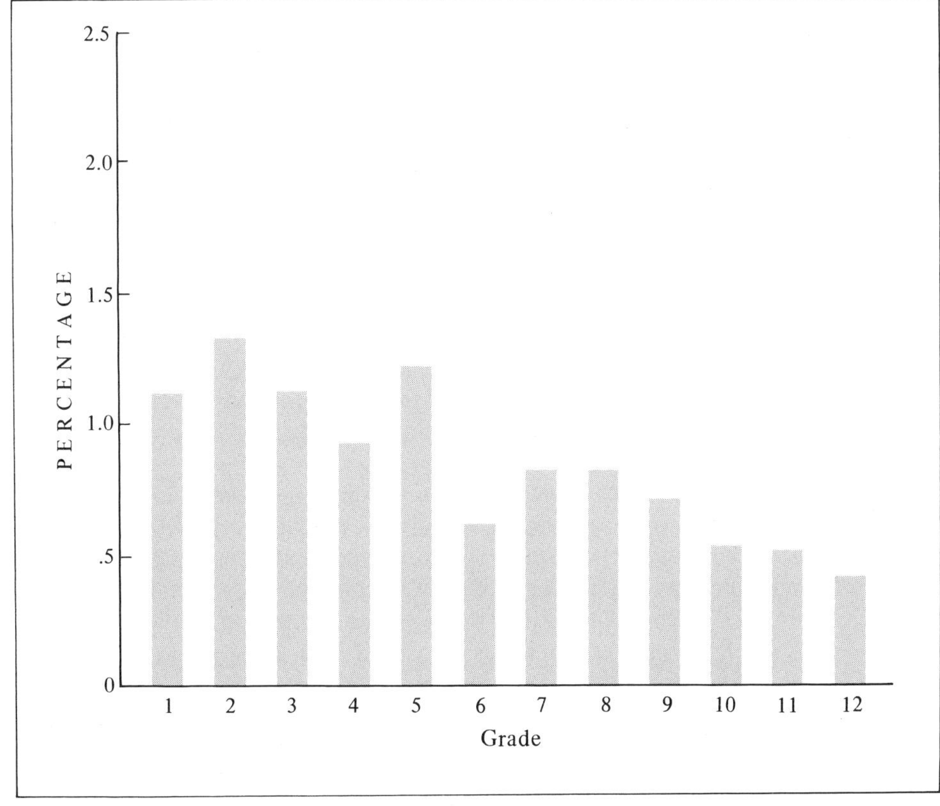

Figure 1–5. Stuttering. (F. M. Hull et al. *National speech and hearing survey interim report* (Project No. 50978). Washington, D.C.: Department of Health, Education, and Welfare, Office of Education, Bureau of Education for the Handicapped, 1969.)

nursing or retirement homes, 90 percent are hearing impaired. Voice problems may not be noted until adulthood, and only those persons who seek help can be counted. Stroke patients are likely to have language and speech production deficits. Again, we have no reporting system for these adults, many of whom could utilize the services of the speech pathologist and audiologist.

THE PROFESSION OF SPEECH PATHOLOGY AND AUDIOLOGY

After this brief description of the nature and incidence of communicative disorders, the logical question is who is responsible for serving this population.

The profession of speech pathology and audiology has the primary responsibility for oral communicative disorders. Its tasks include: (1) evaluation of those with deviations or delay in development; (2) development of programs of intervention to improve the person's communication by minimizing, or eliminating the deficit; (3) development of programs of prevention; (4) research to facilitate clinical work as well as basic research on normal processes of speech, language, and audition.

ASSUMPTIONS

Following are some of the assumptions upon which the speech pathologist bases programs of evaluation, intervention, and prevention for children.

1. The child needs a linguistic system that is functional for him in his many expanding and often changing environments. One out of every five families moves every year. They may move three blocks or three states, but the environment in which a child is born may be quite different from the one in which he attends school. The Black migrant workers' children who move from Georgia up the east coast, or the Mexican American from California into the state of Washington during the different crop seasons are examples of children who must learn to function in many kinds of expanding linguistic environments.

2. The child must develop communication styles for his use within and outside his home, with his own ethnic group and others. If individuals remained within a small, homogeneous neighborhood throughout their lifetimes, there would be no need for a child to learn to use different language styles.

3. There are identifiable standards of language comprehension and use against which the oral communication of individuals can be compared. There are three major standard dialects in the United States: Eastern is the standard dialect of some of the New England states and part of New York, Southern is the dialect of the southeastern states, and General American is the standard for the rest of the country. In addition, there are language characteristics associated with social strata that differ within regions. Numerous nonstandard dialects are acceptable in various ethnic groups.

4. Parents want their children to be skilled communicators. Research based on parent interviews supports this statement. Mothers in low economic families particularly want their children to have more and better education than they had, and they recognize the relationship between education and oral communication.

Adults with communication disorders can be placed in two groups: (1) those who have had communication deficits most or all of their lives and (2) those who have had normal communication skills and have lost them either partially or completely. For these two groups the speech pathologist makes the following assumptions.

1. The need to communicate is present throughout the life of the individual and almost all persons want to be able to communicate.

2. Regular evaluations will help to chart gains and losses for those in group 1. As more effective treatment or intervention becomes available, it can be utilized for them.

3. Immediate intervention when a communication crisis arises will be more beneficial for those in group 2 than delay or no intervention.

CRITERIA FOR NORMAL COMMUNICATION

The criteria for evaluating the level of an individual's communication skill are based on social acceptability. The first question in evaluation is: Does the individual function with adequate linguistic skill in his or her own speech community? If the answer is yes, the next question is: Does the individual function with adequate linguistic skill outside his or her own speech community? If the answer is yes, the third question is: Are there any minor differences in the speech patterns of the individual that contribute to social differences that lead to social devaluation or reduction of status? If the answer is no, the individual's communication can be considered adequate or superior.

If the person cannot function linguistically in his own community, the chances are high that he cannot when he is outside that community. The nature and severity of his deficit will determine the program of intervention that is needed. If the individual functions outside his own speech community with some linguistically different characteristics, those characteristics need to be identified and an appropriate program of intervention provided for him.

EVALUATION

It isn't difficult for most of us to pick out the child who has normal language and communication skills or the one who is severely deficient. It is the child in the middle who presents a problem for many laymen. Unless the child has some additional deficits, his communication skills may not be evaluated until he reaches kindergarten or first grade. Neighbors and relatives may support the parents' comments that "John isn't talking much, but give him time. He's just shy." Or the father may reiterate that he was slow in talking, just like his son or daughter. Parents talk hopefully about a child's "catching up" once he gets into school.

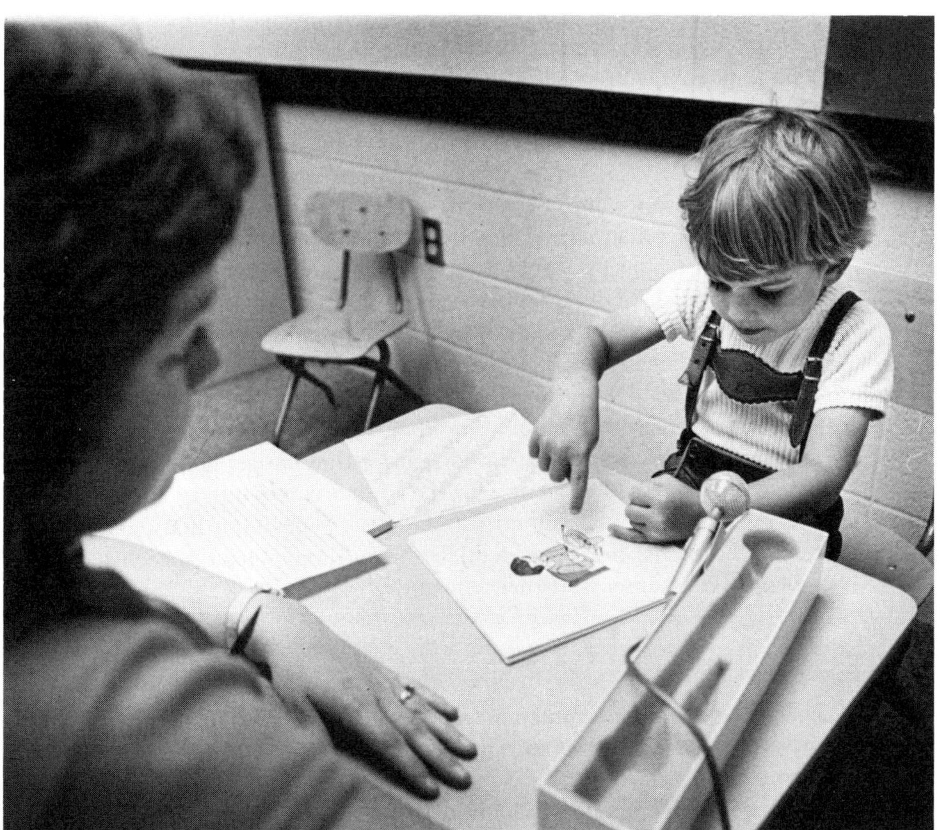

When the speech and language clinician evaluates an individual, he determines specific areas of deficiency in oral communication. He evaluates the language, speech production, and interpersonal exchange. The audiologist provides tests of audition. If either of them questions the cognitive or emotional status of the individual, a referral to a psychologist will be made. If other deficiencies are noted, the speech and hearing specialists will make other referrals—to the family physician for health-related problems, to the dentist for dental evaluation, to the social worker for family financial assistance.

In schools and in clinics teams of specialists evaluate those with severe or multiple problems, share their findings, and agree on a plan of intervention. A team in a school might consist of the speech and language clinician, teacher, psychologist, nurse, and school principal. In a hospital the team that would evaluate an individual with cerebral palsy might include the pediatrician, neurologist, orthopedist, physical and occupational therapists, social worker, audiologist, and speech clinician. A team for a person with a hearing loss should include the audiologist, otologist, and, when appropriate, a teacher of the hearing impaired. The sharing of information and the comprehensive planning that can come from team work can result in more effective intervention.

Evaluation should be an ongoing activity of the speech and language clinician. Some clinicians keep daily records of their clients' progress in therapy. Others do weekly or biweekly testing to determine the amount of learning that has taken place. The improvement or lack of it will change the therapy approach. Since the primary purpose of intervention is to enable the person to establish control of some facet of language, speech production, audition, or interpersonal exchange, the clinician must know when that carry-over or generalization has occurred. The client may do well in the clinical setting, but not in others. The clinician must evaluate progress in as many settings as possible, either directly through testing or indirectly from the reports of others with whom the client associates.

Even after the individual's therapy program has been terminated, there is a need to reevaluate. The client may slip back to old habits, and other conditions may arise to interfere with carry-over. A clinician needs to encourage former clients to check in at periodic intervals for evaluation of the maintenance of the communication skill.

Adults who are gradually losing their hearing or lose their facility in talking should seek evaluations. It is just as important for them to get help early as it is for the child. The main sources of assistance for the adult are community and university speech and hearing clinics, clinicians in private practice, general hospitals, and Veterans Administration hospitals. Some residential nursing homes have speech pathologists and audiologists as members of their consulting staffs.

INTERVENTION

Following the initial evaluation, the clinician must make one of several decisions. One is to initiate a direct therapy program immediately. Another might be to postpone a therapy program temporarily and reevaluate within a particular period of time. A third alternative is to provide information about the nature of the deficit to the teacher or parent and to work with them on procedures for changing the deficiency. Approaches to both clinician and clinician-teacher intervention are presented in Chapter 7.

The clinician's decision will be based upon observations of the communication skills of the individual, testing, information about development obtained from other sources, and the specific criteria she has decided upon.

No one can guarantee that plans of intervention will eliminate the deficits. Some children and adults have such severe communication problems that we can effect only minimal change at present. However, the speech pathologist can help many children and adults to improve their communication skills and some to achieve normal communication patterns. The goal is always the most effective speech for all.

PREVENTION

It is not within the scope of speech pathology to prevent communicative problems at their source. Research in many fields of medicine is concerned with eliminating the original problems from which communicative deficits stem. For example, the development of vaccines has practically eliminated bulbar polio and its aftermath of speech muscle weakness. The development of procedures to identify and treat the metabolic disorder phenylketonuria means that babies who might have been seriously mentally retarded by 18 months now develop normally.

The role of the speech pathologist in prevention is threefold: (1) early identification, (2) early intervention, and (3) dissemination of information about identification and intervention. The goal is to prevent the development of communicative problems and the stabilization of communication deficits.

Early identification involves recognition of symptoms of trouble ahead. High-risk babies and the babies of impoverished ghetto dwellers are examples of children with considerable potential for language delays and deficits. More of them need help with communication skills than children who had normal births and who live above the poverty line.

Some children are born with defective anatomical structures related to normal speech production, such as cleft palates (roof of the mouth), cleft lips, and missing pinnas (the outer ear). Such defects are immediately observable and physicians and parents can plan treatment at once.

Many children who will be classified later as mentally retarded can also be identified at birth or shortly afterwards. The Down's syndrome child has specific facial and other anatomical characteristics. Of the residents in our state institutions for the retarded, 1 in 10 has the Down's syndrome. Microcephaly (abnormal smallness of the head) is another example of a condition involving mental defects which is obvious at birth.

In order to identify children with communicative deficiencies, we need systematic screening evaluations. Such an identification program might consist of screening procedures carried out at well baby clinics or during physicians' regular checkups. In one community mothers of all newborns are invited to participate in a testing plan to determine how their children respond to stimuli. Measures include responses to visual and auditory cues, responses to being held and cuddled, and crying behaviors. Eight out of 10 mothers agree to the testing of their newborns, and many request the examiners to tell them about the results. A report is placed in the child's medical file and is available to the family physician. Specialists in child development hope that such early evaluation will enable them to optimize a child's development.

A screening plan for language and communication might get started when children are 1 year old. Some substantive guidelines have been established for 1-year-olds. Guidelines for children under 1 are less precise, although some public health personnel are administering developmental scales, which include communication items, when children are 6 weeks old. Even though children do not mature at the same rate, longitudinal evaluations would provide opportunities to introduce some intervention or to suggest some modifications in the home talking situation.

If screening on a routine basis for 1-year-olds cannot be provided, such procedures should at least begin when children enter day-care centers and preschools. With the increase in both one-parent families and working mothers, more young children are spending time routinely outside the home. Those children could be tested. In addition, programs offered in these settings could emphasize the development of reasoning and communication skills. Head Start requires speech and hearing screening of all its children. Why not require these services for all?

When children enroll in public schools, they will be given speech and hearing tests if the school has a speech clinician. However, according to the figures prepared by the Bureau for the Education of the Handicapped for 1968–1969 only half of those who needed help were receiving it.

Early intervention can be described as programming that gets started as soon as the problem is identified. It is based on the concept that early treatment will prevent the stabilization of errors and will promote normal communication. It may be either direct intervention, in which the clinician begins working with the individual, or indirect, in which the clinician works with the teacher, parent, or other family members. For instance, Head Start children who receive initial evaluations, may be scheduled immediately for therapy or the nursery school program may be structured to emphasize the language skills needed by those children.

The speech pathologist has a great deal of information to share with the public about communication disorders. In many communities lectures and courses about parenting, including material dealing with language development, are offered as a community service or as a part of a college continuing education program. Parents want information that will enable them to cope more readily with the problems of their children.

Parents need to be reminded of their roles in normal language acquisition. If their child has a hearing loss, the child should receive regular checks by the audiologist. If he needs a hearing aid, he should use it all the time. That means someone must check the batteries to make sure they are functioning. In some communities there are almost no children or adults who stutter. Could it be that these communities have adopted child-rearing practices that are less tension producing for children and more accepting of children's oral communication patterns?

RESEARCH

The fourth responsibility of the speech pathologist and audiologist is research. Not all members of the profession engage in formal research, but each does informal research in testing an individual, determining whether he needs therapy, hypothesizing about the causes of the problem, selecting goals for therapy, carrying out a program, and measuring results.

Research is being conducted to provide information about many aspects of both normal and abnormal language, speech production, and audition. Not all of it is being done by speech and hearing specialists, and so the specialists draw upon the work of the many other professions concerned with aspects of communication.

THE *WHY* OF THINGS

Although the clinician and teacher may not be able to treat the original cause of a language or speech impairment, knowledge of that cause can be essential in planning a program of intervention. For example, the deaf individual should be enrolled in a communication program that will minimize the sensory hearing loss and utilize all facets of his personality in teaching him how to use a normal pattern of communication.

Another example is the child with an unrepaired cleft of the palate. That hole is why he sounds so nasal. He needs either surgical or prosthetic intervention before the clinician can help him. Without closure of the opening, his teacher and his peers will have trouble understanding him.

Clinicians should be aware of etiology also in the interests of research into questions of the relation of certain known conditions to speech and language development. For instance, degrees of deafness seem to be associated with certain kinds of language deficits and even language learning. The knowledge the clinician can derive from his practice can contribute to the work being done in the laboratory and in other fields to chip away at the mountain of ignorance about the relationship of conditions to the resultant communication deficit.

In addition, the clinician deals with parents who want to know why their child has the problem of language delay or deficit and what his future will be. Even though the clinician is not necessarily the one to tell parents, he must have compassion for parents who are struggling with the problems of accepting their child's deficiencies and planning their lives in accordance with the range of development available to their child.

We will never be able to prevent speech and language deficits unless we can understand more of the causes. Today we can indicate that a high-risk baby is more likely to die within a year than a child who has a normal birth. There are some statistics that indicate that 16 out of 100 high-risk babies will have serious learning difficulties, including communication deficits. Why should 16 of the 100 be faced with these problems? It is only through continued research that we may be able to discover why that small number have the problems and others do not.

SOCIAL CHANGE AND ITS IMPLICATIONS

Changing social and educational attitudes and philosophies have a strong influence on the research and clinical activities of speech pathology and audiology. In 1970 the Joint Commission on Mental Health of Children recommended the adoption of the following statement on the rights of individuals.

> The right to be wanted, the right to be born healthy, the right to live in a healthy environment, the right to satisfaction of basic needs, the right to continuous loving care, the right to acquire the intellectual and emotional skills necessary to achieve individual aspirations and to cope effectively in our society, and the right to receive care and treatment through facilities which are appropriate to their needs and which keep them as closely as possible within their normal social setting.

The statement sets forth the basic requisites that society must provide for its newborns. It represents one more example of the obligations we must assume for each person.

The *Basic Education Rights for the Handicapped*, prepared by the National Advisory Committee on Handicapped Children in 1973, includes the following statement: "Each handicapped child must be guaranteed the right to a tax-supported appropriate education. This education must be of high quality and must fit the needs and abilities of each child, no matter the degrees of handicap."

In order to ensure that this guarantee will be met, every state has to document the procedures it is following to accomplish this task by a certain date. Language and communication services are among those that must be provided.

Another influence that is currently determining the activities of the speech pathologist is the philosophy that children and adults with handicapping conditions should be living in the community, rather than in state institutions. The mentally retarded person who has any potential for self-sufficiency is no longer to be placed in the institution where he lives out the rest of his days. Communities must plan how to integrate such persons into the social and employment system. These plans require positive action on the part of the schools and communities. It is not enough to pay taxes to "put them away" any more. Our job will be one of finding the best possible arrangements for a handicapped person to enable him to develop his own self-respect. We must prepare him for the new role he will be able to assume in our communities.

Still another force is the realization of educators that children, once placed in a special class, tend to remain there for the rest of their schooling. In addition, there is scant evidence that such special classes or schools provide any better development of the individual's potential than regular classrooms. Mainstreaming, the placement of children with different types of learning problems within the regular classroom, is one of the current educational movements that will require every teacher and every specialist to develop some different and hopefully more effective ways of dealing with the special child's education. Mainstreaming requires that all classroom teachers be aware of and utilize speech and language programs of remediation.

The teacher actually may have three groups of communication-deficient children in her room. First, there may be children with limited linguistic skills, that is, children who have limited vocabulary, misuse the sounds of our language, and talk either in simple sentences or incomplete utterances. If the language arts curriculum for the school district does not provide adequate listening and speaking activities to improve these skills, the teacher must be able to utilize the speech and language specialist in selecting language enhancement or language development programs for her class.

Second, there may be children whose primary problems have been identified as emotional disturbance, mental retardation, learning disabilities, or physical handicaps. Many of these children also have limited communication skills. It will be essential for the teacher to obtain speech, language, and hearing evaluations for this group and then be able to work closely with the school clinician in a remedial language program if it is recommended.

Third, there may be children whose primary problem is oral communication. These are the children whom the teacher now refers to the speech specialist. The speech and language deficits of these children are the primary responsibility of the speech and language specialists. The role of the teacher, at least at the initial stage of therapy, is limited.

Teachers and clinicians must be able to work together. One cannot administer a successful program of intervention without the other. Selected aspects will be handled by the clinician and by the teacher at different points in the pupil's learning. Neither has the background to accomplish all that is needed alone.

School administrators who mainstream their exceptional children should encourage their teachers to develop guidelines in listening and speaking as well as in reading and writing. These guides should be written by a combination of classroom teachers, special educators, and speech and language clinicians. The input from all three is necessary because each has specific knowledge to bring to the planning.

Although federal support may be diminishing for preschool programs for children from low-income families, many states and local communities are finding funds to maintain these programs. Head Start and day-care centers for children of working mothers have been accepted as a beneficial educational experience. The premise of early educational intervention is well accepted. Even though additional benefits could be gained from further modification of school programs, these preschools have proved their value in many ways.

As we consider all of these and other allied forces at work, we can be sure that more children with special needs will be in clinics and school programs for their communication deficits. The one characteristic that is acknowledged to be the most handicapping is inadequate communication. Parents say, "If you can teach him to talk, everything will be all right," or "He can't hold a job because no one can understand him," or "He doesn't understand me when I talk to him." These comments are heard over and over again. To enroll all these children in remedial programs will be an overwhelming task, unless we can pool the resources, efforts, and knowledge of the community, the school, and the professional communication specialist.

A FRAME OF REFERENCE

Language and speech production are the raw data of this field of study. In order to understand how they emerge and change, it is helpful to have a theory to explain them. McNeill (1971) says that "the acquisition of language can be understood as an interaction between the child's linguistic experience and his innate linguistic capacities." In other words, the infant is born with a capability to learn a language, just as he is born with the potential for developing motor skills such as reaching and walking. His environment will determine which language he masters.

We know that a newborn baby responds to the sounds of adult speech. Condon and Sander (1974) charted the patterns of body movements of infants when an adult spoke to them. To rule out the possibility that the adult modified his rhythm and stress pattern as a result of watching the baby's movements, audiotape recorded material was used. The tape contained tapping sounds, isolated vowels, and Chinese and American English language samples. The babies' movements were synchronous with both language samples, but not with the vowels and tapping. The infants were all under 15 days old, many of them only 1 or 2 days old. They were already in movement when the adult speech started, but they coordinated the movement of body parts to coincide with points of change in the sound patterns of adult speech.

Condon and Sander point out:

> If an infant, from the beginning, moves in precise, shared rhythm with the organization of the speech structure of his culture, then he participates developmentally through complex, sociobiological entrainment processes in millions of repetitions of linguistic forms long before he later uses them in speaking and communicating. By the time he begins to speak, he may have already laid down within himself the form and structure of the language system of his culture.

Not all infants are born with the same capacity for mastering a language. In addition, each environment will interact with whatever capabilities the infant brings to it. The varying forces of capacity and environment shape the quality and quantity of language and speech production. In other words, communication is multiply determined; physical, psychological, and social determinants interact and modify an individual's communication status.

In many instances we cannot tell why a child has a communication deficit. Several factors may contribute to it. The child might have been born prematurely, lacked oxygen, and remained in the hospital for two weeks. He may not have received much attention from parents, peers, and others during the first few months. He might even have been a battered child. During the early critical years of life, he might have been exposed to little personal communication, but much uninterrupted television. There are several dimensions of the physical, psychological and social determinants to which this child has been exposed. We cannot attribute a speech and language deficit to any one of these, because of their interrelated effects.

We can cite instances where children have had all of these negative experiences and yet have no measurable speech or language deficit. Some children are able to adjust to the family's life-style and circumvent its potentially negative effects. Others cannot adapt and we do not know why. We can give you examples of children whose histories show a multitude of adversities concentrated in one of the three determinants; and have strong clinical evidence to suggest a positive relationship between the determinant and the language deficit. The child who has been deaf from birth or shortly afterwards is an example.

SUMMARY

In this chapter we have described normal and abnormal communication. We have discussed the extent of the problems of communication and introduced you to the responsibilities of the speech pathologist and audiologist. We have indicated why we need to know about the causes of communicative disorders and have discussed some of the social forces that are actively influencing the profession of speech pathology and audiology. Finally, we have outlined our theoretical frame of reference, which emphasizes the role of determinants in acquisition and use of communication.

REFERENCES

Condon, W. S., and Sander, L W., Neonate movement is synchronized with adult speech. *Science*, *183*, 99–101 (1974).

Hull, F. M., Miekle, P. W., Timmons, R. J., Willeford, J. A. *National speech and hearing survey interim report* (Project No. 50978). Washington, D.C. Department of Health, Education, and Welfare, Office of Education, Bureau of Education for the Handicapped, 1969.

Marge, M. The general problem of language disabilities in children. In J. Irwin and M. Marge (Eds.), *Principles of childhood language disabilities*. New York: Appleton, 1972.

McNeill, D. *The acquisition of language*. New York: Harper & Row, 1971.

National Advisory Committee on Handicapped Children. *Basic education rights for the handicapped* (DHEW Publication No. (OE) 73-24000). Washington, D.C.: Department of Health, Education, and Welfare, 1973.

Trager, G. L. Paralanguage: A first approximation. *Student Linguist*, *13*, 1–12 (1958).

THE STRUCTURE AND FUNCTIONS OF LANGUAGE Chapter 2

Language is a set of symbols that a community has agreed upon to designate and describe people, objects, actions, concepts, and relationships of all kinds. The symbols are organized and arranged according to principles that permit an infinite number of combinations. Each language has its own structure and the structures have many functions. In this chapter we shall discuss the structure and functions of the English language.

STRUCTURE

The linguistic structure of English has four basic components. Phonology deals with the phoneme or sound system. Examples of phonemes are [b] and [a]. Morphology is concerned with the smallest identifiable language unit that is grammatically pertinent—a word or word-forming element. An example of a morpheme is the word *book;* another is the phoneme [s] which is added to words to indicate plurality, as in *books.* Syntax is the orderly and meaningful grouping of words within a sentence or phrase. For example, *John is a big boy,* is a syntactically correct sentence. Semantics deals with the meaning of the words or combinations of words we use. A word can have one or more referents. The word *circle* may refer to a round enclosed plane, a group of people with a common goal, or an action, as in *The police circled the block.* The precision of our definition and the actual meaning of a word or group of words will vary as a function of the situation in which we use them.

1. PHONOLOGY—the sound system
2. MORPHOLOGY—words and word-forming elements
3. SYNTAX—word order of an utterance
4. SEMANTICS—meanings of an utterance

Figure 2–1. Components of a language.

PHONOLOGY

Phonology is the study of the distinctive and contrastive sounds that make up a language and the rules that govern their use. A phoneme has psychological reality. In other words, it is perceived by its user and by the listener as different from all other phonemes. Phonemes convey semantic differences. In the following examples we can check their distinctive and contrastive character at the beginning of the words: *b*oat, *c*oat, *d*ote, *g*oat, *m*oat, *n*ote, *t*ote. Each of the initial phonemes is different from the others. The change from a [b] to another phoneme signals a change in meaning, even though the rest of the phonemes remain constant.

There may be several variations in the way a specific phoneme or sound family is produced. These variations are called *allophones* of the phoneme. Even if we pronounce a phoneme such as [s] in a manner slightly different from other people, it is still within the same sound family if it is understood and accepted by the listener as [s] and if it does not indicate a change in meaning. One person may produce the [s] phoneme with more or less air expulsion or more air may be emitted between missing front teeth or directed out the sides of the mouth or through the nose.

In addition to individual differences in the way people produce a sound, other factors contribute to some changes in the production. We perceive the [s] as the same in *sea*, *ask*, *store*, and *bus*, but in reality each is somewhat different. The production is influenced by its position in the word and by the sounds on either side of it.

In a country as large and as socially diverse as the United States, we would expect variations in pronunciation of words. Linguists who have compared the use of selected phonemes of speakers in urban centers have predicted the presence or absence of phonemes on the basis of social stratification. Labov (1966) found that clerks who worked in New York department stores tended to use pronunciation that was more similar to that of their customers than to that of sales persons in general in New York City. For example, he found the sales persons used the [r] phoneme in ways that could be predicted from social strata of the store's customers. Those who worked in the stores that catered to the upper-income group used the [r] phoneme in certain test words and those who were employed in the stores which attracted the low-income group did not use the [r] in the test items.

Regional differences in pronunciation account for another modification of phonemes. In the preceding chapter we listed the three major standard dialects—Eastern, Southern, and General American. As we listen to a speaker from one part of the South, we may note that a word like *father* is pronounced with a prolonged vowel, [ɑ]. In addition he may not pronounce the *r* at the end of the word. Many such examples can be identified in analyzing speech from different areas of the country.

Phonetics is the description and classification of the speech sounds of a language. In order to facilitate our description and classification of the sounds, we have adopted the symbol system of the International Phonetic Alphabet (IPA). The English language does not have a single written symbol for each sound. In addition, there is only partial consistency between the written letter and its sound. The symbol *b* always represents the same sound and no other one. However, others, like the written symbol *s*, may have the sound of *z*, as in *rose*, or *sh* as in *sugar*. In the IPA, each phoneme has its own symbol. Consistent phonetic symbols from the Roman alphabet, such as *b* and *t*, have been retained; some, such as *c* as in *cat* or in *cent*, have been dropped; and additional ones have been devised, such as [ʃ] for the initial sound in the words *shoe* and *ship*.

There is some variation in the number of phonemes identified by different phoneticians. Fairbanks (1960) lists 44; Denes and Pinson (1973) list 38. Phoneticians point out that the number can be increased considerably if we utilize more precise differences as the criteria for each phoneme. Not all the phonemes are used in the three major standard dialects; and, of course, there is some individual variation in the production of the phonemes.

For our purposes we identify 43 phonemes that are typical of General American

Table 2–1. List of Phonemes in General American English

Consonants			Vowels		
Phonetic Symbol	Dictionary Symbol	Example	Phonetic Symbol	Dictionary Symbol	Example
p	p	*pin*	i	ē	h*e*
b	b	*bin*	ɪ	i	h*i*m
m	m	*me*	e	ā	ch*a*otic
t	t	*to*	ɛ	e	m*e*t
d	d	*do*	æ	ă	c*a*t
n	n	*no*	ɑ	ä	f*a*ther
k	k	*key*	ɔ	ȯ	*a*ll
g	g	*go*	o	o	*o*bey
ŋ	ng	ri*ng*	ʊ	u	p*u*t
f	f	*fee*	u	ü	f*oo*d
v	v	*vie*	ʌ	ə́	h*u*m
s	s	*see*	ə	ə	sof*a*
z	z	*zoo*	ɜ	ər	b*ir*d
ʃ	sh	*sh*oe	ɚ	ər	moth*er*
ʒ	zh	mea*s*ure	ɔɪ	ȯi	b*oy*
tʃ	ch	*ch*ew	ɑʊ	ɑü	*ou*t
dʒ	j	*j*ust	eɪ	ā	t*a*ble
θ	th	*th*umb	oʊ	ō	c*oa*t
ð	th	*th*is	aɪ	ī	h*i*de
h	h	*h*ome			
l	l	*l*ie			
r	r	*r*ed			
j	y	*y*ellow			
w	w	*w*ing			

English, 19 vowels and diphthongs and 24 consonants. Table 2–1 gives the phonetic symbol, the dictionary symbol, and an example for each phoneme. It is difficult to choose examples for the vowels, because they are produced with some variations within General American English. The student should listen to his instructor's production of the phoneme and then determine whether he himself utilizes that phoneme as in the example or changes it slightly. In addition he should determine whether Table 2–1 includes all the phonemes he uses and whether there are some that he rarely pronounces.

The placement of sounds in phonemic categories is one functional way to study them. We have already classified the phonemes in Table 2–1 as vowels or consonants. If a phoneme is a vowel, it cannot be a consonant simultaneously. We must keep in mind that all phonemes are produced by a speech mechanism that is not absolutely fixed and is constantly being modified because of the flexibility of its structures. In addition, in continuous speech we move from one sound to another without a break in between. Production of the vowels and consonants will be described in Chapter 4.

Consonants can be classified according to the place and manner of articulation and voicing. The phonemes listed as consonants in Table 2–1 have been classified by these three means in Table 2–2.

The place of articulation may be the lips (labial), teeth (dental), lips and teeth (labiodental), alveolus or teethridge (alveolar), hard palate (palatal), velum (velar), or glottis (glottal).

The manner of articulation may be plosive, fricative, affricate, liquid, nasal, or semivowel.

The third means of classifying consonants is voicing. Each consonant is either voiced or voiceless. A voiced phoneme is produced with the vocal cords vibrating; an unvoiced phoneme is produced with the folds apart.

As you examine Table 2–2, remember that the vocal mechanism is flexible and that the sounds that precede and follow a consonant modify its production slightly. During

Table 2–2. Classification of Consonants by Place of Articulation, Manner of Articulation, and Voicing

Place of Articulation	Manner of Articulation						Voicing
	Plosives	Fricatives	Affricates	Liquids	Nasals	Semi-vowels	
Bilabial	p						No
	b				m	w	Yes
Linguadental		θ(th)					No
		ð(th)					Yes
Labiodental		f					No
		v					Yes
Alveolar	t	s					No
	d	z		l	n		Yes
Palatal		ʃ(sh)	tʃ(ch)				No
		ʒ(zh)	dʒ(j)	r		j(y)	Yes
Velar	k						No
	g				ŋ(ng)		Yes
Glottal		h					No

conversation we may be articulating more than 600 phonemes a minute or 10 a second. Such fast speech production requires rapid adjustments of the total mechanism.

In the preceding section we have used the classical categories of consonants and vowels and have listed them by manner and place of articulation. However, the phonemes of a language can be classified in other ways. Jakobson, Fant, and Halle (1952) were interested in finding a set of universal and natural features that could be used to analyze all the languages of the world. In their system they describe a phoneme as a bundle of distinctive features. They have identified nine features which have specific acoustic and articulatory characteristics. The features are contrasts—if a phoneme has one, it does not have the other. The nine contrasts are: consonantal-nonconsonantal, vocalic-nonvocalic, tense-lax, nasal-oral, continuant-interrupted, strident-mellow, grave-acute, compact-diffuse, flat-plain.

To demonstrate how phonemes can be classified using a distinctive feature approach, let us consider two of the above binary contrasts, vocalic-nonvocalic and nasal-oral. In the speech science laboratory the acoustic features have been identified for each class by studying their spectra. All vowels and two consonants—[r] and [l]—are vocalic. All the other consonants in Table 2–2 are nonvocalic. There are three phonemes that fit the description for the nasal in contrast to the oral feature. These are [m], [n], and [ŋ]. All others are oral.

Critics have noted several weaknesses in this system. Fant, who helped to develop it, has said that it is not precise enough (1962). Others have questioned the validity of a contrastive approach. And some have pointed out that the acoustic and other correlates of each feature are not clear enough for others to use in experimental work. We have mentioned the system here because some evaluation and therapy programs utilize this approach. Many texts include tables which list the distinctive features of English phonemes (an example of such a table is included in the Appendix). In using this system we must accept the judgments of those who devised it in determining the presence or nonpresence of the features.

PROSODIC FEATURES

In the above descriptions and categories of phonemes, we have been concerned with the phonetic units that follow one another in a successive pattern. These are called segmental phones—*b* ʌ *k* is an example. When analyzed, they are the segmental phonemes.

Prosodic features of length, loudness, tone, and junctures occur simultaneously with the production of segmental phonemes. It is possible to contrast the varied productions of vowels and consonants and identify their prosodic features.

Length refers to the elongation of a phoneme. For example, some speakers will stretch the production of [i], as in *he*, while others will clip it.

Loudness is dependent on the force with which air is expelled from the lungs and the energy used in articulating the phoneme. In a word like *admit*, there is a secondary stress on the first vowel and a primary stress on the second. We might then say that first vowel is produced with *weak* loudness, in contrast to the strong loudness of the second vowel.

Tone is a function of the tension of the vocal folds and their rate of vibration.

Deviation from what is considered a normal tone of voice to comparatively higher or lower pitches on some phonemes emphasizes those phonemes. In the sentence *I want it now*, we can change our tone for *I* or for the vowel in *now*. The meaning of the sentence shifts, depending on where we change our normal tone.

The fourth prosodic feature deals with the *junctures* or *terminal points*. Phonemes can be run together in different ways and an utterance can end in several different ways by a combination of changes in volume and pitch. In both cases the meaning conveyed can be affected. For example, in the familiar *I scream for ice cream* did the speaker say *ice cream* twice or was the sentence said as it is written? Did the child say *here some water* or *here's some water?* Did the juncture obliterate the contracted *is* or did the child omit it? The terminal point is in the way we end an utterance. For example, saying *on the table* with rise in pitch, with a falling pitch, or a sustained one each conveys a different meaning.

MORPHOLOGY

Morphology is the study of words. Since words are made up of sounds, we can say that morphology is concerned with sequences of phonemes that have meaning. The word *park* is such a sequence, and it is a morpheme. Morphemes are the smallest units of language that are grammatically pertinent.

There are two general classes of morphemes.

1. Roots—words that cannot be broken down into smaller units. Other terms for roots are *morphs* and *stems*.

   Examples: *park, boy, dress*

2. Affixes—prefixes, infixes, and suffixes that are added to the root to indicate some kind of change. Another word for affixes is *inflections*.

Examples:	Root	Affix
	park	park*s*
	boy	boy*s*
	dress	dress*es*
	do	*un*do
	success	success*ful*
	goose	*gee*se

We will discuss only the major principles governing morphemes, although there are others that apply in special cases (Gleason, 1965).

The information we have about adult morphology has come about through the study of speech samples. Phoneticians and others try to determine the principles that govern a person's use of roots and additions. What features of meaning and expression are common to speakers of General American English? Once we have found clusters that follow certain rules, then we have a more manageable body of knowledge with which to work.

We have some guidelines about four sets of roots or morphs: nouns, verbs, adjectives, and pronouns. These are also referred to as parts of speech.

Nouns are used primarily to indicate one or more than one object, person, or quality. You can think of hundreds of nouns that you use everyday—*shoes*, *house*, *school*, *umbrella*, *papers*, *pen*, *children*, *hunger*, *food*. Count nouns, like *pen* and *shoes*, can be either singular or plural. Mass nouns, like *hunger* or *courage*, are used only in the singular form.

A singular noun is changed to a plural by using a plural inflection or morpheme. The inflection we use is $[-Z_1]$; it may take several forms, which are called allomorphs of the $[-Z_1]$ inflection.

Allomorphs are variants of a morpheme which are appropriate as affixes for certain words but not for others. All have the same meaning, all serve the same purpose, but they have different distributions. For example, the most frequently used allomorphs of the $[-Z_1]$ inflection are listed below. Say these words aloud, remembering to use the sound of the phonetic symbol.

1. [z], [s], or [əz] added to the root or morph

Root	+ [z]	Root	+ [s]	Root	+ [əz]
cab	cab [z]	cap	cap [s]	maze	maz [əz]
ride	ride [z]	light	light [s]	grass	grass [əz]
rug	rug [z]	park	park [s]	inch	inch [əz]
sofa	sofa [z]	cliff	cliff [s]	wish	wish [əz]

2. [z] or [əz] plus a change in the final consonant of the root

knife	kni *vz*
house	hou *zəz*
mouth	mou *ðz*

3. [ən] with or without additional changes

child	child *rən*
ox	ox *ən*

4. Replacives

man	m*e*n
foot	f*ee*t
mouse	m*i*ce
woman	wom*e*n

5. No change (indicated by the symbol ∅)

sheep	sheep
deer	deer

From these examples you can derive the most important principles that govern which allomorph is to be used to change the noun from singular to plural. We add [z] to nouns whose stem ends in a voiced sound—a vowel or one of those listed as voiced in Table 2–2. There is one exception, however. If the noun ends in a voiced sibilant like [z], [ʒ], or [dʒ], it requires [əz] as the plural form. The allomorph [s] is added to nouns whose stems end in the voiceless consonants. Here, too, there is an exception. If the singular form of the noun ends in [s], [ʃ], or [tʃ], the plural form is [əz]. The rule for adding the allomorph [əz] then involves words that have one of the sibilants as the final phoneme. These are [z], [s], [ʃ], [ʒ], [tʃ], and [dʒ].

Those nouns that take the allomorphs listed in 2, 3, 4, and 5 above are irregular in the way they are pluralized. Each of these categories must be memorized as individual plural forms. There is no principle that states that the noun *child* should change in the way it does to form the plural or to explain why other nouns with a similar ending, like *cold* or *mold*, do not form the plural the same way. We talk about *colds* and *molds*, but *children*. These are the vagaries of the English language to which children must adjust. They do adjust when they use these plurals by overgeneralizing the usual rule to the irregular nouns. They'll talk about *childs* and *sheeps* until they have memorized these individual differences.

The context is important in interpreting whether some words have one or two morphemes. Compare the following uses of the word *deer*.

1. The deer is cute.
2. The deer are cute.

The first is a single morpheme, but the second has two morphemes. In the second example no phoneme is added or changed on the word *deer*, but the plural form of *deer* is indicated by the change in the form of the verb *are*. As we said earlier in this section, morphemes are described in terms of phonemes. However, additional phonemes are not always required to change a word from the singular to the plural, as this second example indicates. There is no change in the phonemic structure of the morph *deer* in sentence 2, but it has changed in meaning.

To indicate possession the morpheme [-Z_2] is used. Its several allomorphs are the same as the allomorphs of the plural inflection. The most frequently occurring forms are:

FORM	ROOT	POSSESSIVE
[z]	boy	boy' [z]
[s]	park	park' [s]
[əz]	dress	dress' [əz]
0	parks	parks' (no change in pronunciation)

The possessive forms are written differently from the plural forms, but sound the same. The form which represents what the speaker intends can be determined only by the context. For instance, in the sentence "The boys are home," we know that *boys* is a plural form because of its relationship to the plural form of the verb *are*. In the sentence "The boy's car is here," we know that *boy's* is the possessive form because we're talking about someone's car.

VERBS

A verb is a word that expresses an action, such as *go*, *drive*, and *eat*, or a state of being, such as *feel* and *be*. A verb can be classified as a main, a secondary or an auxiliary verb according to its use. Main verbs have expressed or implied subjects.

1. Go to the store for me.
2. You'll go to the store for me.

In the first example the subject of the verb is implied—*you* go. In the second the subject is expressed.

In the following examples the verb *go* is utilized as a secondary verb and has no subjects.

1. *Going* to the mountains will be difficult.
2. I want *to go* to the mountains.
3. *Going* to the mountains, he wrecked his car.

In the first example *going* functions as a noun and is the subject of the sentence. A verb form which functions as a noun is called a gerund. In the second example *to go* functions as a noun. The verb is used in its infinitive form (the preposition *to* plus the main verb form). In the third *going* functions as an adjective and is considered a present participle.

Auxiliary verbs are those that assist a main verb in forming voice, mode, and tense. They include the verbs *be*, *have*, *do*, *shall*, *will*, *may*, *can*, *must*, and *ought;* and their inflectional forms, such as *was*, *had*, *did*, or *might*. It is possible to combine several auxiliaries with the main verb, as in the following examples: *may have gone*, *will have been taken*.

Main verbs have many characteristics, some of which are expressed by inflections. The characteristics are:

1. Number
   singular: he *eats*
   plural: they *eat*
2. Person
   first: I *eat*   we *eat*
   second: you *eat*
   third: he, she, it *eats*   they *eat*
3. Tense
   present: *go*
   present progressive: *is going*
   past progressive: *was going*
   future: *will go*
   past: *went*
   present perfect: *have gone*
   past perfect: *had gone*
   future perfect: *will have gone*
4. Voice
   active: The bear *ate* the bread.
   passive: The bread *was eaten* by the bear.
5. Mood
   indicative (to express a fact): *We drive a truck.*
   imperative (to express commands and requests): *Drive to the Corner*.
6. Requires auxiliaries for different forms
   modal: will, can, must—*he must drive* or *he can drive*
   progressive tense (form of the verb *be* plus the inflection *ing* added to the main. verb): *was eating*
   perfect tense (form of the verb *have* plus the perfect tense form of the main verb): *have eaten*

passive voice (form of the verb *be* plus the perfect tense form of the main verb): *was eaten*

7. Transitive or intransitive
   transitive (takes a direct object to complete the meaning): *he takes a walk*
   intransitive (makes an assertion without requiring an object): *he went to the store*

The verb *be* requires some additional consideration. It can be a main verb, a secondary verb, or an auxiliary. When it is the main verb, it is called a *copula*. We have only one in English. It connects a subject to a noun, pronoun, or adjective in the predicate: they *are* the books, the book *is* mine, the books *are* heavy. As a main verb it is always intransitive. As a secondary verb it is most likely to be found as an infinitive: to paraphrase Hamlet, *to be* or not *to be* is the question. As an auxiliary it is a part of another verb and may or may not be contracted: *he's coming* home tomorrow, he *is going* to school, the children *were playing* on the street.

Three of the characteristics of main verbs require special inflections: person, number, and tense. Only one inflection is needed to express person and number because a change in the verb form is limited to the third person singular, present tense. The inflection [-Z_3] indicates both the person and number and has three allomorphs, [z], [s], and [əz]. These allomorphs follow the same phonological principles as those associated with [-Z_1]. Examples would be:

[z]	[s]	[əz]
he hide*s*	walk*s*	toss*es*
he carrie*s*	stop*s*	watch*es*
he send*s*	sleep*s*	judg*es*

There are three inflections to differentiate the three tenses. The inflection [ɪŋ] indicates present progressive tense and is constant across all verbs. It is always used in this form and has no allomorphs. [-D_1] is the inflection for the past tense and has many allomorphs. [-D_2] is the inflection for the perfect tense and usually has the same allomorphs as [-D_1].

Eight major sets of allomorphs for tense inflection are listed below.

	Root	[-D_1]	[-D_2]
1. [d]	hurry	hurry [d]	hurry [d]
	pull	pull [d]	pull [d]
2. [t]	kick	kick [t]	kick [t]
	jump	jump [t]	jump [t]
3. [əd]	treat	treat [əd]	treat [əd]
	fold	fold [əd]	fold [əd]
4. ∅	hurt	hurt	hurt
	cost	cost	cost
5. Vowel change only			
	swing	sw*u*ng	sw*u*ng
	meet	m*e*t	m*e*t
	feed	f*e*d	f*e*d

6. Vowel change plus addition of [t]

sleep	slep*t*	slep*t*
keep	kep*t*	kep*t*

7. Vowel change plus final consonant change

catch	*caught*	*caught*
bring	br*ought*	br*ought*

8. Final consonant change: [d] changes to [t], [v] changes to [d]

send	sen*t*	sen*t*
spend	spen*t*	spen*t*
have	ha*d*	ha*d*

When the inflections for [-D_1] differ from those for [-D_2], the verbs are classified as irregular verbs. Some typical examples are:

Root	[-D_1]	[-D_2]
ride	r*o*de	r*i*dd*en*
know	kn*e*w	kn*own*
tear	t*o*re	tor*n*
give	g*a*ve	g*i*v*en*

The verb *be*, whether it is a copula or an auxiliary, is very irregular. It does not conform to the usual inflection rules, and therefore we must learn its unique individual forms.

I Root	[-Z_3]	[-D_1]	[-D_2]	[Iŋ]
be	am	was	been	being
	is	were		
	are			

ADJECTIVES

Adjectives are used to describe a person, event, or object: a *clever* person, a *big* event, a *small* object. Each of these descriptors is a morpheme.

Only two suffixes used as inflections for adjectives are described here: *er*, to indicate comparison of a quality, and *est*, to indicate the highest degree of a quality. The following examples show how these two inflections are used.

Root	Comparative Inflection	Superlative Inflection
great	great*er*	great*est*
small	small*er*	small*est*
big	bigg*er*	bigg*est*
tall	tall*er*	tall*est*

We draw your attention to one extensively used, but highly irregular, adjective. Its forms are:

good	better	best

There is no rule for such changes, so the forms must simply be learned.

PRONOUNS

There is no adequate way to classify all the pronouns or to provide inflectional rules. One group, the personal pronouns, can be identified, however. Because we use them so often, we must be prepared to learn or to teach them without a set of structural guidelines. Table 2–3 provides a complete list of the personal pronouns, organized according to use (as a subject, object, or possessive) and number. Instances of similarity in form are self-evident.

A few of the other types of pronouns with some examples are demonstrative (*this*, *that*), interrogative (*who*, *which*, *what*), reflexive (*myself*, *herself*), and indefinite (*another*, *everything*, *no one*).

Because there are so many different ways in which these words can be used as nouns and modifiers, it is difficult to prepare a list that is inclusive and accurate, but at this point you have sufficient examples to recognize the complexity involved in defining a pronoun. For now we will describe a pronoun as a word or combination of words that stands for, refers to, or takes the place of a noun. In most cases, except for the personal pronouns, we must have the context in which the pronoun is utilized before we can be sure of its classification. In the following sentences the italicized words are types of pronouns.

This is the ball *I* found.
Everyone went home.
Who came with *you*?
Both are possible candidates.
The book *that you* have is *mine*.

In spite of our difficulty in finding adequate procedures to organize pronouns, we use a great many of them when we talk. In fact, Denes and Pinson (1973) found that of the ten most frequently occurring words in adult speech samples, four were pronouns—*I*, *you*, *he*, and *it*.

OTHER AFFIXES

Although we have concentrated on the inflections of selected classes of words, there are many suffixes and prefixes added to morphs. Some morphs can have both a prefix and a suffix. The English language, unlike Hebrew and Arabic, has no infixes. Infixes are placed in the middle of a morph to change its function in some way.

Prefixes and suffixes may or may not change the classification of a word. In the

Table 2–3. Personal Pronouns

	Singular					Plural		
Person	First	Second	Third			First	Second	Third
Subject	I	you	he	she	it	we	you	they
Object	me	you	him	her	it	us	you	them
Possessive	my	your	his	her	its	our	your	their
	mine	yours	his	hers	its	ours	yours	theirs

following examples you can determine in which instance the function of the morph has changed as a result of its new structure.

MORPH	SUFFIX	PREFIX
success	successful	unsuccessful
know	known	unknown
possible	possibility	impossible
easy	easily	uneasy
relevance		irrelevant
apply		reapply
force	forceful	
cooperate	cooperation	
red	redness	
hazard	hazardous	
pain	painless	

SUMMARY

Morphology, the study of words and their affixes, must be viewed within a framework of two types of rules. The first is the phonological change and the second is content. The preceding deals with phonemic arrangements that are observable because of acoustic and articulatory characteristics. The second is concerned with the new meaning or classification of the word as a result of the phonological change.

The study of roots or morphs can be intriguing for those who enjoy reading. To teach and to understand morphs and all their affixes require that we define as many rules as possible in order to make the learner's task an easier one. These rules are probably finite, but unfortunately we have deduced only some of those that apply to Standard English.

SYNTAX

Syntax is the study of the orderly arrangement of words in an utterance and the rules that govern the order. We combine words in many different ways to explain the same phenomena and to construct new messages. The sentence *The cat scratched the dog* can be rephrased as *The dog was scratched by the cat*. Both statements provide the same information. If we add *The dog then bit the cat*, we've generated a new message.

PRESENTENCES

When a child begins to put two words together, he tends to arrange them in ways that show appropriate relationships. For instance, he may point to the cookie he wants as he says *that cookie* or he may indicate he wants *that book*. He may refer to daddy in ways such as *daddy car* or *daddy work*. In looking at a book he may say *here a boy*, *here a truck*, *here a man*, and so on.

At the initial two-term phase he may combine a few key words with many different ones. This arrangement has been called pivot-open grammar by McNeill (1970) and the pivot-look by Brown (1973). Whether such two-term expressions should be considered within the framework of a grammar is a matter of opinion. Most children demonstrate some pivots, such as *that*, *daddy*, and *here* in the above paragraph, and many attachments to them that would be labeled *open*, such as *boy*, *truck*, and *man*.

Not all two-term utterances fit the category of pivot-open. Many might be called open-open arrangements. Two appropriate words are strung together to convey an idea, such as *car dirty* or *me sick*. The child is using morphemes in a meaningful fashion to fit a particular situation. He may or may not use *car* or *me* as pivots.

SENTENCES

Most adults use utterances that are either sentences or partial sentences. The sentence is a series of words consisting of hierarchical units that we identify as subject and predicate. A partial sentence or phrase is a series of related words which does not contain units identified as a subject or a predicate. It is a reply to or an echo of what the first speaker has said. For example, in answering the question (a sentence) "Where did you put my books?" you might use the sentence *I put them on the table* or the partial sentence *On the table*. If you were surprised that your friends rode a bus, you might echo that part of the utterance and say *On the bus?*

Sentences have two linguistic structures. *Surface structure* is concerned with the grammatical relationships in the sentence. An utterance is separated into phrases, and the phrases then are classified grammatically as subject and predicate. The *deep structure* of a sentence refers to its underlying semantic relationships. It is analyzed not in terms of subject and predicate, but in terms of the basic meaning of the sentence. Here are two simple sentences, the first of which can be neatly separated into a subject and a predicate.

1. John wants a dog.
2. John wants out.

In the first we know that *John* is the subject, *wants* is the action or process verb, and *dog* is the object. In the second sentence what do we do with *out?* Is it an adverb or a part of the verb? We "know" what each sentence means—the surface structure of the first is simple, but we must consider the deep structure to understand the second.

In a sentence like *Visiting friends can be a pain*, the word order alone is not sufficient to clarify the meaning. Does the sentence mean that to visit friends is sometimes unpleasant or that friends who visit are sometimes unwelcome? To make the appropriate interpretation, we need to know the context in which the remark was made, something about the personality of the speaker, and perhaps the intonation and stress pattern on the words themselves. This type of ambiguity is an example of a surface structure that has two distinct deep structures.

Even though we can identify a subject and a predicate in the following examples, the sentences do not have meaning.

1. The man appears lamb.
2. The man is a bus.

They are grammatical in style, but nonsense in meaning. We could say:

1. The man appears to be lamblike.
2. The man has a bus.

Certain characteristics of words—whether they are animate or inanimate, process or state verbs, or verbs that can also be descriptive adjectives—must be known by the speaker. Otherwise, we generate inappropriate sentences.

If we know the underlying semantic meaning of a sentence, we have no difficulty with sentence pairs like the following:

1. The dog bit the man.
2. The man was bitten by the dog.

The surface structure is different, but the deep structure, the underlying meaning, is the same.

Analyses of children's early utterances indicate that they know the basic sentence relationships from the beginning (Brown, 1973). They generally express a subject and predicate for sentences, supply objects for the verbs, and place the words for the subject and the object of the verb in the correct position. Other writers and observers of children speaking American English have found few errors or reversals in these sentence relations.

GRAMMAR

Grammar is a description of a language. Many linguists have studied the speech of children and adults in order to deduce the general principles which speakers of a language demonstrate when they talk. In this section we will describe three approaches to the study of the grammar as it is applied to syntax—phrase structure, transformational generative, and case.

Phrase structure grammar permits us to analyze the surface structure of the sentence. We can separate even the longest sentence into its constituents. A constituent is a morpheme or a set of morphemes that go together. In the sentence *The girl wears a pretty dress* the entire string of words may be considered a constituent. *The girl*, *wears a pretty dress*, and *a pretty dress* are all constituents because they are phrases which are coherent and have meaning. The string of words *wears a* does not fit the definition of a constituent. Each morpheme in a sentence is also a constituent—the roots as well as the verb inflection.

Phrase structure grammar also provides the rules for segmenting a sentence into its two major parts—the noun phrase and the verb phrase. In this instance we have the following:

Noun phrase: *the girl*
Verb phrase: *wears a pretty dress*

At one time a different set of terms and categories was used.

Subject: *the girl*
Predicate: *wears*
Object: *a pretty dress*

In current practice the predicate and object are identified as parts of the verb phrase.

There is also another way of identifying the same constituents. The constituents are labeled in terms of their function.

Agent: *the girl*
Action: *wears*
Object: *a pretty dress*

The functional arrangement is more dynamic and shows the relationships of words to one another.

As we said earlier, the morphemes of an utterance must be arranged so that they denote a meaning. Linguists have provided types of linear and hierarchical patterns to help us to understand how we have internally analyzed the syntactic rules. In Figure 2–2 we can observe the required ordering of the words in this sentence and also one type of a hierarchy.

If the linear order—the left to right arrangement on paper—is changed, we no longer have a grammatical sentence. The word order cannot be reversed to read:

1. Girl the wears a dress pretty.
2. A pretty dress wears the girl.

The branches of this open triangle diagram the hierarchical pattern, that is, which words are the key words and which words go with each of the key words. *Girl*, *wear*, and *dress* appear at the end of the three main branches, and the morphemes which go with each key word appear on subsidiary branches.

Figure 2–3 diagrams the phrase structure arrangement of the sentence and also gives the part of speech of each morpheme. The tree diagram divides the sentence (S) into its major constituents, noun phrase (NP) and verb phrase (VP), and then divides it further into its smaller constituents.

A third, and the simplest, way to describe the sentence is given in Figure 2–4. It shows the functions of the constituent units. The relationships of the agent, action, and object of the action are clearly noted, with no concern for parts of speech, phrases, or hierarchies.

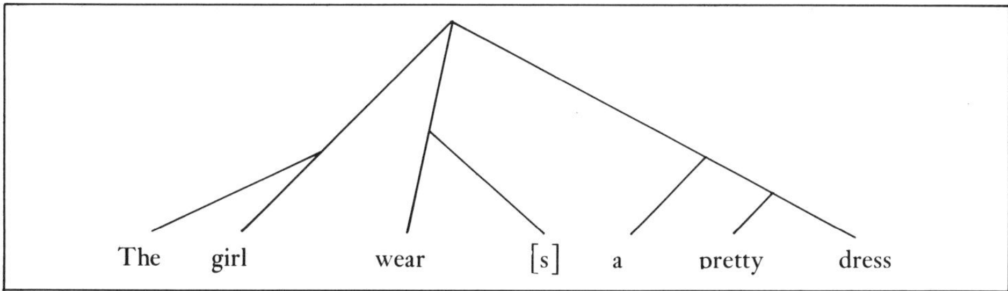

Figure 2–2. Linear and hierarchical arrangements.

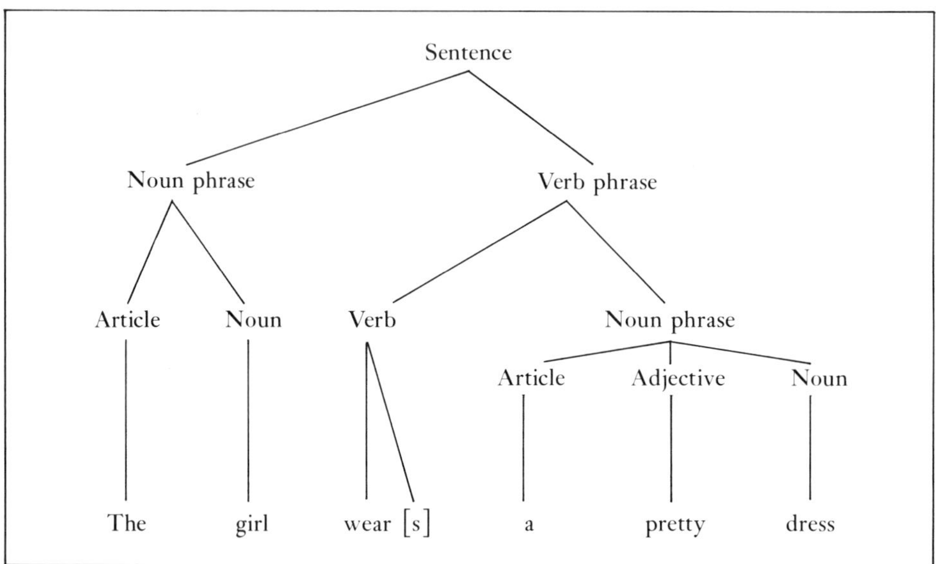

Figure 2–3. Phrase structure arrangements of a sentence.

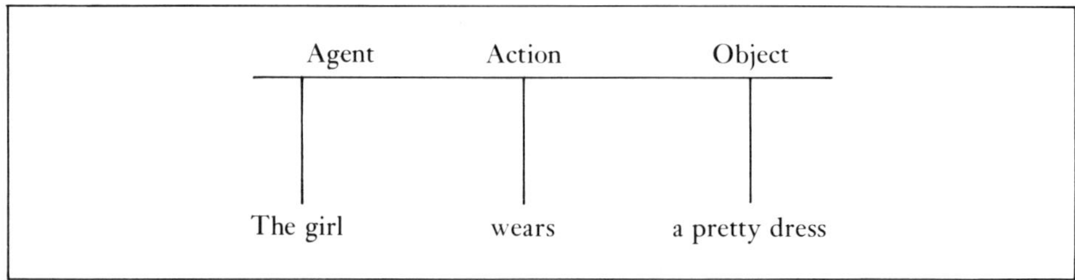

Figure 2–4. Relationships of agent, action, and object.

Some constituents are superfluous. In the sentence *The book that he wanted is in the library*, the word *that* is not needed. It does not add anything to the sentence. Its omission does not change the structure or the meaning.

Young children tend to use the word *and* to string together series of ideas and events. Such outpourings as *I got up and I washed my face and I dressed and then I had breakfast* are common at certain stages of language development. Later, they use recoding or embedding to rephrase the chunks of information included in each short phrase. Some adults continue to talk in such strings, but such construction is likely to lose the attention of the listener. The above sentence can be recoded in the following ways without losing its basic lexical information.

1. After I got up, I washed my face, dressed, and then had breakfast.
2. I got up, washed my face, dressed, and had breakfast.

In addition to using excess verbiage when we talk, we also use sentences that are ambiguous. In the example given earlier, *Visiting friends can be a pain*, we found that we needed additional information about the context, personality of the speaker, and intonation to interpret the statement correctly. This type of string requires consideration of deep structure. Arrangement of the phrase structure depends on more than the actual words in the utterance.

Phrase structure grammar rules do not account for all the variations in the sentences we use. However, they do permit us to examine and to group words within a hierarchy.

The concept of *transformational generative grammar* was described by Chomsky (1965). He recognized that more than a phrase structure grammar is necessary to explain all the sentences we generate and the variations within them.

Transformational grammar is a set of rules or principles that permits us to rearrange, add, delete, and change elements of a sentence. It enables us to generate or create an infinite number of utterances. If we want to change the statement *Mary wears a pretty dress* to a question, the arrangement becomes *Does Mary wear a pretty dress?* Or if we wish to deny the nature of the dress, we can say *Mary isn't wearing a pretty dress*. Linguists who have written grammars have gone into great detail to specify the transformations the children are using. Brown (1973) found that a 34-month-old child, using utterances that were on the average less than three morphemes in length, had 24 transformation rules. For example, he used the rule for agreement of subject and verb in person and number, elliptical possessive forms such as *yours*, and deletion of the subject in imperative sentences. (We will discuss the order of acquisition of transformation rules in the next section.)

Case grammar as Fillmore (1968) describes it is semantically based. In both phrase structure and transformational grammar theory the constituents of the sentence are related to grammatical units such as subjects, objects, agents, and action and, depending upon the linguist (Bloom, 1970), may or may not be coordinated with word order. In Fillmore's case grammar the semantic roles are not tied to grammatical relations. He analyzes the deep structure of a sentence into a proposition and a modality. The proposition has a verb and one or more nouns that are associated with the verb in a case relationship. The verb and the nouns are not ordered. The modality constituents contain the markers for the sentence as a whole, such as question, negation, tense, and mood. Some of the most important cases are given in Table 2–4.

Objections can be raised about all three of these approaches to the study of rules that children must be following when they create their own sentences. Perhaps the phrase structure concept is too simplistic and the transformational generative, not sufficiently complete. Case grammar is by far the most complex system of the three. When Bowerman (1973) applied it to the children whom she studied, she found it inadequate in accounting for the competence underlying children's utterances.

COMPETENCE AND PERFORMANCE

A grammar according to Chomsky is "a description of the ideal speaker-hearer's intrinsic competence" (1965). The adult who has mastered his language has absolute,

Table 2–4. Fillmore Case Grammar

Case Name	Description	Example
Agentive (A)	Animate, perceived instigator of the action	*Mary* hit John. John was hit by *Mary*.
Instrumental (I)	Inanimate force or object causally involved in the state or action named by the verb	The *door* slammed.
Dative (D)	Animate being affected by the state or action named by the verb	He hit *John*. *She* has a house.
Factitive (F)	Object or being resulting from the state or action named by the verb	John built a *wall*. John is a *boy*.
Locative (L)	Location or spatial orientation of the state or action named by the verb	Tom drove to *school*. *Los Angeles* is smoggy.
Objective (O)	Anything representable by a noun whose role in the state or action named by the verb depends on the meaning of the verb itself	Tom opened the *book*. It is a *coat*.

Source: Adapted from C. J. Fillmore. The case for case. In E. Bach and R. T. Harms (Eds.), *Universals in linguistic theory*. New York: Holt, Rinehart & Winston, 1968.

complete knowledge of the linguistic structures. In this sense competence is an abstraction, for we cannot be sure there is such an ideal adult speaker-hearer.

Performance is concrete and measurable. It is an individual's application of linguistic rules and an empirical measure of competence, that is, we infer what linguistic competence a speaker has from how he talks. When the child says *That mine*, we deduce that he does not yet have the concept of the verb *to be* as a copula. If occasionally he says sentences like *That is big*, in which the verb is used correctly, we say his performance indicates that the rules for the copula are emerging, but are not yet established.

The fact that a speaker does not demonstrate specific linguistic rules is not proof that he does not "know" them. It merely indicates that he is not using them. The lack of use may be attributed to many variables. There may not be a need for the person to say much in his environment and thus he may not do much talking. Or he may elect not to talk for a variety of reasons. The child who is usually not understood when he talks may limit his conversation to the briefest sentences or phrases.

SUMMARY

Syntax is the orderly arrangement of words that represent the application of grammatical rules for the construction of sentences. There are many ways to show relationships between words and between the parts of sentences. Phrase structure grammar and transformational generative grammar are the two current approaches that seem most useful in explaining language use. Case grammar, which utilizes a discrete semantic approach, seems less applicable. Competence and performance have been described in relation to linguistic theory.

SEMANTICS

The semantic aspect of language deals with the relationships between referents and the words we use for them; and the changes in the meaning of words. The words, phrases, and expressions we use are the linguistic symbols. The referents are the objects and concepts which the symbols represent. The words *book* and *blue* are descriptors—the first refers to a particular object and the second to an attribute. When we hear the phrase *that blue book,* we call to mind what the words stand for.

MEANING

Meaning is assigned to words by those who use them. When people talk or write, they use verbal symbols whose meanings will be understood by the receiver of the message. The words and phrases must have common denotations in order to have communication. Of course, different languages have different symbols for the same referent. Frenchmen use the term *vous* in conversing with one another, but Americans use its English equivalent *you*. The French say *C'est la vie*, but Americans say *That's life*. Even within one language, problems of denotations arise.

Words and phrases can have multiple meanings, depending on the intent of the user and the context in which the words are employed. As we indicated earlier, we can refer to a *circle* versus a square or a circle of friends. We can *change* a tire or pay for the coke with some *change*. We *back* into a garage, carry the sack on one's *back*, or put the coat *back* in the closet.

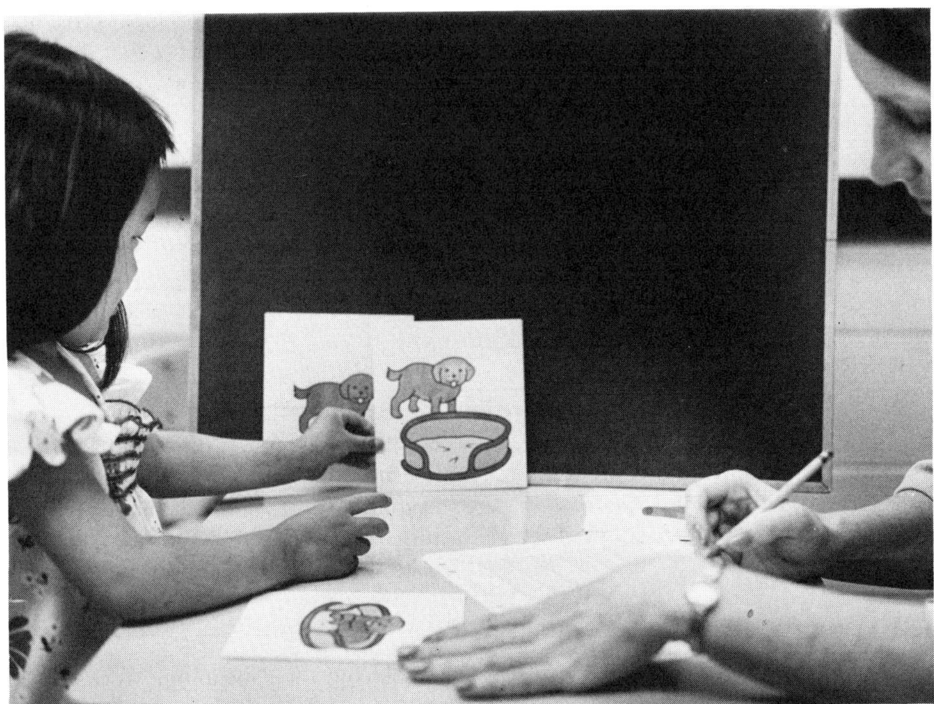

Words are used in new ways as occasions and social interactions dictate. We develop idioms like *dig* that song and *really neat*. The phrase *it's cool* can refer to the temperature of the air, the emotional climate of the room we enter, or the rise in our adrenalin activity triggered by something or someone who clicks with us.

Words take on connotative or emotive meaning beyond their referential meaning. The feelings associated with the symbols may assume greater importance than the dictionary descriptions indicate. For instance, the word *baby* is the linguistic symbol for a young infant. To parents who have waited for months for the arrival of their own baby, the term has added meaning. It's *their* baby and their feelings are now a part of the way they conceptualize and say the word *baby*. The verbal symbol generates feelings in the user of the symbol beyond its stated definition.

A child may use his blanket as a symbol which signifies his bed. His bed provides warmth, protection, pleasant experiences of many kinds. He holds onto his blanket as a sign of his not wanting to be separated from the comforts it signifies. *Blanket* to him has an emotional meaning that extends beyond its naming function.

CONCRETE AND ABSTRACT REFERENTS

A verbal symbol can be thought of as having either a concrete or an abstract referent. *Concrete* means it is capable of being perceived by the senses; and *abstract* means it cannot. Although *concrete* and *abstract* are used as opposites or antonyms, referents are only relatively concrete or abstract. Concrete refers to real, specific, particular things or events. Abstract refers to concepts that are theoretical, impersonal, detached, having limited pictorial representation. Words like *dress, book, coat, shoes* are names given to actual objects, and so we refer to them as concrete. Many process verbs, like *jump, run, open*, and *hit*, denote actions that are also concrete. Adjectives that describe an object, such as *blue, big, tall*, and *pretty*, fall into the same category.

A concrete symbol may also have a general referent, such as *animal, tree*, and *country*. Each of these concrete categories can be made more specific and more concrete by combining it with descriptors or attributes, such as *a carnivorous animal, a canine animal, the animal is a French poodle*.

Words with abstract referents can also be nouns, verbs, or adjectives. Examples are nouns such as *truth, beauty, theory*, and *idea*, stative verbs such as *seem* and *be*, and adjectives such as *unusual, interesting*, and *creative*.

BORROWED SYMBOLS

Most languages have borrowed words from other languages. When a word like *garage* was needed for a referent and the English language did not have a counterpart, Englishmen incorporated the French term into their language. Trade names like *Coke, hamburgers*, and *Cordon Bleu* have become a part of many languages of the world. Americans have adopted several terms that are related to greetings, such as *bon voyage* and *aloha*.

SUMMARY

Semantics is the study of verbal symbols and their meaning. Words are given meanings by the community of language users and the meanings change over time. Dictionary meanings are denotative—they describe or point. However, some words take on emotional or connotative implications that overlap or supplant the denotation. Children first use words as pointers and later to replace the referents when the objects are no longer in view. Words have been classified as relatively concrete or abstract. Some concrete nouns are more general than others, but all can be made specific by the use of qualifiers. We supplement our ability to communicate with others by borrowing words from other languages.

FUNCTIONS

Since language is a system of symbols that people in a community use and understand, we would expect that it could serve many functions. The more symbols we comprehend and utilize, the greater the likelihood that our language will serve multiple purposes. In this section we shall consider the functions of language as they relate to its structure.

PHONOLOGY

There are two principal functions of the phonologic structure. The first is to enable the speaker to combine phonemes to create words of all kinds. It is possible to make an almost infinite number of combinations of the English phonemes. However, there are limits to the actual number because of production and acoustic variables. Some arrangements are too difficult to produce and others would require fine acoustic modulations which we find difficult to differentiate.

The second function is related to the morphologic structure. The affixes we discussed earlier in the chapter are phonemes that are attached to or imbedded in words, and the affixes have special functions.

MORPHOLOGY

The functions of the morphologic structure can be considered in two parts—those related to the morphs or roots and those related to inflections. Words are the basic units of the language and as such convey multiple meanings. These words have functions related to their classifications as nouns, pronouns, verbs, adjectives, adverbs, prepositions, conjunctions, and articles. A morph can be utilized as a noun in one context and as a verb in another, for example, a *pound* of sugar and to *pound* the table.

As children begin to talk, they first utilize words as referents. Among their first words are *this*, *that*, *bye*, *mommy*, *daddy*, and *doll*. The first two may be accompanied by gestures that either designate or locate what they want. As they say *bye*, usually they are also waving with their hands or arms. The other three are names, but children may use them along with many gestures and body movements to reveal a wide range of needs, explanations, or just simple pleasure. The number of referents grows at a fantastic rate during the early years; as we are exposed to more and more experiences, we learn more referents.

The naming function is important not only to the user of language, but to his listener as well. We can get as frustrated as the gnat in *Alice in Wonderland* when he bemoaned to Alice, "What's the use of them having names if they won't answer them!" Alice replied, "No use at all, but it's useful to the people who need them, I suppose. If not, why do things have names at all?" (Carroll, 1954).

The second function of morphology is related to the inflections added to words to transform them and their significations. For instance, there are the inflections that express plurality; possession; verb tense, number, and person; comparative and superlative forms of adjectives. Other inflections change meaning from a positive to a negative (*careful*, *careless; successful*, *unsuccessful*). Still others change the function of the word from that of a noun to that of an adjective and vice versa (*work*, *workable; big*, *bigness*).

SYNTAX

The functions of the order of words in utterances can be viewed in relation to the length of the presentence and complete sentence. Two-term utterances identify the following relationships (Brown, 1973).

1. Agent and action: *boy go*
2. Agent and object: *daddy car*
3. Action and object: *throw ball*
4. Action and location: *go home*
5. Entity and location: *mommy store*
6. Entity and attribute: *pretty girl*
7. Possessor and possession: *my bike*
8. Demonstrative and entity: *that boy*

The functions of these two-term units have been expressed as relationships that children need to convey in this stage of development. They can manage only two-word utterances in the early presentence phase, and the words they use must be key elements. There is no extra verbiage, no embellishment. These are the "bare bones" that will culminate shortly in sentences.

These relationships eventually are expressed within sentences. Most sentences are declarative-affirmative in nature. Thus we could say that the function is unitary—the sentence makes or expresses a declaration that is affirmative. However, we can identify three separate functions of the declarative-affirmative sentence.

1. To inform or report
2. To describe
3. To refer to people, events, or things

To inform or report involves statements about an idea or the facts of a situation. To describe may or may not be part of informing or reporting. The referential function may be considered a way of considering people, events, or things in a temporal relationship.

The sentence serves three other functions.

4. To ask questions
5. To give commands or directions
6. To negate an action or idea

Function 6 can be combined with the other functions of a sentence, so that we can ask a question in a negative fashion or tell someone not to do something, for example, *Which book don't you want? Don't do that.*

SEMANTICS

Since semantics deals with verbal symbols and their meanings, we might have placed some of the functions related to syntax under semantics. However, the ordering of the words contributes to the purposes of utterances, and for this reason we tried to isolate the functions related to syntax.

In discussing semantic aspects, we must consider some of the general functions of language. The first is categorization. A young child perceives and calls the thing that races around him or chases him a *dog*. He will try to pull its tail, climb on top of it, or hug it. As the child has more experiences involving different animals, he or she begins to recognize features that are common to groups of animals, for example, to sort out those that bark from those who say meow. This phenomenon can be observed in many situations.

Young children may, at first, use the term *dada* to refer to anyone who plays with them. At a further level of differentiation they perceive that there are a father, a mother, and other big people and that each has its own characteristics. Young children also like to explore and examine things they see and touch. They will not only put a spoonful of peaches in their mouths to eat, but also may try a spoonful of the dog's food or a spoonful of soap powder. Two-year-olds may try to put their fingers in electric plug recepticles. As yet they have not learned which substances they can and cannot eat nor which holes are dangerous or not dangerous. The process of classifying perceptions continues as long as the individual is exposed to new experiences or conceptualizes old experiences in different ways.

In order to utilize the thousands of bits of information accumulated over the years, the individual must classify them. Each person stores data related to number, color, time, position, family, clothes, furniture, professions, and so on. As we perceive and organize the concrete world and develop our concepts, our original classifications are broadened and new ones emerge. We find commonalities among things and ideas and can share them with others with greater facility than we could share the parts and pieces.

Language functions as an aid to memory, reasoning, new learning, and fantasy. First let us consider memory. The 12-month old perceives only what is in his direct line of vision. If his ball is covered with a blanket, he will not be able to find the ball, even if he has watched it being covered. He may indicate that it is gone, but he will not try to find it. It may be many months before he will talk about his ball or blanket when those objects are out of sight. The concept of remembering involves skill in placing events in time, use of accurate referents, and sometimes a correct sequence. Several witnesses to a car accident may give different versions of the event even at the scene. A few weeks later many of the details of the accident may have become blurred to the point that the viewer has difficulty reconstructing it. We sometimes say our memory plays tricks on us. We forget what we've promised to do tomorrow, that we've already written that letter, that we took the coat to be cleaned, or where we stored last summer's bathing suit. Some children do not remember that they burn their fingers each time they put them on the hot stove.

Although we can learn by doing alone, language in an asset. Luria's (1961) experiments with Russian children indicated that tasks were learned faster when the children received oral instructions as they carried out a task. By the time children are in third grade, they are expected to learn a great deal of the school subject matter through reading. Since we can read faster than we can listen to "talking" books, the reader has a greater chance of acquiring more information than the nonreader.

Reasoning or problem solving, particularly at abstract levels, requires a symbol system. Language facilitates thinking and permits the user to consider alternative actions, to weigh arguments on several possible solutions, and reach some defensible positions.

The expression of fantasy and imagery is a less frequent, but nevertheless important function of language. The poet selects ideas and experiences from many sources and freely creates a poem. Imagery is a part of our best fiction and nonfiction, of the songs that tell a story, but only occasionally of our oral language. Loban (1963) reported that he found very few examples of metaphor, irony, simile, or personification in the oral language transcripts of elementary school children. He suggested that we do not encourage this form of oral language, and therefore it is not prevalent. Emphasis placed on the technical and scientific aspects of school subjects may also contribute to the paucity of figurative expressions.

SUMMARY

In this chapter we have defined language as a symbol system that has been developed and is understood by those in a community. We have considered its structure and functions. The structure has four major components: phonology, morphology, syntax, and semantics. Each has been described as it applies to the English language.

Each of the four components has special functions, which may overlap, and these have been identified. We have associated the most general of the functions with the semantic aspect of the language. Language used with appropriate structure, but with no meaning for the speaker or listener serves no function. It is a meaningless string of nonsensical items.

REFERENCES

Bloom, L. *Language development: Form and function in emerging grammars*. Cambridge, Mass.: MIT Press, 1970.

Bowerman, M. *Early syntactic development*. London: Cambridge University Press, 1973.

Brown, R. *A first language The early stages*. Cambridge, Mass.: Harvard University Press, 1973.

Carroll, L. *Alice's adventures in wonderland and Through the looking glass*. New York: Dutton, 1954.

Chomsky, N. *Aspects of the theory of syntax*. Cambridge, Mass.: MIT Press, 1965.

Denes, P. B., and Pinson, E. N. *The speech chain*. Garden City, New York: Anchor Press, Doubleday, 1973.

Fairbanks, G. *Voice and articulation drillbook*. New York: Harper & Row, 1960.

Fant, G. M. Descriptive analysis of the acoustic aspects of speech. *Logos, 5*, 3–17 (1962).

Fillmore, C. J. The case for case. In E. Bach and R. T. Harms (Eds.), *Universals in linguistic theory*. New York: Holt, Rinehart & Winston, 1968.

Gleason, H. A. *An introduction to descriptive linguistics* (Rev. ed.). New York: Holt, Rinehart & Winston, 1965.

Jakobson, R., Fant, G. M., and Halle, M. *Preliminaries to speech analysis* (Acoustics Laboratory Technical Report 13). Cambridge, Mass.: MIT Press, 1952.

Labov, W. *The social stratification of English in New York City*. Washington, D.C.: Center for Applied Linguistics, 1966.

Loban, W. D. The language of elementary school children. *NCTE research report No. 1*. Champaign, Ill.: National Council of Teachers of English, 1963.

Luria, A. R. *The role of speech in the regulation of normal and abnormal behavior*. New York: Liveright, 1961.

McNeill, D. *The acquisition of language The study of developmental psycholinguistics*. New York: Harper & Row, 1970.

Minifie, F., Hixon, T., and Williams, F. *Normal aspects of speech hearing and language*. New York: Prentice-Hall, 1973.

LANGUAGE ACQUISITION AND LANGUAGE DEFICITS Chapter 3

This chapter deals with two aspects of language—normal language acquisition and deficits in language. In the discussion of normal acquisition we describe the communication interactions, the procedures that are utilized for teaching and learning in the early acquisition phase, the stages of language acquisition, the general characteristics, and the relationship of comprehension and production. In the section on deficits we describe and classify abnormalities that may occur in the structure of language and provide some guidelines for determining whether language is delayed, deviant, or different.

NORMAL LANGUAGE ACQUISITION

THE COMMUNICATION INTERACTIONS

In Chapter 1 we indicated that the newborn reacts to the mother's voice through synchronous body movements. Even when only a few days old, she will stop her total body activity and substitute a rhythmic pattern in tune with the speech she is hearing. The infant is already aware of her auditory environment.

The learning process through which the child achieves a language system includes exposure to thousands of experiences, including units of language. Adults and other children give the child opportunities to participate in new experiences, listen, practice, and finally consolidate the new learning with the old. Figure 3–1 outlines this process.

The child attends to and actively participates at her level of capability with other people in her environment. During the early stages it may only be through looking at

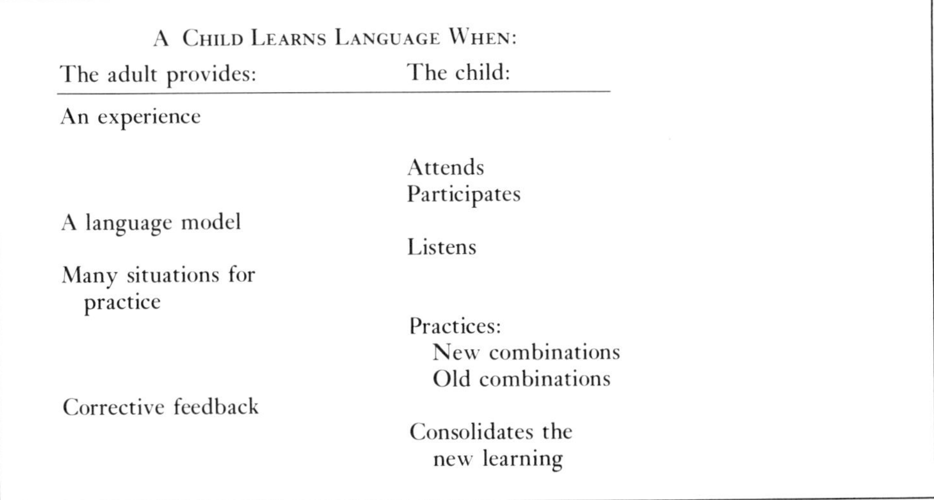

A CHILD LEARNS LANGUAGE WHEN:

The adult provides:	The child:
An experience	
	Attends Participates
A language model	
	Listens
Many situations for practice	
	Practices: New combinations Old combinations
Corrective feedback	
	Consolidates the new learning

Figure 3–1. Process of learning a language system.

the individual, smiling, or making a few noises. When the adult provides a language model, the child listens. As she is given opportunities to use language, she practices, whether an adult is present or not. She makes mistakes, corrects them, and finally acquires a whole set of rules to match those of the people in her environment. The process of learning is gradual and continuous. It begins in the home, continues in school, and in the neighborhood and terminates only when all learning stops.

THE EARLY ACQUISITION STAGE

PROCEDURES FOR TEACHING

There are some universal procedures that parents and others utilize in teaching language. Figure 3–2 identifies and describes them. Until we are able to read, we obtain most of our information through *modeling*. Parents talk to their young children a great deal. They explain what they are doing, provide the names for things, problem-solve aloud, tell stories, and so on. When the children are able to reply, mothers model on the same topic or on a different one. The best learning situation is the one in which the adult listens to the child's reply.

Many of the child's early attempts to use language are incorrect. Parents help by *expanding* the child's remark, either by correcting the grammar or by providing appropriate vocabulary. Studies by Brown (1973) indicate that mothers are more likely to utilize semantic expansion than grammatical expansion. They are not as sensitive to grammatical errors of their children.

1. Modeling—adult engages in conversation with the child
   - Antecedent—adult initiates or continues a conversation with the child
     - Example: *Adult:* I'm going to make a cake. Do you want to help me?
   - Subsequential—adult comments on the child's reply without correcting or repeating the child's statement
     - Example: *Child:* Yes, I like to help you.
       Adult: Good. Then get me the pans from the cupboard.
2. Expansion—adult corrects the child's remark and may add another one
   - Grammatical—adult corrects the grammar
     - Example: *Child:* Yes, I likes to help you.
       Adult: I like to help you. Get me the pans.
   - Semantic—adult corrects the lexicon
     - Example: *Child:* Here are the pans.
       Adult: No, they're not cake pans; they're for baking cookies.
3. Echoing—adult echoes the child's remark, but replaces an unintelligible part of the remark with a wh- word (what, when, where, who)
   - Example: *Child:* I ate the (unintelligible)
     Adult: You ate the what?

Figure 3–2. Teaching procedures.

At first the child's comments may be partially or completely unintelligible. The parent who understands even a part of the comment may use the technique of *echoing*. The parent gives the child the feeling of partial success by showing that some of his communication unit was understood. Many parents utilize this procedure even when they are "guessing" at what the child has said, with the hope that the shorter response that is necessary from the child will enable them to comprehend more easily and perhaps help them to fill in the rest.

Sometimes the parent will echo the child's statement with a rising intonation. The child says, "I don't want anymore," and the parent repeats, "You don't want anymore?" The parent may be surprised by the remark or may be questioning it to be sure that the child's meaning is understood.

Wyatt (1969) reported some observations of mother-child interactions that run the gamut from ideal to overwhelming. In a conversation between Lisa, age 4, and her mother, the modeling is both antecedent and subsequential, with short but complete sentences used by the mother and slightly shorter sentences and phrases utilized by Lisa. Here is an excerpt.

MOTHER	LISA
1. What happened to your toe? Did you rock on it?	No, I bent it (examines her toe).

2. Is it all right now?	Yes. (She finds another picture in her book.) Look at the man. He's writing on the thing.
3. That's a typewriter. He's writing on the typewriter.	(Rocking back and forth) See the fence. He can't climb over.
4. No, the fence is too high.	A kanagaroo could jump over the fence. See me jump (laughs and jumps twice).
5. You'd make a good kangaroo.	

In Lisa's second comment to her mother she uses the word *thing*. The mother provides a more accurate description of the *thing* by supplying the word *typewriter*. This is an example of a semantic expansion. The child must learn names of things and parents or others provide the words. The mother might have expanded Lisa's comment "He can't climb over" by saying "He can't climb over it." Such a correction would be an example of a grammatical expansion.

In another of Wyatt's observations of a mother and her 4-year-old daughter, the mother did all the talking. There were only three speeches—the mother used 99 words in the first one, the daughter replied in a statement of 11 words, and the mother continued her modeling with another comment of 56 words!

When we talk, we stress some words more than others. Mothers use paralinguistic structures such as increased loudness and pitch change to focus the child's attention on selected parts of a comment. Experiments by Blasdell and Jensen (1970) and others demonstrated that young children, 28 to 39 months of age, use the primary stress pattern of the speaker to comprehend what is being said. In the examples in Figure 3–2 adults would stress the words which they want to emphasize in the expansion procedure. The same investigators also noted that the position of a word in an utterance is important. The final word is the one the young child is most likely to remember and repeat back.

There is some evidence that mothers and fathers have different communication patterns for their sons and daughters and for older versus younger children. Hubbell, Byrne, and Stachowiak (1974) reported that when parents were teaching their children how to put some puzzles together, both parents talked more to their 3-year-olds than to their 6-year-olds. Fathers talked more to their sons than to their daughters, and mothers were more active with their daughters than with their sons. In addition the parents used a greater variety of and more complex comments when they talked with their older children. Since parents perceive the needs of children of varying ages differently, they react to suit what they consider to be the appropriate level for their children. In dealing with 2- and 3-year-olds middle-class mothers increase the syntactic complexity of their speech according to the age of the child and what they think he'll understand, even though they are not aware of the modifications.

Models such as those on television programs are also important. *Sesame Street* and similar shows have provided opportunities for children to watch, listen, and participate in learning experiences. One of the dangers of too much exposure to most television is that it does not provide any opportunity to talk about a program or what it means. Children who only watch and listen never become participants in the experiences that are being featured, do not assimilate the information, and do not learn the language of the speakers. The same situation occurs in the wards of institutions where radios and record players blast the ears of the residents and the workers. They become immune to the noise and cannot tell anyone what is being played. The music becomes a part of the background, and even the ads are tuned out.

PROCEDURES FOR LEARNING

The procedures for teaching are initiated by the adults and others who are talking to the child. How does the child learn? Initially, he learns through listening to those in his environment, being a part of the situations, and imitating what he hears. During the first year, he listens to someone say *momma* as he is picked up. Then he produces his version of the word. He listens to his mother say *goodbye*, while he simultaneously waves and says *bye*.

Imitation is a process whereby a behavior is acquired through copying the behavior of a model. Just as the child imitates the visual pattern of the motor act of waving an arm, hand, and fingers to indicate *goodbye*, he copies the verbal label. He does not reproduce the waving actions of the adult at first, but over time he changes his movements to match more closely those of his model. His speech likewise is his version of what he hears. He gets a mental representation of the modeled words and begins to imitate.

The many phonological errors a child makes in early imitation may be due to faulty perception or memory of the entire word or sequence. Ingram (1974) has provided us with examples of words produced incorrectly by the child but certainly understood by the adults. A child hears the word *elephant*, but says *hefənt*. The child's imitations are not exact copies of the models, but what he perceives the model to be. His perceptions are influenced by the stress pattern the speaker has used and the length of the utterance, as well as other as yet undefined variables.

What we have said about imitation at the phonological level applies also at the morphologic and syntactic levels. He has heard his mother tell him to *drink* his milk or his mother's remark that the cat *drinks* his water. At first he may imitate each verb inflection correctly, but later he may mix them up. He learns some modeled units as separate entities.

McNeill (1970) reported that only 10 percent of the speech of children 28 to 35 months of age represented direct models. As his repertoire increases, the child must organize what he is hearing into some kind of a system. He is now entering the second phase of his language learning which is the *induction of rules*. He continues to imitate selectively, but also engages in generative creation, that is, he tries out combinations he has not actually heard in his environment. For example, when Tom was showing his father his toy tractor, he said, "him breaked it." When his mother asked Gary the name of his teacher and did not understand his reply, she tried guessing, "Is it Beth? Ted?" Gary replied, "He not a boy. My teacher a girl." There could never be sufficient time for any child to learn through imitation all of the specific verbal responses he will produce in his lifetime. Somehow he must develop rules to help him to generate responses for millions of situations.

Incidental learning takes place also. The child internalizes much of what he hears, practices, and combines the new with the old forms. There may be a combination of what he has imitated completely or selectively, memorized words and grammar forms, and utterances based on construction rules that he has figured out for himself.

STAGES OF LANGUAGE ACQUISITION

The stages of language acquisition will be considered in relation to the structure of a language. We have organized this material in relation to the phonologic, morphologic, syntactic, and semantic aspects. Because the information comes from a wide variety of sources, we have reviewed the sources first.

SOURCES OF INFORMATION

Our knowledge of language development is based on information gathered in many different ways. The sources include orthographic and phonetic transcriptions of children's speech, tape recordings and transcribed records of children talking in a natural environment, tests and tasks designed to answer specific research questions, interviews, and anecdotal reports prepared primarily by parents. The data obtained in carefully controlled studies agree across investigators for the most part, in spite of the limitations of the specific procedures.

In the days before quality tape recorders were available, investigators, such as McCarthy (1954), transcribed in words and symbols the spontaneous speech and elicited responses of preschool children. Irwin and Chen (1946) phonetically transcribed utterances of young children from 1 to 30 months old. These procedures required well-trained ears and hands, because there was no permanent record to which the investigators could return to verify what a particular child had said.

Tape recordings of children as they talked in their homes began to be gathered in the period after World War II. The most widely known tapes are those obtained by Brown and his students on Adam, Eve, and Sarah in the 1950s. Tapes were transcribed and morphemic analyses were made of the utterances. About 78 percent of the utterances were sufficiently intelligible to be transcribed. The degree of intelligibility of tapes is dependent on several factors such as amount of background noise, type of equipment used for recording, placement of the microphones, and the intelligibility of the speech of those being taped. These factors must be considered in evaluating the findings of an investigator.

Tests and tasks have been designed to determine which structures a child comprehends or is expressing. Even though many of the tests of grammar have not been adequately standardized, they do provide some guidelines about a child's status.

Mothers who bring children to well baby clinics or to physicians may be asked about the language milestones that interested Gesell (1940) and others. The information obtained in such interviews may be gross because mothers do not necessarily remember exact dates and may have widely varying interpretations of the milestones. For example, most case history forms ask the age of the first words of a child. But there is no way to know how a parent defines a word. If a father picks up his infant daughter and she says *da da da*, he may think the child is using the word *daddy*. However, if the baby also says *da da da* when her mother fondles her, those sounds may be her utterance for any person. Or the two or three syllable utterance may be nothing more than random vocal activity with no meaning. In any event, the investigator has no way of knowing whether the utterance has the lexical meaning that adults have given the word *daddy*. This same problem of interpretation applies to anecdotal records. The information must be viewed with caution, unless it can be verified in some other way.

PHONOLOGY

The first cries of newborn infants herald the beginning of the sounds they will use during their lifetime. Crying and reflex noises infants make during the first few months are the preliminary to the language phase. Although they do not stop their crying, it diminishes as they grow, just as the reflex noises disappear. During the first six weeks infants begin to turn toward the sound of household noises and they attend briefly to voices and music. Horowitz (1974) reported that although 5- and 6-week-old infants stopped attending to a repeated visual stimulus, their attention was regained when music was paired with the visual stimulus.

Early Phoneme Production. The early sound-making of children has been reported by Irwin and Chen (1946). Irwin phonetically transcribed the spontaneous

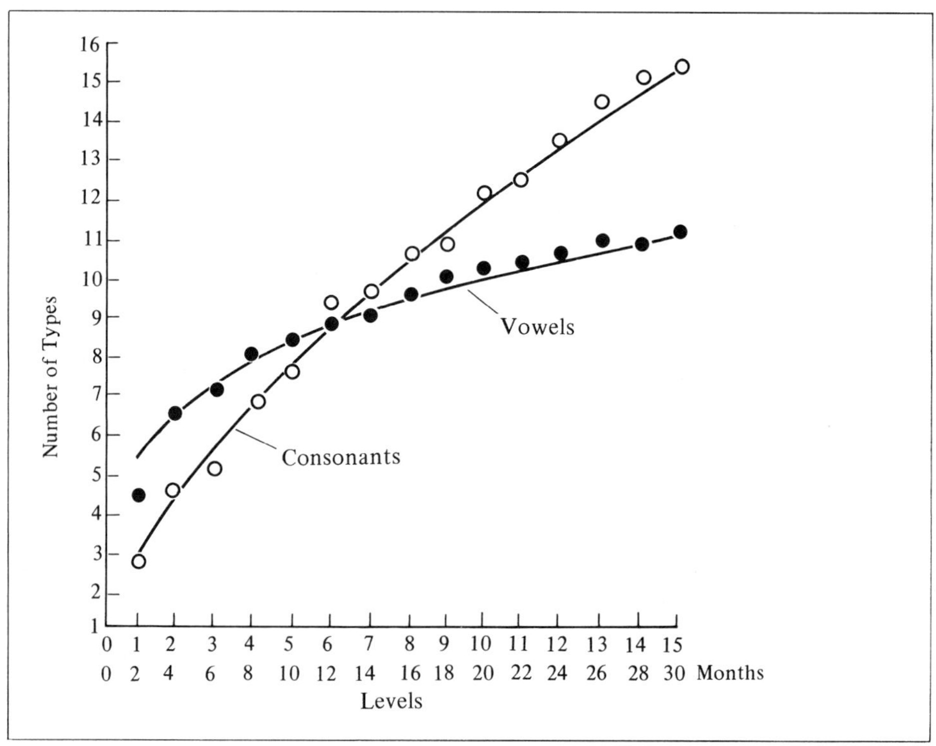

Figure 3–3. Types of vowels and consonants. (H. P. Chen and O. C. Irwin. Infant speech: Vowel and consonant types. *Journal of Speech Disorders*, *11*, 27–29, 1946.)

utterances children made in each of 30 breath units or exhalations. He transcribed breath units that contained noncrying sounds. The units were not necessarily consecutive because of the difficulty he had in writing as fast as the children uttered sounds and eventually words. He began his transcriptions when the children were 1 to 2 months of age and continued with them until they were 30 months old. He analyzed the sounds in many ways, but we will mention primarily the type and frequency data.

Irwin was able to distinguish a total of 44 different phonemes in the speech of the children. These included 28 consonants, 3 of which are not a part of the adult standard English phoneme system, 11 vowels, and 5 diphthongs. Figure 3–3 shows the mean number of phonemes as they appear over time. There is a steady increase from 7 at level 1 (1 to 2 months age group) to 27 at level 15 (29 to 30 months age group). Not all children at each level used the same phonemes; and even at 30 months they were not all producing within the 30 breath units all the possible 44.

The mean frequency of sounds for those at level 1 was 62; at level 15 it had risen to 156. During the first few months the most frequently appearing vowels were [I], [ɛ] and [ʌ]; [k], [g], [h] and [ʔ] were the consonants most frequently used. By age 30 months the frequency of vowels and consonants approximated that of the adult. The increment in frequency can be noted in Figure 3–4.

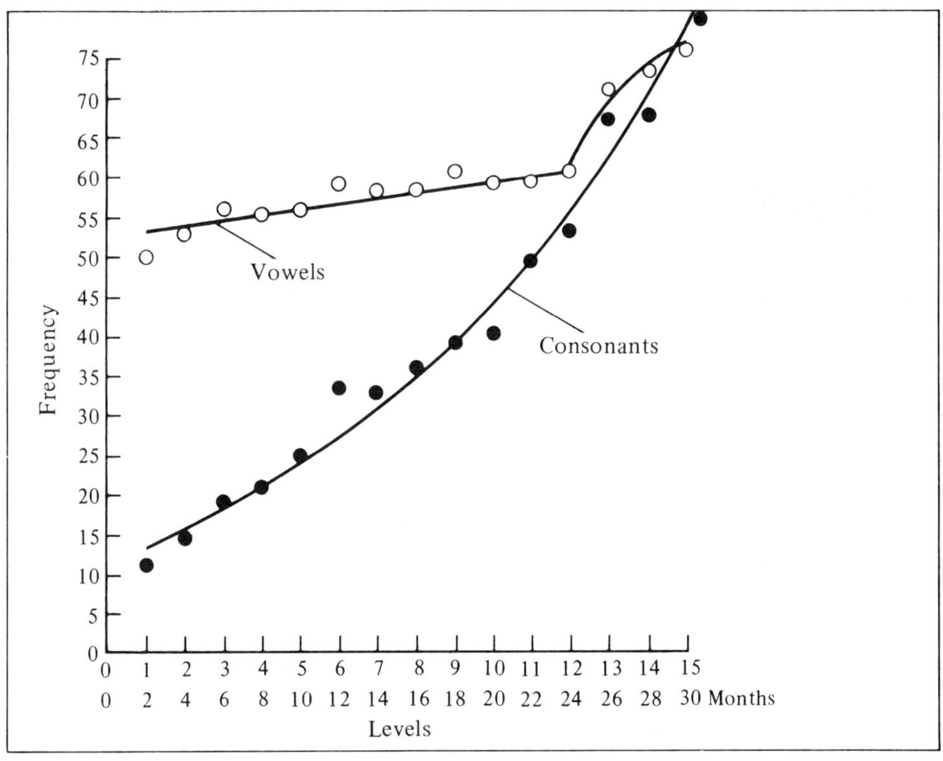

Figure 3–4. Mean frequency of vowels and consonants. (O. C. Irwin and H. P. Chen. Infant speech: Vowel and consonant frequency. *Journal of Speech Disorders, 11*, 123–125, 1946.)

When Irwin (1947a) considered the relative proportion of vowel categories over time, he noted that front vowels, so prominent in the newborn, decline; mid vowels stay about the same; and back vowels increase in frequency. Among the consonants the glottals decline, the velars remain about the same, and the labials, dentals, alveolars, and palatals increase. Analyses of the proportion by manner of articulation over the age levels (Irwin, 1947b) showed that fricatives decline in frequency, plosives remain high, nasals increase gradually, and liquids and semivowels remain the same.

Winitz and Irwin (1958) analyzed the vowel and consonant composition of the words of children divided into three age groups—13 to 14 months, 15 to 16 months, and 17 to 18 months. The frequency of occurrence of vowels and consonants in these three groups is given in Figures 3–5 and 3–6. The vowel [ɑ] as in *father* predominates in all three age groups. Consonants [b] and [d] have the highest percentage of occurrence

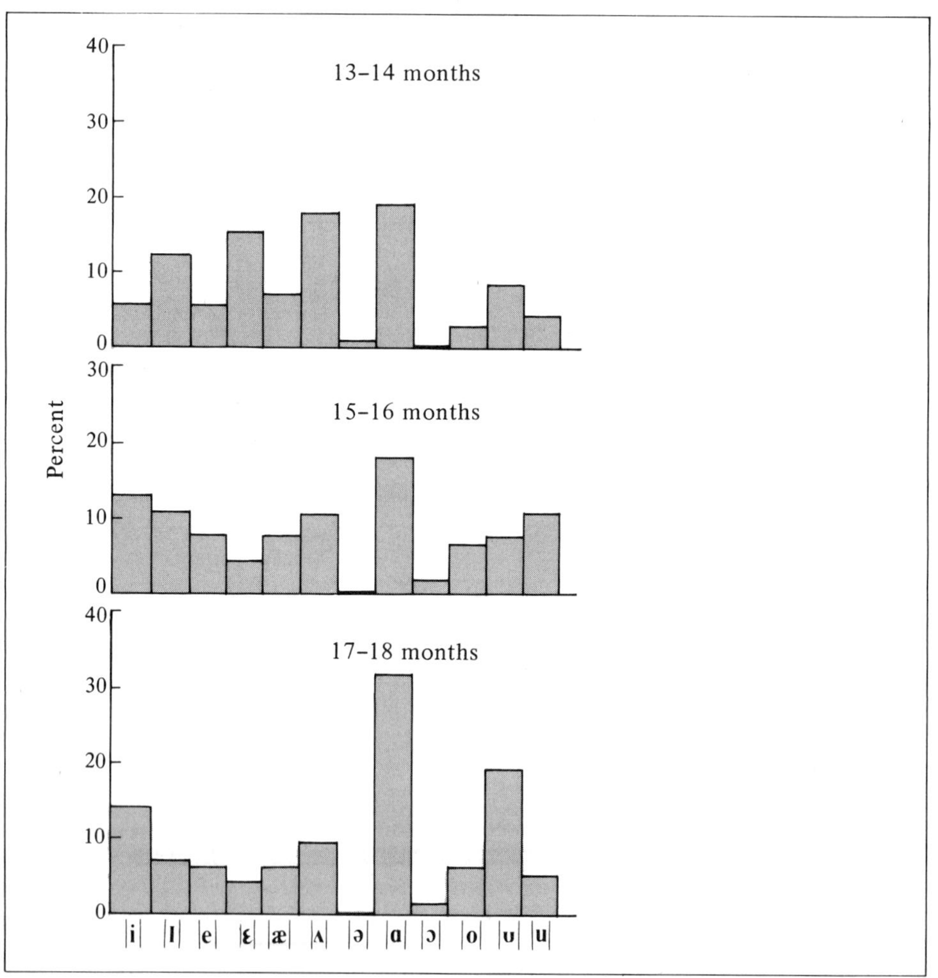

Figure 3–5. Vowel percentages in infants' words. (H. Winitz and O. C. Irwin. Syllabic and phonetic structure of infants' early words. *Journal of Speech and Hearing Research, 1*, 250–256, 1958.)

across the groups. In the youngest group note that only 13 consonants have appeared, 5 additional appear in the second age group; and even in the oldest group 8 are still not in use in words.

MASTERY OF THE PHONEMES. Although phonetic sounds are being produced almost from the beginning of life, complete mastery is not attained until 7 or 8 years. By 7 years 75 percent of the girls are using the two- and three-consonant blends in words such as *school* correctly, as well as the single consonants, vowels, and diphthongs; 75 percent of the boys have achieved that level by age 8 (Templin, 1957).

Mastery of vowels and diphthongs is achieved by most children by age 3. Metraux (1950) recorded and transcribed phonetically the speech production of more than 200 children between the ages of 18 and 54 months. The children were enrolled in a

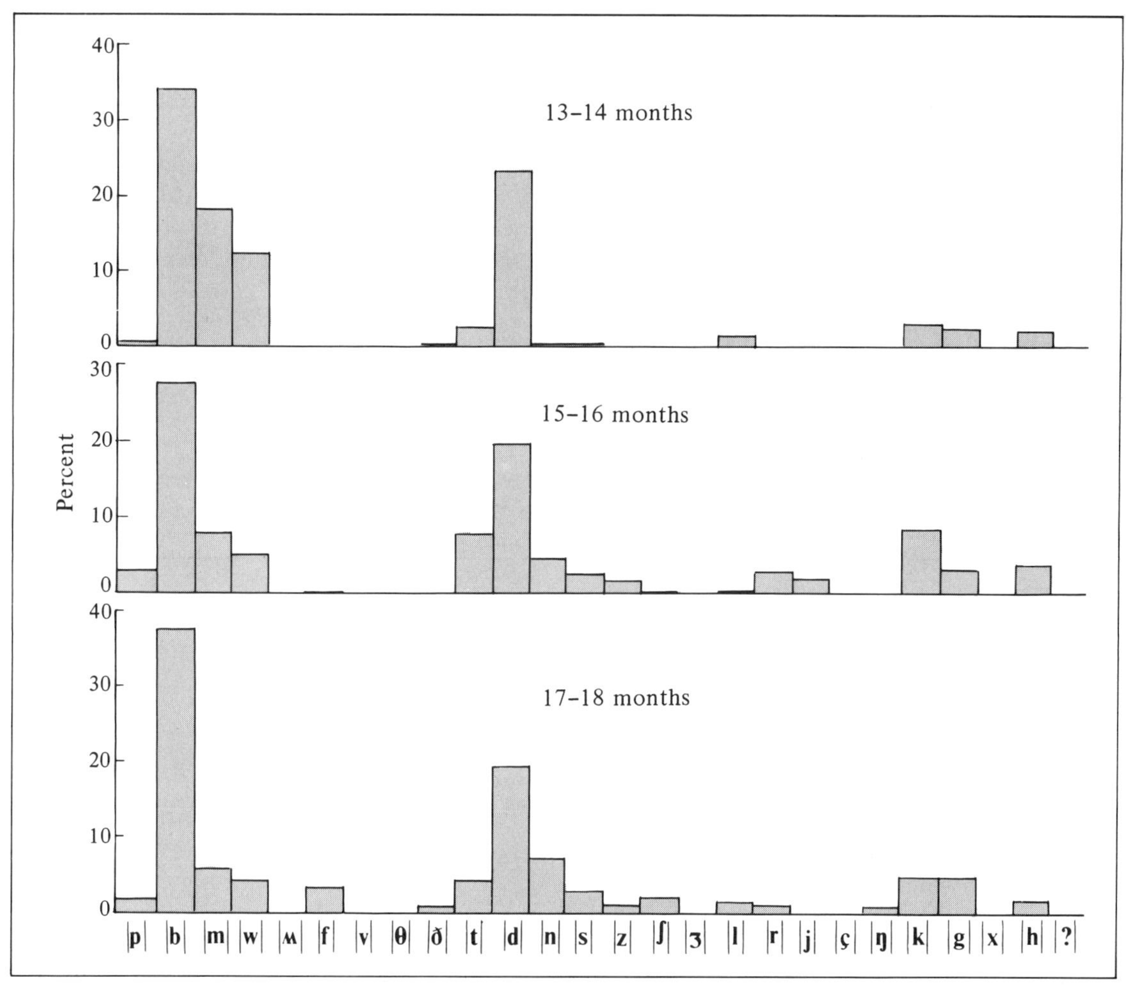

Figure 3–6. Consonant percentages in infants' words. (H. Winitz and O. C. Irwin. Syllabic and phonetic structure of infants' early words. *Journal of Speech and Hearing Research*, *1*, 250–256, 1958.)

nursery program at Yale University, and all had either average or above average intelligence. After analyzing the data on these children, Metraux reported that their vowel production was more than 90 percent correct by 30 months.

In a more controlled study Templin (1957) reported similar findings. She tested 60 children at ages 3, 3½, 4, 4½, 5, 6, 7, and 8 years. There was an equal number of boys and girls. The proportion of children in different socioeconomic categories was similar to national proportions. Templin identified the age at which 75 percent of the children used each phoneme correctly and used that age as a guide. More than 95 percent of the 3-year-olds were using 4 of her 5 tested diphthongs and 10 of the 12 vowels correctly. Since she did not test children below age 3, we do not know whether 75 percent of 2-year-olds, for instance, would have passed her vowel and diphthong test. However, we can be confident in using age 3 to indicate the upper age limit for mastery of most vowels and diphthongs.

There have been many studies of the age of acquisition of consonants. The most recent (Prather, Hedrick, and Kern, 1975) involved children 24 to 48 months of age. They were Caucasian, lived in the Greater Seattle area, and were drawn from high, middle, and low social classes. The children had normal hearing and normal language development.

The basis for determining the age of acquisition of a phoneme was the responses to a picture test of 25 consonants. Each consonant was tested in the initial and final position in words. For instance, [s] was evaluated as being correct or incorrect as it was used in the word *sun* (initial position) and *bus* (final position). The age of acquisition was set as the one at which 75 percent of an age group produced the phoneme correctly in both the initial and final positions. Table 3–1 lists the consonants that were tested and the age of acquisition. By 4 years of age 20 of the 25 had been acquired; 3 consonants, [s], [r], and [l], were utilized by an earlier age group, but then showed a regression to a lower percent correct in one older age group.

Table 3–1. Earliest Age in Years and Months at Which 75 Percent of the Children Produced the Phoneme Correctly

Phoneme	Age of Acquisition	Phoneme	Age of Acquisition
m	2–0	g	3–0
n	2–0	s	3–0
h	2–0	r	3–4
p	2–0	l	3–4
ŋ	2–0	ʃ	3–8
f	2–4	tʃ	3–8
j	2–4	ð	4–0
k	2–4	ʒ	4–0
d	2–4	dʒ	4+[a]
w	2–8	θ	4+[a]
b	2–8	v	4+[a]
t	2–8	z	4+[a]
		hw	4+[a]

Source: E. M. Prather, D. L. Hedrick, and C. A. Kern. Articulation development in children aged two to four years. *Journal of Speech and Hearing Disorders*, *40*, 179–191 (1975).

[a] Not produced correctly by 75 percent of the children in the oldest age group.

The fact that 20 out of 25 consonants are accurate in these preschool children is one indicator of the rapid growth in mastery of the consonants of the language. The slippage in three consonants may indicate lack of stability in correct production for a period of about eight months.

The Templin (1957) study provides information about consonant singles and blends as well as vowels and diphthongs. Table 3–2 gives the ages at which 75 percent

Table 3–2. Earliest Age at Which 75 Percent of the Children Studied Produced Each Tested Sound Correctly

Chronological Age in Years	Position of Consonant		
	Initial	Medial	Final
3	m	m	m
	n	n	n
		ng	ng
	p	p	p
	t		t
	k	k	
	b	b	
	d	d	
	g	g	
	f	f	f
	h	h	
	w	w	
3.5		s	
		z	
			r
	y	y	
4			k
			b
			d
			g
	s		
	sh		sh
		v	
	j		
	r	r	
	l	l	
4.5			s
		sh	
	ch	ch	ch
5		j	
6		t	
	th (*th*umb)	th	th
	v		v
	th (*th*is)		
			l
7		th (fea*th*er)	th (smoo*th*e)
	z		z
			j
8	Most 2 and 3 blend elements		

Source: Based on data from M. Templin. *Certain language skills in children.* Minneapolis: University of Minnesota Press, 1957.

of the children had mastered the consonants. Before the children were 3½ years old, 75 percent of them were using half the consonants in at least one position in the test words. They had mastered 5 of the 12 in all positions and the other 7 in two positions. Within another year 8 additional consonants were being utilized. In other words, by age 4 most of the consonants, including those that appear most frequently in our spoken language, were being produced correctly. Only 3 additional ones were left, and these were used by 75 percent of the 6-year-olds. By 8 the two- and three-consonant blends had emerged. In the short span of 8 years most children had learned the phonology of American English.

Table 3–3 has been constructed from the raw data of the Templin study. Using the data, we can compare the ages at which 75 percent and 90 percent of the sample showed correct responses. Of the 20 phonemes mastered by 75 percent of the 4-year-old or younger groups, 4 ([r], [s], [l], [ʃ]) were slow in reaching 90 percent criterion. For this sample of children, we can say that if they did not master these phonemes early, another two years would go by before an older group would show almost complete correct production. One consonant, [tʃ], was utilized correctly by 75 percent of the 4½ year olds, but it was not until the 7-year-old age group that 90% of the children used it accurately. We recognize that the Templin 5- and 6-year-old

Table 3–3. Templin Speech Sound Normative Data: Age at Which Children Produced Phonemes Correctly

	75% Correct Responses			90% Correct Responses		
Phoneme	Initial	Medial	Final	Initial	Medial	Final
m	3	3	3	3	3	3
n	3	3	3	3	3	3
ŋ	—	3	3	—	4.5	6
p	3	3	3	3	3	4
f	3	3	3	3.5	4	4
h	3	3	—	3	3.5	—
w	3	3	—	3	3.5	—
j	4	5	—	4	4	—
k	3	3	4	3	3	6
b	3	3	4	3	3	6
d	3	3	4	3	4	6
g	3	3	4	3.5	3	6
t	3	6	3	3	—	7
s	4	3.5	4.5	7	8	8
r	4	4	3.5	7	6	6
tʃ	4.5	4.5	4.5	7	7	7
ʃ	4	4.5	4	7	7	7
l	4	4	6	6	6	7
v	6	4	6	7	6	8
dʒ	4	5	7	5	6	—
θ	6	6	6	7	6	7
z	7	3.5	7	7	7	—
ð	6	7	7	7	8	8

Source: Based on data from M. Templin. *Certain language skills in children.* Minneapolis: University of Minnesota Press, 1957.

samples might not have been a random sample and therefore not representative of the population. However, there is evidence from a different source that supports our interpretation. School speech clinicians report that children in their articulation therapy programs have errors primarily on these five phonemes: [r], [s], [l], [ʃ], and [tʃ]. At first-grade level and above clinicians are teaching these phonemes to many of those children who were in the 25 percent of the younger age groups who had not achieved correct production.

MORPHOLOGY

At the same time that the phonemes of a language are being mastered, children are combining them appropriately to express the roots or morphs and the inflections. Let us consider first the morphs that are used and their characteristics.

The first words of a child are short and are related to his immediate environment. Some of those first words are *this*, *that*, *here*, *no*, *more*, *daddy*, *mommy*, and *bye*. Their phonemic structure is simple, only a few phonemes are used, most are consonant-vowel-consonant arrangements, and all utilize the feature of voicing.

FIRST WORDS. Darley and Winitz (1961) reviewed the published research to determine the age of acquisition of first words. They found that because many different definitions of first word had been utilized, it was difficult to arrive at a specific age. Their work showed that two principles were employed in a general way in identifying a child's first words: (1) consistent use of an utterance as the label for an object or action; (2) form or structure of the utterance similar to the adult English form. Both of them are difficult to apply, particularly when we cannot gauge how systematically the children used an utterance like *dada* only to refer to *father* and what standard the parents and others used to decide that *dada* was similar to the adult form. In spite of the difficulties in interpretation Darley and Winitz's review showed that the age for first words ranged from 9 to 19 months for normal children. Some handicapped children did not have words even at 60 months. The age for the handicapped was dependent on the degree of retardation, physical involvement, and environment.

On the basis of this report we can conclude that the normal child will be using a word or two by the time he is 12 months old. If he has no words by the time he is 18 months, we should consider possible reasons for the delay. If a child has no words by 24 months, parents should consult a speech pathologist.

The child's first words have been called *holophrastic* by McNeill (1970). A holophrase is a single word used to express a more complex idea. In order to interpret the word correctly, information about the situation which generated its statement is necessary. The more cues a child provides, the greater the likelihood his idea will be understood. For example, at bedtime, when a child brings her father a book, opens it, hands it to him with a smile, and says *book*, the father deduces that his daughter wants him to read the story. If the father misinterprets, his child will usually "tell" him he has made a mistake by using other words, such as *no*, or by providing a gestural cue.

The single-word utterances of children tend to express a major idea. The contentives—nouns, verbs, adjectives, adverbs, and pronouns—dominate the speech of most young children for months. Only at a later time do they use the functors—

prepositions, articles, and conjunctions. When children say something like *a daddy*, the expression may be one word perceptually to them, rather than two words. Brown (1973) has referred to these as monomorphemes. Children do not separate or segment the two as adults do.

Case history and anecdotal studies indicate that the first words of children are *mama*, *daddy*, and *bye*. However, research indicates that more functional words than these appear first. In the Zonshin (1974) study of middle-class Hebrew boys the first words elicited by the mothers in the home were *here*, *this*, *that*, *no*, and *food*. Many other investigators have provided similar reports. These words, along with a gesture or two, will solve many of the children's problems at age 12 months. They use locators and designators (*here*, *this*) and a word for negation. The frustrated mother can go through a list of 20 names of objects that she thinks might represent what her child wants, and all he has to do is say *no* to each one!

Zonshin found that some of the boys used a word for *mother* and *father* when they were 15 months old. They had also added the names of several objects in the homes, such as *car*, *wheel*, and *fire*. By the time these same boys were 18 months of age, they had acquired many additional names, a few verbs, and words for *hello*, *yes*, and *more*.

Individual differences make it difficult to quote a reliable figure for how many words children are using by 24 months. Records show some children with a vocabu-

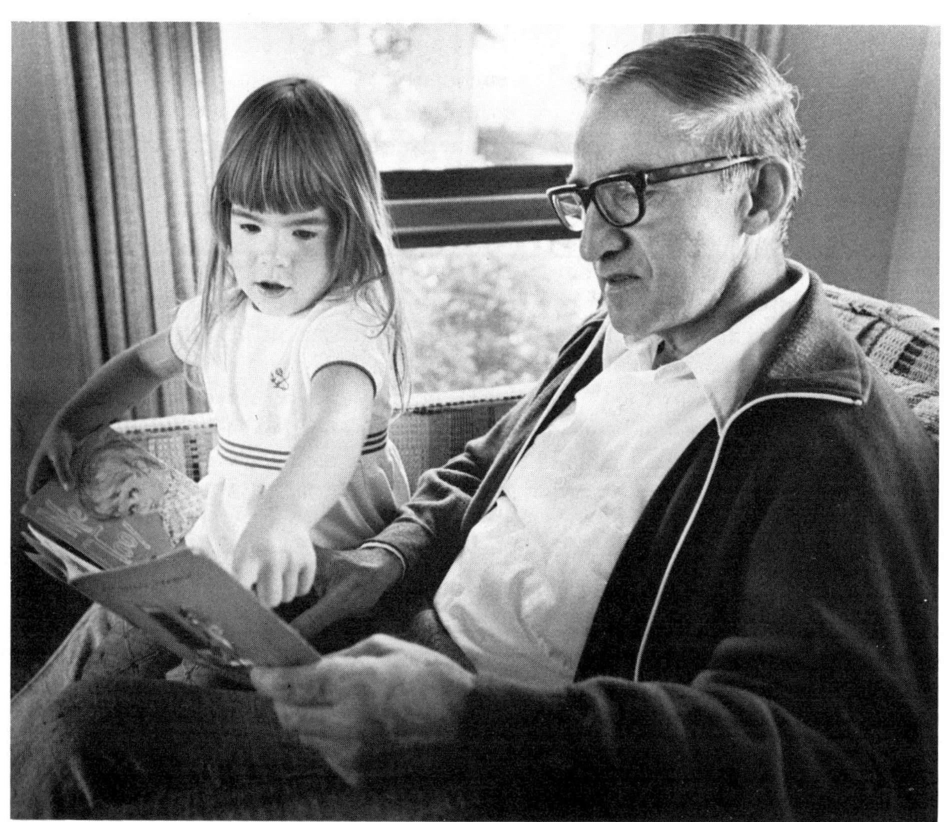

lary of less than 5 and others with repertoires of more than 150 words. However, as we have already said, by that age there should be some words as defined in the Darley-Winitz review. The child's goal should be the comprehension and use of many, so that his communication can proceed to the next phase.

INFLECTIONS. English has one of the simplest inflectional systems. Inflections are used to signify noun plurality and possession, verb tenses, some subject-verb agreements, and comparative and superlative forms of adjectives. Other languages have special additional endings for gender and case, others for adjective-noun agreement, noun markers for quality and action, and so on. However simple the system may seem, the child must still learn to choose the correct ending from among several possibilities.

Few mistakes are made in expressing the present progressive tense, because English has only one ending, *ing*, to add to the verb to form that tense. But for all other inflections, the child must first acquire general inflectional rules, determine whether particular words are regular or irregular, and then select the appropriate endings. Some inflections learned correctly as a part of vocabulary may be used incorrectly at a later stage as the child begins to differentiate inflectional rules. For example, a child who has learned to use the verb *went* as a vocabulary item may at a later time say *goed* because he has learned the [d] ending for past tense for so many verbs.

Studies of inflections have provided us with the order in which they are used correctly by children. Berko (1958) reported the percentage of correct production and used this information to rank the inflections in the order of acquisition. Brown (1973), on the other hand, considered that an inflection was acquired only when his subjects used the correct inflection in 90 percent of the cases in which it is obligatory.

The Berko study (1958) is one of the best known of the early works. She tested the abilities of preschool and first-grade children to form 10 plurals, 1 progressive, 3 past tenses, 3 third person singular verbs, and 6 possessives. Her procedure for eliciting the responses involved the use of drawings and nonsense words, as illustrated in Figure 3–7. She found that for 25 of the 28 inflections the first-grade children had higher

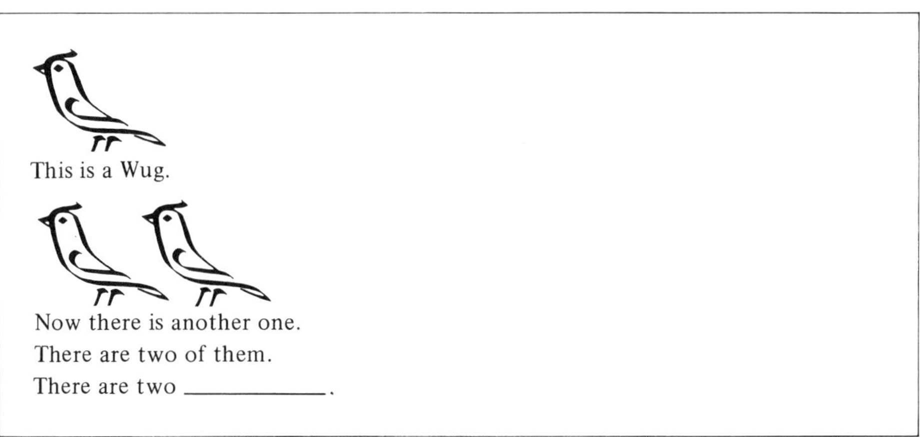

Figure 3–7. Sample drawing and nonsense word used to elicit inflectional responses. (J. Berko, The child's learning of English morphology. *Word, 14*, 150–177, 1958.)

percentages of correct responses than the preschool group. This finding indicates that learning of these inflections is still continuing among the younger children. Table 3–4 provides a ranking of the inflections she studied for the two age groups, with the percentages of correct answers.

In addition, she found a wide range of percentages of accuracy for her combined sample of preschool and first-grade children, particularly among the plurals and the verb tenses. The range for plurals was 28 to 91 percent, depending on the required allomorphs. With the exception of the non-nonsense word *glasses*, which had the highest percent of correct responses, those nonsense words which required a [z] allomorph were more likely to be accurate. The range for them was 79 to 91 percent. The allomorph [s] was correctly applied 79 percent of the time, and [əz] less than 36 percent of the time. Of the three verb tenses she studied, the present progressive form

Table 3–4. Age Differences on Inflectional Items

Item	Percentage of Correct Preschool Answers	Percentage of Correct First-Grade Answers	Significant Level of Difference
Plural			
glasses	75	99	.01
wugs	76	97	.02
luns	68	92	.05
tors	73	90	—
heafs	79	80	—
cras	58	86	.05
tasses	28	39	—
gutches	28	38	—
kazhes	25	36	—
nizzes	14	33	—
Progressive			
zibbing	72	97	.01
Past tense			
binged	60	85	.05
glinged	63	80	—
ricked	73	73	—
melted	72	74	—
spowed	36	59	—
motted	32	33	—
bodded	14	31	.05
rang	0	25	.01
Third person singular			
loodges	57	56	—
nazzes	47	49	—
Possessive			
wug's	68	81	—
bik's	68	95	.02
niz's	58	46	—
wugs'	74	97	.02
biks'	74	99	.01
nizzes'	53	82	.05

Source: J. Berko. The child's learning of English morphology. *Word, 14*, 150–177 (1958).

ranked first. The ending was used correctly by 90 percent of the children. The range of correctness for allomorphs for past tense was 17 to 78 percent, with [əd], [t], and [d] in that order. The third person singular verb ending of [əz] was correct 48 to 56 percent of the time.

Such data make it possible to establish a hierarchy of trends, but we still cannot state rules for the acquisition of inflections, such as pluralization always precedes past tense. For these two inflectional groups the nature of the allomorph makes a difference. Therefore, we can only report the order of accuracy for the allomorphs in each instance.

Brown's data (1973) are based on the speech of three children, Adam, Eve, and Sarah, who were tape-recorded in their homes over a period of months. Brown set up stages of development, based on the mean length of utterances (MLU) in morphemes and the highest number (upper bound) of morphemes in an utterance. Essentially, each root or morph and each inflection was given a point, and the utterances were considered to belong to one of the five stages, according to the figures in Table 3–5. From the large corpus of material he had for each child, he drew 700 consecutive complete utterances for each of these five stages. When he analyzed his material, he included all categories of morphemes. He found that 14 morphemes had achieved a 90 percent level of accuracy in obligatory contexts. The mean order of acquisition is given in Table 3–6. These included, in addition to certain inflections, two prepositions, the

Table 3–5. Mean Length of Utterance (MLU) and Upper Bound in Morphemes of Brown's Five Stages of Language Development

Stage	MI U	Upper Bound
I	1.75	5
II	2.25	7
III	2.75	9
IV	3.50	11
V	4.00	13

Source: R. Brown. *A first language: The early stages.* Cambridge, Mass.: Harvard University Press, 1973.

Table 3–6. Mean Order of Acquisition of 14 Morphemes Across 3 Children

1. Present progressive
2. *in*
3. *on*
4. Plural
5. Past irregular verb
6. Possessive
7. Uncontracted copula
8. Articles
9. Past regular verb
10. Third person regular verb
11. Third person irregular verb
12. Uncontracted auxiliary
13. Contracted copula
14. Contracted auxiliary

Source: R. Brown. A First language: The early stages, Cambridge, Mass.: Harvard University Press, 1973.

articles, the copula, and the auxiliary. The present progressive verb inflection was at the top of the list. Plurality, regardless of allomorphs, was the next inflection. Irregular past tenses were acquired before the regular past, but third person regular verb forms were acquired before third person irregular forms.

These same data are presented in a different way in Table 3–7. The age and mean MLU of each child is considered in relation to the 14 morphemes. This arrangement of the data shows the amount of individual difference among the three children. At age 2 years 2 months Eve had acquired 6 of the morphemes, but neither Adam nor Sarah had any. Eve had acquired all 14 by the time she was 2 years 3 months, in comparison to Adam who was 2 years 6 months before he had acquired even the present progressive.

Since both noun and verb inflections have several allomorphs and since there is evidence that some allomorphs are learned before others, it is appropriate that we look further into both groups of inflections. Solomon (1972) had hypothesized that the correct plural allomorph would vary as a function of the final consonant of a word. In other words, the ending of the stem or morph would be the primary factor in the

Table 3–7. Age and Order of Acquisition of 14 Morphemes by Adam, Sarah, and Eve

Stage[a]	Adam	Sarah	Eve
I	2–3[b]	2–3	1–6
II	2–6 present progressive *in*, *on*, plural	2–10 plural *in*, *on* present progressive past irregular possessive	1–9 present progressive *on*
III	2–11 uncontractible copula past irregular	3–1 uncontractible copula articles	1–11 *in* plural possessive
IV	3–2 articles third person irregular possessive	3–8 third person regular	2–2 past regular
V	3–6 third person regular past regular uncontractible auxiliary contractible copula contractible auxiliary	4–0 past regular uncontractible auxiliary contractible copula third person irregular contractible auxiliary	2–3 uncontractible copula past irregular articles third person regular third person irregular uncontractible auxiliary contractible copula contractible auxiliary

Source: R. Brown. *A first language: The early stages.* Cambridge, Mass.: Harvard University Press, 1973.
[a] Stage based on mean length of utterance in morphemes: I, 1.75; II, 2.25; III, 2.75; IV, 3.50; V, 4.00.
[b] Chronological age in years and months.

frequency of correct pluralization. She devised pairs of nonsense words, with each pair having one of the endings given in Table 3–8. She then asked 5- and 6-year-olds to give her the plural form for each of her "words." As the data in the table show, she too found that children have not mastered pluralization by the time they enter first grade. Words requiring the [z] inflection are more likely to be correct than words requiring [s] or [əz]. Children may surmise that a word like *bis* is already plural and therefore fail to supply the [əz] inflection. However, failure to supply the [s] to the stems ending in the five voiceless phonemes cannot be explained on this basis. Perhaps their rule is that words ending in voiceless plosives as well as voiceless fricatives do not require an additional voiceless fricative for pluralization. We can not be sure because no one asked the children why they did what they did, and even if they were asked, we are not sure that they could tell us.

The fact that nonsense words were the stimuli in both the Berko and Solomon studies should not have been the reason. Words such as *wug* and *cra* sound like English words; in fact, Berko reported that some children thought that the nonsense words were real ones they had not yet learned. In any case, they failed to make the correct generalizations about the plural inflections in many instances.

In an attempt to add to the limited information about correctness of verb inflec-

Table 3–8. Percentage of Correct Responses by Consonant Ending and Age

Stem Ending	5-Year-Olds	6-Year-Olds
Allomorph [z]		
m	85	88
r	80	85
l	78	93
w	78	85
j	78	88
n	75	83
b	73	78
d	73	85
g	70	93
v	65	68
ŋ	63	63
ð	30	25
Allomorph [s]		
k	70	83
p	70	88
t	68	73
θ	45	33
f	43	55
Allomorph [əz]		
ʃ	25	8
ʒ	25	5
tʃ	25	8
dʒ	23	10
s	15	5
z	15	3

Source: Adapted from M. Solomon. Stem endings and the acquisition of inflections. *Language Learning*, 22, 43–50 (1972).

tions, Moran (1977) selected for study 10 classes of verbs based on inflectional change and 3 tenses. She took photographs of children engaged in activities to represent present progressive, future, and past tense. She used 5 examples for each of the 10 classes—a total of 50 verbs. She presented her pictures to 27 7-year-old and 33 8-year-old normal children. As she pointed to each picture, she asked each child to tell her what the child in the picture was doing. She would say, for example, "These are pictures of *swim*. Tell me what the child is doing." The child would respond, for example, "He's swimming," "He will swim," or "He swam." All the children gave correct responses for the present progressive and future tenses for all 50 verbs. Since there is only one way to show these two verb forms, the task was easy and the children made no mistakes. When they expressed past tense, however, they reached a criterion level of 90 percent in only two of the allomorphs, [t] and [d]. For verbs that form the past tense through the addition of [d] or [t], such as *climb* and *rake,* the children were almost 100 percent correct. The range of the number of correct responses in other categories was 124 to 241, approximately a range of 41 to 80 percent correct (Table 3–9). A considerable amount of learning must take place with normal children. At the stage at which they were tested, the children in Moran's study had the concept of past tense, but the application of correct allomorphs to all verbs was still to be mastered. As we might expect, their most typical errors were overgeneralization of the two regular allomorphs [d] and [t] and the zero allomorph.

The use of the phonemes [s] and [z] reflects how quickly children induce rules that apply to regular forms. The phonemes [s] and [z] are the markers for plurality, possession, and the third person singular verb form. These three inflections appear very early in the speech of children. Adam, Eve, and Sarah were using all of them correctly within a year of the appearance of any one of the three. The marker itself carries a different meaning depending upon whether it signifies plurality, possession,

Table 3–9. Number of Correct Responses for 10 Sets of Verb Inflections

Inflection	Verbs	Number of Correct Responses (300 = 100%)
1. [d]	climb, pull, play, open, scare	300
2. [t]	rake, jump, fix, lick, wash	299
3. [əd]	trade, dust, paste, paint, fold	241
4. No Inflection	hit, cut, spread, shut, put	238
5. Vowel change + [t]	sweep, sleep, leave, feel, feed[a]	209
6. Vowel change	tear, ride, write, choose, break	180
7. Vowel change	string, dig, swing, win, spin	154
8. Final phoneme changes to [t] or [t] is added	burn, spend, bend, build, send	145
9. Vowel change	ring, drink, sing, swim, sink	133
10. Vowel change + final consonant change	catch, bring, teach, fight,[a] buy	124

Source: M. Moran and M.C. Byrne. Verb inflections of normal and learning disabled children. *Journal of Speech and Hearing Research, 20,* 529–542 (1977).

[a] No change in final consonant.

or a verb form. Therefore, children have to learn these meanings, thus attaching to the phoneme a semantic character that depends on its specific use.

Grammatical forms can be grouped in two categories: those that require only one inflection, like *ing* for all present progressives, and those that have multiple inflections, like [s], [z], [ɪz], and others for plurality. The rules for the first category are simple, and the inflections reach a degree of stability early. The rules for the second category are more difficult for the child to sort out and thus require a longer time span to be learned and applied correctly.

We see these principles in operation with the children in classes for the learning disabled to whom Moran (1975) presented her verb inflection tests. Like the normal children they did not make errors on the present progressive or future inflections. They had multiple errors, however, on the past tense inflections, more than the normal children in regular classes.

SYNTAX

PRESENTENCES. By 2 years of age many children are stringing words together in an orderly fashion. They continue to use one-word utterances, but as vocabulary expands and the need for more productive communication increases, they begin to use words in sequence. The arrangement of words is orderly and governed by rules. These utterances are the precursors of the sentence. Some can be considered noun or verb phrases and others can be interpreted by the listener as incomplete noun phrase–verb phrase combinations. Some are like the partials to which we referred in Chapter 2. A few are greetings that are just like those of adults.

In a language sample of 50 consecutive comments of a 27-month-old boy, we noted that half were single-word utterances and the rest were combinations of two or three words. Following are some examples:

1.	bye Daddy	**7.**	I fine
2.	in there	**8.**	it mine
3.	on there	**9.**	all mine
4.	hi, Daddy	**10.**	my car
5.	Oh, Mommy	**11.**	I go car.
6.	more car	**12.**	I want ball.

Items 6 and 10 could be considered noun phrases; 2, 3, and 9 may be parts of the verb phrase; 7 and 8 have a noun phrase and a verb phrase, with the verb missing; 1, 4, and 5 are greetings; 11 and 12 are sentences.

Here are other examples from the speech of children. The utterances may be incomplete or incorrect, but the listener knows what the child means. In some utterances the verb may be omitted, for example, *nose not wet*, *it on the table*, *mine not hot*, *you five years*. In the following no subjects are expressed: *ate it all*, *like my milk*, *cut it up*. There is both a subject and a predicate in the following, even though the verb form does not agree with the subject: *he give it me*, *I wipes it up*, *the big hammer do*. In the following the incorrect form is used for the subject: *her hit me*, *me saw car*.

Reports in the literature indicate a wide range in the number of such presentences by 30 months. Some children have only a few and others as many as a thousand, but it is generally expected that normal children will have acquired at least a few hundred by the time they are 30 months.

Sentences. The sentence emerges as a key landmark in language acquisition. By 3 years of age most children are demonstrating the principle for construction of a simple affirmative-declarative sentence. They are telling us something by putting together a noun phrase for a subject and a verb phrase for a predicate. These basic relationships are evident in the following examples from the conversation of a 3-year old.

1. That is mine.
2. The big boy jump high.
3. He roped him.
4. He want the black horse.
5. Oh, it broke.
6. I put the airplane here.
7. He fit in this car.
8. Me can make them like this.

Even though there are subject-verb agreement errors in sentences 4 and 7, and an incorrect personal pronoun in 8, the utterances demonstrate the basic relationships needed for a sentence.

The basic units of the sentence expand in many ways. Modifiers are used for the subject and objects are included in the predicate. In the above examples, sentence 2 has an article-adjective-noun combination as the subject. Sentences 3, 4, and 6 have objects as part of the predicate. The construction of a sentence also expands with the acquisition of morphemes. The uninflected verb form can be supplanted by the present progressive and past tenses: I *go*, I *going*, I *went*. Then the copula *be* and the auxiliary *be* are utilized: he *is* big, I *am* John, he *is* eating, he *is* putting on his 'jamas.

The next step in the development of syntax is the use of embedded or subordinate clauses. Children continue to use simple sentences that are appropriate, but also add a new dimension to their speech. Clauses appear for some by 4 to 4½ years. Here are some examples.

That's the one that's broke.
Everytime I heard the noise, I had to drop a block right there.
I don't want that one 'cause it's too small.

Another indicator of syntactic expansion is the use of conjunctions in the noun phrase, in the verb phrase, and between main clauses. One four-year old girl told the clinician:

Johnny and Jimmy are at home.
I got one truck and one car.
I go home and change my school clothes.

Some 4-year-olds are also using *but* and *because*. The following is an example of the presence of both in a series of comments a child made. The visitor asked where the boy's wagon was and the child answered, "*But* I just told you. It's in my basement. I can't bring it here, *because* it's too big to carry up here."

Some mothers report that their 4-year-olds use many *and's* when they want to tell about an experience that has been particularly exciting to them. After watching a fire, one child said, without stopping, "The fire engine got there and a helicopter got there and they started the water and the house burned down anyway."

Children will join together clauses that are not additive. For instance, in the above sentence the four conjoined clauses are reported in a temporal order. An older child who has learned about cause-effect relationships might say, "When the fire engine got there, the fireman started the water, but the house burned down anyway," or "Even though the firemen started the water right away, the house burned down."

SENTENCE TRANSFORMATIONS. As children learn to utilize simple affirmative-declarative sentences, they also learn how to use sentence transformations. These are procedures which enable them to change word order and to add to or replace words to express grammatical classes. Table 3–10 lists the transformations that appear early. Negation is first, followed by question. In the speech of many children all of these are utilized occasionally by the time they are using three- and four-word responses. Some of the detailed analyses of children's speech indicate they are all being developed at the same time and appear simultaneously.

You will recall that children have some form of *no* very early in their speaking careers. They have heard mothers say it over and over again. Negation is the earliest transformation to appear. At first children shake their heads to indicate *no* or just push their half-filled dishes away to show they do not want anymore. When they begin to express *no* orally, they use it as a one-word response or put *no* or *not* in front of the phrase: *no play*, *not play*, or *no eat now*. A little later they introduce negation between the noun phrase and verb phrase: *He not going home*, *My daddy not take the car*, *He not a boy*. The next step is the use of *not* or a contraction between parts of the verb in conjunction with the verbs *can* and *do*: *He isn't going*, *I can't find it*, *Daddy didn't build mine*. The negative-imperative sentence also begins to appear: *Don't do that*, *Don't put it in my milk*, *Don't pound my blocks*. The negation is added to the auxiliary verb *do*.

In learning the rules for placement of the negation term, a common mistake is the use of a double negative: *I don't want no milk*, *No, you can't have no more*. Even adults sometimes use the double negative, occasionally for greater emphasis, but usually as an inappropriate grammatical statement.

Children learn to ask questions in an order similar to the learning of negation. A

Table 3–10. Sentence Transformations That Appear Early in the Speech of Children

Transformation	Example
Negation	I am not.
Question	Who is it?
Contraction	That's my hat.
Got	He's got my hat.
Verb auxiliary *be*	The dog is licking the milk.
Do	I do want it.
Infinitive complement	She wants to read.

question may at first be expressed simply by a rising intonation. They may say *huh* or *no* or make a statement like *you want me* with a gradual rise in the pitch. The second stage involves placement of an interrogative (who, what, where, which, why) in front of a word, phrase, or complete sentence: *who that*, *what this*, *What you have for me*, *Why you crying*.

The third stage is the application of the principle of inversion, that is, placing a verb form of some kind before the subject: *Is daddy outside? What's he doing?* The principle of inversion is then combined with the use of the auxiliary verb *do*: *Do you want mine? Does he go in the car?*

Of course, some children just ask *why* or *how* or *what* as a reply to what someone has said to them. When mothers say, "Put your toys in the toy box," children, particularly at age 3, reply *Why?* Tag questions like *You have one, don't you?* or *They went to play, didn't they?* appear a little later.

The contracted forms of the copula and *be* auxiliary are among the morphemes on Brown's list (Table 3–6). The contraction is also heard on other auxiliary verbs, such as *have* (*I've* been good) and *will* (*He'll* get it). The verb forms *do* and *got* appear as early as age 3; and the infinitive complement by age 4.

As syntactic structures become more complex, many transformations are used within the same utterance. No one has listed all the possibilities–children and adults will continue to generate some new ones.

SENTENCE TYPES. Loban (1963) and O'Donnell, Griffin, and Norris (1967) classified the syntactic structures that students used routinely from kindergarten through twelfth grade. Table 3–11 is a composite of these types. O'Donnell indicated that 85 percent of the sentences in his samples of speech of children in elementary school were either types 1 or 2, the subject-verb-object types. Types 6 and 7 are rarely heard. Type 10 appears more frequently in written work. Fragments or partials are

Table 3–11. Types of Syntactic Structures Used by Children from Kindergarten Through Twelfth Grade.

Types	Examples
1. Subject-verb	John went.
2. Subject-verb-object	John jumps rope.
3. Subject-verb-predicate nominal	John is a big boy.
4. Subject-verb-predicate adjectival	John is big.
5. Subject-verb-indirect object-direct object	John gave Mary his book.
6. Subject-verb-object-object complement	He considers Mary his friend.
7. Subject-verb-object-object adjectival	He considers Mary pretty.
8. Expletive-verb-subject	Here comes John.
9. Any question	What is that?
10. Use of passive voice	John was given a book.
11. Commands or requests	Give it to me.
12. Partials	Any incomplete unit

Source: Compiled from: Loban, W. D. *The language of elementary school children* (Research Report No. 1) and O'Donnell, R. G., Griffin, W. J., and Norris, R. C. *Syntax of kindergarten and elementary school children: A transformational analysis* (Research Report No. 8) Champaign, Ill.: National Council of Teachers of English, 1963 and 1967.

characteristic of all speech, including adults'. Typical answers to a question about where someone has been are *to the store*, *to the movie*, *to the office*.

Children and adults both get into word tangles as they talk. We start to say one thing, change our minds, and put in unnecessary words. Here is an example from the spontaneous speech of a 4-year-old: "Yes, they—I told them—go. I told them not to bump me; and I go,—you bump me; and I told them, told them that." These word tangles or mazes decrease with age, but they rarely disappear completely except in the highly skilled speaker. The garble makes it difficult to follow what the speaker is saying. Listeners tend to cut off the speaker whose sentence is so entangled that they cannot follow his intent. Inaccurate grammar and imprecise use of words combine to reduce the intelligibility of the message. Even in these tangles, however, the ordering of the subject and predicate is generally correct.

SEMANTICS

Development of the Verbal Symbol. Stages in the development of the verbal symbol system can be identified in young children. Meaning evolves from their experiences and their activities. The child listens and imitates some of the words he hears and then begins to associate the sounds with his environment. For example, he perceives that the word *milk* seems to "go with" his cup or bottle of white liquid, but not with the clear liquid he sometimes gets. He begins to associate the word *milk* with the white liquid and uses the word when he sees milk. Later, his concept of milk becomes attached to the verbal symbol; at this point he can yell for his milk when he is hungry, even if no milk is visible. He has moved a step further along in his development of a referential relationship. Words are no longer only pointers, but become symbols for objects or activities outside his visual field.

The child says *milk* because it conveys an idea of a special content, even though he does not perceive all elements of the content. This content is the referent of the symbol. The verbal symbol represents a concept which he has now equated with the word he is using.

During this early phase of language development we must be careful not to attribute meaning to a child's words that other observers cannot corroborate. If we are to classify words, we must have as much information about the situation in which the words are spoken as possible. That will be the only way to avoid misinterpretation. The little girl who says *dolly* may simply be naming an object. If she says *dolly* with tears in her eyes and we note that the dolly's legs have come unglued, we might with a degree of confidence fill in the words the girl left out and surmise that she is telling us that the doll is broken or the doll's legs are broken, or something similar. On the other hand, if we have watched her break the doll's legs before she said *dolly*, we might surmise that she is telling us that she broke the doll and, since she is crying, that she is sorry.

Children sometimes use the wrong symbols while they are learning the language. Here are two examples: I got it *from* Christmas and girl has brown on top of *his* head. The child grasps concrete concepts such as objects and place long before he can grasp abstract concepts such as time. Therefore, names of objects and place words appear earlier in the vocabulary and are used more accurately than words with abstract referents. Words like *this*, *that*, and *here* are among the first used; *yesterday* and *tomorrow* appear much later and may be used inappropriately. Children often ask, "Is it tomorrow yet?" and yesterday may represent any time—a day, a week, or a month—before the present.

Children tend to learn routine expressions early—greetings, such as *hi* and *bye bye*, and names of people close to them, such as *mommy*, *daddy*, and proper names of selected people. These have high semantic value and are words to which children are exposed hundreds of times.

Among the first of the personal pronouns to be used is the self-referent, *I* or *me*. Many young children will substitute *me* for *I* when they are still mastering the personal referent, but they give the correct meaning to the words themselves. Children are discovering themselves and their worlds and *I* or *me* enables them to express *their* wishes.

It is difficult to estimate how large a vocabulary a child should have at various points in his development. Such estimates must be based on the total verbal output of a random sample of children at different age levels, involved in many different but appropriate situations. The task of recording, transcribing, and counting is so overwhelming that no one has done it, but, what is more important, such counts provide only one kind of information. They do not tell us how the words are used, for how many referents the same word is spoken, or whether the count is a truly complete record that applies to children at the different age levels.

Bloom (1974) reported that her daughter Allison used more than 50 words at least twice by the age of 14 months, but did not say them again for several months. These words referred to recognizable objects or people. In addition, she said a few words many times, including *no*, *more*, *up*, *down*, *away*, *there*, and *stop*. Each of these was syntactically functional and had meaning for the child.

Within a few months Allison was using 150 substantive words, mainly nouns. Most were referents for things and people, but others were used as objects of an action or as the agent for an action. For instance, Allison might say *mamma* as she closed the door to hide her mother or she might say *mamma* as her mother was cleaning the floor. Bloom interpreted these utterances as indicating *Allison hides mamma* and *mamma cleans the floor* respectively.

Weir (1962) tape recorded all the utterances of her son Anthony as he talked to a favorite toy and blanket in his crib just before he fell asleep. His entire set of remarks, gathered over a period of two months when Anthony was 26 to 28 months old, has been transcribed and analyzed in many different ways by his mother. From the list of words and their frequency (Table 3–12) we can make some generalizations: (1) Anthony talked a lot; (2) his speech included not only four of the five types of contentives, but two functors as well; (3) of all the possible verbs, only the copula *is* was utilized more than 100 times.

Weir reported that there were 5500 running words in Anthony's recordings. Of these about 80 percent were contentives and the rest were functors. She also found that of the contentives about 38 percent were nouns and 27 percent were verbs—a total of 65 percent of all the words Anthony spoke. In these monologues he used a total of 675 different words, a sizeable number. However, Anthony's mother said that his vocabulary in the monologues was quite limited in comparison with what he used during the day!

Table 3–12. Words Appearing 100 or More Times in Anthony's Monologues

Category	Words and Frequency
Nouns and pronouns	Bobo (132), blanket (125), it (103)
Verbs	is (167), go (90),[a] jump (31),[a] get (20)[a]
Adjective	that (121)
Article	the (394)
Conjunction	and (105)

Source: Data compiled from R. Weir. *Language in the crib.* The Hague: Mouton, 1962.
[a] These were included because of their designations of actions even though they did not occur 100 times.

In contrast to Anthony's verbal output at less than 2½ years, the following is the entire repertoire of a 3-year-old encountered in a clinical situation.

General: *no, yes, hi, ok, allgone, hey, there, back*
Nouns: *baby, dog, rabbit, fly, flower, milk, house, head, wagon, phone wheel, chicken, fire, shoes, mama, dadda, light*
Pronouns: *you, I, one*
Adjectives: *pretty, yellow*
Verbs: *cut, sit, look, want, go, know*
Two-word combinations: *hey look, mama back, hey go, I donno*

The child did not pronounce the words as written here, but according to her parents and clinician she used close approximations of correct pronunciation. By using the child's accompanying gestures and vocal pattern and the context of the utterances, her parents were able to understand her part of the time. Her nursery school teacher, however, not as familiar with her and not accustomed to interpreting what children like this one are saying, did not understand her.

The linguistic environment makes available to children the vocabulary they can assimilate. The environment may be of extended or limited size and depth. The children may or may not learn to use the available vocabulary, depending upon many variables. They may learn about opposites, like *hard-soft, big-little, light-dark,* and use them appropriately. They may develop a sense of humor which permits them to describe people and situations in unusual ways. They may develop problem-solving skills which they demonstrate in the language they use.

Books and reading skills open up wider horizons for children. Even books that parents show and read to their very young children are valuable. Once children can read, they can select books that teach them subject-related vocabularies and enable them to practice their use. Experiences in school continue to increase their facility in language use. The farther along they go in an intellectual environment, the greater exposure they have to words and their meanings. The process of increasing skill in the use of words in meaningful arrangements should be continuous throughout life.

CHARACTERISTICS OF LANGUAGE ACQUISITION

There are some general characteristics that we can identify in the child's language acquisition. It is evident that language learning is cumulative and hierarchical. The child builds his linguistic system much as adults build a house or a bird builds a nest. He uses the language he hears with modifications at first, and only by age 12 years will he be mastering an infinite variety of correct utterances.

He can store a minimal number of features at first. As a result his first words are short and may have multiple meanings that depend on the situation for interpretation. Among the first features that he demonstrates is *order*—order of phonemes and order of words in presentences and eventually in sentences.

The child learns all four aspects of the structure of language simultaneously. We can observe a gradual mastery of the phonology, morphology, and syntax. The semantic component, however, continues to develop throughout life and is probably never fully realized (Figure 3–8).

Overgeneralization of the rules of morphology is characteristic. Because of the number of inflections and the number of regular and irregular noun and verb forms, the child has difficulty sorting out the rules he should follow. There are many mistakes during the preschool and primary grades.

INDIVIDUAL DIFFERENCES IN LEARNING

There is a great deal of individual difference in the rate of acquisition of language. Regardless of the measures being utilized to study comprehension and verbal output, one conclusion is obvious—not all children at a particular age will be performing at the same level. Sharf (1972) analyzed seven tape recordings of each of 13 children who were evaluated at two- to four-month intervals. He found that all his linguistic measures reflected development, but that none predicted the individual's rate of language acquisition. There was no smooth learning curve that was applicable to each child in his sample.

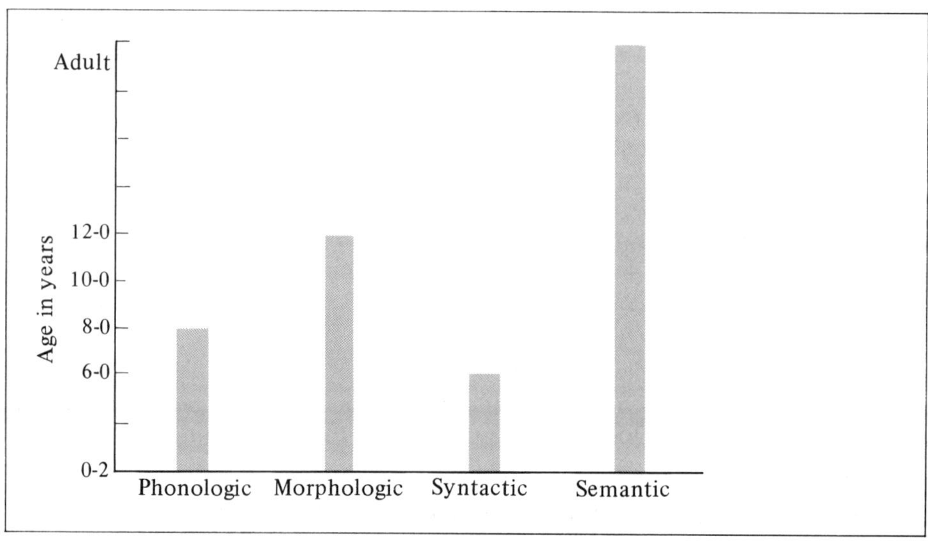

Figure 3–8. Age of acquisition of the four aspects of language.

When Sharf began this longitudinal study, the average age of the children was 21 months. All of them were using at least single words. Over a span of 13 to 14 months some children were using utterances averaging less than two words and others had a mean length of utterance of almost five words. The length of the utterance at the initial recording was not a predictor for what that child would be doing later. Some made slow but steady progress, others regressed temporarily and then spurted ahead, and others made fast progress from the beginning.

These same comments apply to the three children whom Brown (1973) followed for months. Eve at 18 months had a mean utterance length (MLU) in morphemes of 1.50 and within ten months, at the age of 28 months, reached a mean of 4.20; Adam and Sarah started at age 27 months with MLUs of 2.0 and 1.75 respectively and reached Eve's MLU of 4.20 only when they were 43 months of age.

COMPREHENSION

Comprehension is a cognitive skill that is even more important than the use of oral language. There is controversy about whether comprehension precedes or follows the use of language. We know from observing examples of incorrect application that children utilize some words which they do not understand. At the same time, we know that they often understand words which they cannot use. For example, a 3-year-old child is able to carry out two or three consecutive verbal orders. A 2-year-old may be able to follow directions such as "Bring me a dry diaper and the powder" or "Give Daddy your hand while we cross the street." We do not know to what segment of the utterance the child is responding, but he carries out our wishes. Yet he cannot produce these commands in words or with word order that is comparable to the model.

Psychologists and others have reported that the adult vocabulary of use is quite small in comparison with the vocabulary of comprehension. An individual may use only two or three thousand words in verbal exchanges, but may comprehend ten or twenty thousand words. The sight vocabulary is even larger.

Much of the information we have about the development of comprehension is based on the results of tests and tasks. It has been easier to construct measures of comprehension than of production. We can identify what children have understood by asking them to point to the correct picture for an item or to act out a set of directions. The major limitation of such tests, however, is that only grammatical forms and vocabulary that can be pictured or acted out can be studied.

One of the earliest attempts to obtain information about several aspects of language comprehension resulted in the Test of Auditory Comprehension of Language (Carrow, 1973). The test assesses a child's understanding of 101 lexical, morphologic, and syntactic items. It was given to children ages 3 through 6 years. The data were analyzed to provide the age at which 75 percent and 90 percent of the children in an age group passed each item. Since the test items were standardized on low socioeconomic children, many of whom were from bilingual homes, we can say that at least for this group we have some information. Thirteen of the items, including some in each of the lexical, morphologic, and syntactic categories, did not reach the 75 percent correct criterion. More than half of the items were correct by age 4½ years. Items that reached the 75 percent correct criterion among 3-year-olds included pointing to *bicycle*, *on the table*, *fattest*, *the girl is sewing*, *who is by the table*, and *find the cat with no eyes*. Items that were too difficult for even the 6-year-olds included *Find the one that is neither the ball nor the table*, *pair*, *Here is a star*, *Point to the bottle on the left*.

There are only a few studies of comprehension of syntactic order. One by De Villiers and De Villiers (1972) suggests that young children will accept an incorrect order of words and demonstrate comprehension by acting out the speech's intent correctly. Older children will correct the word order and also act out the speech. Only short sentences have been used in this type of study, however.

C. Chomsky (1969) studied comprehension of syntactic structures of 5- to 10-year-old children. She presented a set of four sentences for each child to act out. The first, *The doll is easy to see*, was designed to probe their understanding of the syntactic structures in the sentence. She put a blindfolded doll in front of the child and asked, "Is the doll easy to see or hard to see?" If the child replied, "It's hard to see," she asked why. The typical answer was "Because you covered her eyes." Only 25 percent of the 5-year-olds and 75 percent of the 7-year-olds gave the correct answer. By age 9 all of them understood the syntax. One explanation for their failures is their inability to transform the sentence. The transformation would have enabled them to reorder the sentence as *It is easy to see the doll*, thus recognizing that *doll* is not the subject of the copula *is*.

Tests by Sanders (1971) indicate that adults are still learning syntactic comprehension. When the syntactic structure is complex and tricky, one out of three adults fails. For example, the reply to the order "Ask me which block to take" should be "Which block do you want me to take?" or "Which block should I take?" Any other reply is an indication that the listener did not know the rule to apply and did not make the appropriate transformation.

COMPREHENSION VERSUS PRODUCTION

Fraser, Bellugi, and Brown (1963) investigated the relative difficulty of imitation, comprehension, and production in an assessment of grammatical contrasts. They selected contrasts such as affirmative-negative, subject-object in the active voice, and present progressive-future tense. They presented these contrasts in the form of picture stimuli to 12 children who were between 3 and 3½ years of age. They had learned that younger children did not attend to this type of task and were therefore not testable and that 4-year-olds and older children performed most of the tasks correctly. The results indicated that on most of the tasks the children did best when they imitated and that they comprehended better than they produced the syntax. Also, it was possible to order the tasks in terms of least to most difficult for this group. The task that was easiest for them to comprehend was the affirmative-negative contrast, followed by the distinction between subject and object in the active voice, and present progressive versus future tense. Only a few children correctly identified the subject and object in passive voice and the indirect and direct objects. Even though this study had some methodological difficulties, it was the first one to attempt this type of comparison and has provided a pattern for many others.

When Monroe (1971) tested the comprehension and production abilities of 40 normal children aged 2 through 5 years on selected inflections, she found that comprehension either preceded or was developing at the same time as production for the most part. Table 3–13 gives the mean percentages of errors for each inflection for each age. Of the five inflections that she studied, only the regular plural had fewer production than comprehension errors. However, when we add the mistakes on the expressive regular and irregular plurals together, the percent of error would be about the same as on comprehension.

The Monroe data indicate that comprehension improves from the younger to the older group. Five-year-olds comprehended the inflections to a greater degree than 2-year-olds. Also, some inflections are more difficult to comprehend. The progressive verb seems the easiest and superlative adjectives the most difficult. It is also important to note that there were some errors on each inflection even at the age of 5 years.

The Northwestern Syntax Screening Test (Lee, 1971) has a format like the one used by Fraser (1963). It consists of 20 pairs of sentences that the subjects must identify by pointing to the correct picture and 20 pairs that they must produce in response to pictures. The lexical structures evaluated are the same for both the comprehension and production sections. The test provides information about knowledge of subject-verb agreement, prepositions, pronouns, question-statement contrasts, verb tenses, *wh-* questions, negation, possession, passive voice, indefinite pronouns, grammatical confusions, direct-indirect object, and singular-plural contrasts. It is suitable for children between 3 and 8 years of age.

The results show that scores for comprehension of these structures tend to be

Table 3–13. Mean Percentage of Errors for Each Inflection by Age Groups

	Age Group			
Inflection	2 Years	3 Years	4 Years	5 Years
Plural noun				
receptive	72.5	43.8	47.5	40.0
expressive regular	80.0	8.8	5.6	0.0
expressive irregular	96.3	97.5	92.5	76.3
Past tense verb				
receptive	56.3	51.3	43.8	27.5
expressive regular	97.5	72.5	48.8	10.0
expressive irregular	100.0	100.0	93.3	93.3
Progressive verb				
receptive	68.8	28.8	16.3	5.0
expressive	85.0	26.3	18.8	0.0
Comparative adjective				
receptive	61.3	41.3	20.0	7.5
expressive regular	98.8	88.8	67.5	30.0
expressive irregular	100.0	95.0	90.0	70.0
Superlative adjective				
receptive	78.8	66.3	30.0	13.8
expressive regular	100.0	92.5	70.0	27.5
expressive irregular	100.0	100.0	85.0	50.0

Source: N. Monroe. Concept learning in the acquisition of inflectional endings. Doctoral dissertation, University of Kansas, 1971.

higher or the same for production. In addition, there is a gradual increment in the number of correct items as the children get older. The items that are most difficult for the children are those that require knowledge of the rules for direct-indirect objects and passive voice.

When children do not comprehend a language, they can imitate the words, but they do not have meaning for them. We see the effects of lack of comprehension in deaf children who do not use speech until they have had special training. Because of their hearing losses they do not understand what is being said to them and cannot produce appropriate answers. As adults exposed for the first time to a foreign language, we experience similar problems.

SUMMARY ON LANGUAGE ACQUISITION

Language learning is a dynamic process which requires active participation on the part of the learner. A child learns the language of his environment, whether it is English or one of the other thousand spoken languages of the world. He is listening to and comprehending some of what he hears before he begins to talk.

The structure of English is such that some parts are used correctly from the beginning and others are mastered over time. Syntax, or the order of words in an utterance, is correct from the beginning. The length and the complexity of the utterances increase over time. Phonological aspects are mastered by age 8 years, and morphological units by 10 or 12 years. The semantic, particularly the ambiguous aspects, are being learned throughout life.

The role of comprehension is crucial to both children and adults. It generally develops prior to or concurrently with related aspects of production. Adults continue to broaden their comprehension skills.

LANGUAGE DEFICITS

DEFINITION

We can define a language deficit in several ways. We can decide that all those who have scores on specific tests or measures that are below a predetermined point are deficient for their age and social milieu. For instance, a speech clinician can administer the Illinois Test of Psycholinguistic Abilities (Kirk, 1968) to a group of students and identify as deficient those whose scores fall two or three standard deviations below the mean. These would be the pupils who score approximately at or below the 30th percentile. The clinician can administer a test of articulation, like the Templin-Darley 50-Item Screening Test (1969), and compare the students' scores with the cut-offs that the authors of the test suggest are indicative of a need for a therapy program. Such tests are ways of defining differences in an empirical fashion.

A second way to define a language deficit is to consider the relationship of a person's language to his purpose and to the group with whom he lives. The individual has a language deficit when he has consistent difficulty in comprehending others or his listeners do not understand what he says. His social group sets criteria for normal language with respect to his age.

Neither of these is completely satisfactory. The first compares the student with a hypothetical "normal" population. The second leaves a great deal to specific environments which may be atypical and not ones in which the students will remain. In addition, some people who have a single deviation, like a lisp, are very conscious of their speech and consider it a handicap. If we want to obtain any job that requires much oral communication, then we will have to demonstrate competency in Standard English. Therefore, our goal should be achievement of Standard English, at least by the time we have completed high school.

Regardless of the criteria set for a language deficit, there are ways we can describe the language use of a person. In this section we will first consider ways of classifying deviations in the phonologic, morphologic, syntactic, and semantic aspects of the structure. We shall then describe the language characteristics of groups such as those with learning disabilities or mental retardation.

CLASSIFICATIONS OF ERRORS

PHONOLOGIC DEVIATIONS

Errors in the sound system of the language fall into four groups: (1) substitution, (2) omission, (3) addition, and (4) distortion. The most frequent among a school aged population is substitution. Although it is possible for an individual to substitute any phoneme for any other one, only a few phoneme substitutions generally occur. The most frequent are listed in Table 3–14. In general, children tend to substitute one voiced phoneme for another voiced phoneme, and unvoiced for unvoiced.

There is no general rule concerning the manner or the place of articulation in selection of substitutions. Sometimes one fricative will replace another, [s] for [ʃ], or a plosive for another plosive, [t] for [k], but a plosive may also be used instead of a fricative, [b] for [v]. Substitutions of phonemes by place of articulation are found in the category of alveolars. There we note errors such as [t] for [s] and [d] for [z].

It is not unusual for a child to substitute [θ] for [s] in the word *sun* and [s] for [ʃ] in *shoe*. His problem is not inability to produce the phoneme correctly, but rather inability to select the appropriate phoneme for a word.

Table 3–14. Most Frequent Phoneme Substitutions

Substitution	Example
[w] for [r] and [l]	in *r*ed, *l*amp
[θ] or [t] for [s]	in bu*s*
[ð] or [d] for [z]	in *z*ebra
[f] for [θ]	in *th*umb
[d] for [ð] and [g]	in *th*is, *g*o
[t] for [k]	in *k*itten
[b] for [v]	in *v*alentine
[s] or [tʃ] for [ʃ]	in *sh*oe
[l] for [j]	in *y*es

Omissions occur among all the phonemes, depending upon the age of the child. A word like *daddy* may come out as *dæi*, with the [d] in the second syllable omitted, when children begin to use words. Parents report that their young toddlers say *that* without the final [t] when they are first pointing to something they want. Omissions decrease during the first three years. Most children ready for preschool rarely omit phonemes. If they do, the omissions tend to occur at the end of the word. The consistent omission of most or all final phonemes would be considered a severe problem. The more omissions there are, the more difficult it is to understand the speech of the child.

Additions are rare, but do occur. In the early stages of speech therapy children sometimes add the error phoneme following the correct one or add the new sound they are learning in inappropriate contexts. For instance, as they learn to replace their [f] with the [θ] in *thank you*, they add the [f] after the [θ]. They may also add the [θ] after the [f] in words such as *four* and *five*.

Distortions are more likely among the plosives and fricatives, according to Templin (1957). A phoneme is classed as distorted if the production of the sound is perceived by the listener as either visually or acoustically different from standard, but still has the basic characteristics of the phoneme. For example, some children produce [s] so that air is emitted from the sides of the mouth, rather than through the middle. This distortion is referred to as lateral emission of the phoneme.

Some clinicians do not specify the nature of the error in the production of phonemes. They indicate that the sound is either correct or incorrect. It is much easier to obtain agreement among clinicians using the right-wrong category than the nature of the error. For beginners such a dichotomy is very acceptable if the person has only a few errors and is consistent in the errors. Classroom teachers with limited or no training in listening for the sounds accurately refer children to school clinicians for evaluation of sound productions. For purposes of referral that is all the information that is needed. For those persons with multiple errors, however, the clinician may wish to make a distinctive feature analysis. Then the type of error must be specified. In the distinctive feature analysis the number of correct productions of each phoneme is utilized, whether the phoneme is appropriate in the test word or is a substitution. Thus, the number of times the individual uses the feature of voicing versus nonvoicing (correct use of [b] plus substitution of [b] for [p]) is an indication of the presence of the feature of voicing. Further analysis may indicate that the person uses no voiceless phonemes or only a few. This type of analysis is made for each of the major distinctive features.

The concept that consonants can be classified according to their position at the beginning, middle, or end of a word is controversial. Classification by position is based on the definition of the phoneme as the smallest unit of sound. Using this definition, we can say, for example, that the word *sun* has an initial [s] and a final [n] or that *potato* has an initial [p] and two medial [t]s. Adherents of this view use tests to evaluate the production of phonemes in the three positions.

Other speech specialists consider the syllable the smallest unit of production. Consonants serve to release or arrest a syllable. Therefore, there is no such entity as a phoneme in the medial position. According to this concept the word *potato* would be analyzed as having three syllables, with the consonants [p] and [t] serving as releasers. In the word *potatoes* the phoneme [z] would be an arrester of the syllable. Both of these approaches have merit and can be utilized in describing the nature of the errors in phonology.

MORPHOLOGIC DEVIATIONS

When we deal with morphology, we are concerned with morphs or words and the inflections. A deficit in morphs can be defined in terms of the number a person has. A speech analyst would not actually count the morphs, but would make a judgment about whether the individual has enough to express his thoughts or ideas and whether the number is appropriate for his age. He may have no morphs, only a few, or an adequate supply.

Inflectional errors can be classified as those of omission, substitution, or addition. Inflections and their uses with nouns, pronouns, verbs, and adjectives have been described in the preceding chapter. Some individuals do not inflect nouns to show plurality in the usual fashion. They may omit the ending completely and say, for example, *two dress*. Other individuals may use *dress* as the plural form because they mistake the stem ending of the word for the plural inflection. In the former group, however, the zero inflection may be characteristic of their use of plurals regardless of the stem ending. Other common errors are the omission of the inflection for the third person singular of a verb, *go* for *goes*, and the use of the uninflected form of a verb for other tenses, *I swim yesterday*.

Substitution is the use of the wrong inflection and occurs most frequently in words which take irregular endings, for example, *childs* instead of *children*. It is not unusual for children of 6 or 7 to say *swimmed* instead of *swam* or *rided* instead of *rode*. Some linguists explain this error pattern as one of overgeneralization of a rule. The individual learns to use certain inflections with many words and then uses those endings with any verb or noun even if they are not appropriate. For example, children may add the comparative ending learned for the word *big* to the word *good*, so that they say *gooder*.

Addition is another type of inflectional error. Individuals may use two forms of the same inflection with one word, for example, *bedses* rather than *beds* or *swamd* rather than *swam*.

Many errors of addition, omission, and substitution of inflections can be heard in the speech of preschool and early elementary school children. They have so many choices that it is not surprising that some are still making errors in adulthood.

SYNTACTIC DEVIATIONS

Errors in syntax can be classed in the following ways: (1) no syntactic structures present in the speech, (2) limited number of syntactic structures, (3) grammatically incorrect structures; and (4) omission of structures.

Such errors are appropriate when a child is first learning a language. We do not expect a 1-year-old to use more than single-word utterances. However, the absence of syntactic structures, such as noun or verb phrases, at the age of 30 months would be considered a syntactic error. The child would be considered slow in mastering this phase.

A child who has only a few syntactic structures and does not join them to make a sentence by age 3 would be considered below average.

Many sentence types are characteristic of our speech. We have referred to these earlier in this chapter and listed the most frequent ones. The individual who has only a limited repertoire of sentence types can express himself in only those forms. We expect first graders to be using many different types of sentences, with both embedded and coordinated clauses.

There are several ways in which a sentence can be grammatically incorrect. These include incorrect word order and lack of subject-verb agreement. Incorrect word orders are associated primarily with questions. Some questions require a partial reversal of the position of the subject and the verb, others also require an auxiliary verb, and still others use a tag at the end in which the subject and verb are reversed. These transformations should begin to appear in children's language as soon as they have mastered two- and three-word phrases.

Lack of subject-verb agreement is characteristic of the speech of young children and may even be a problem for some adults. We hear such sentences as *Bobby and Mary is coming*, *They wants some more milk*, and *She do the dishes tonight*. Such misuse of verb forms may be due to a failure to realize that a compound subject requires a plural verb form or that the inflection for the third person singular is different from that for the first person singular. Number and person must be taken into account in matching the subject with the verb.

Another type of error is omission. In early language use children leave out the functors—the prepositions, articles, and conjunctions. They also omit the verb or part of it. We understand what Susan is telling us when she says *book table,* because she says it as she puts the book on the table. We fill in many words for young children and sometimes even think they have used them. A typical omission is the auxiliary verb. Two- and 3-year-olds will say *I going to the store*. By 4 they should be using not only the auxiliary, but also the contractions to say *I am going* and *He's giving a party*.

SEMANTIC DEVIATIONS

Deficits in the semantic aspect of speech are viewed in relationship to the social code of the individual's community. The meanings attached to words and word groups evolve in a society, and the members of the society help to establish, moderate, and change meaning.

We shall consider the deficits in terms of: (1) reception or comprehension and (2) expression or use. When a person listens to a speaker and is required to respond, an inadequate or inappropriate reply may represent a failure in comprehension. His comprehension of the symbols of the speaker must be viewed along a continuum from no decoding to partial decoding. For example, a child who is asked to point to his eyes may give no response. Is his lack of a response due to failure to understand the total syntactic unit or the symbols *point* or *eye?* Another child, given the same command, may put his finger close to the eyes of the examiner. Did this child have only partial understanding of the speaker's symbols?

Comprehension can be measured to some degree by tests that require nonverbal responses. Like all such tests, however, they represent only part of the total repertoire of language as symbols.

Deficits in expression are also viewed along a continuum from none to partial. An individual's symbols may be: (1) nonexistent, (2) incorrect, (3) inappropriate, or (4) limited. Of course, age is an important factor in evaluation. What is considered as abnormal at one period may be standard at another age. We do not expect a child to have expressive symbols at 6 months, but we do at 24 months. We accept the use of the symbol *cat* to designate a dog at 24 months, but not at 36 months. In clinical evaluation one 5-year-old child had many such in-class errors; he used the terms *bed clothes* for *pajamas*, *noise* for *drum*, and *comb* for *brush*. Another child, when asked about *rakes*, called them *pocketbooks*.

An example of an inappropriate use of symbols is the following. An examiner, meeting a child for the first time, asked, "What's your name?" The child replied, "That's a dinosaur." The child was looking at the examiner when she gave her answer, and there were no pictures or toys in sight to which she could have been responding. Another example is the child who, when shown a picture of a boy eating his breakfast, said, "Daddy don't eat baby."

Use of symbols can also be measured by tests. A person's use would be interpreted as limited on the basis of age-related norms for the test.

Aram and Nation (1975) found that children with semantic problems were more likely to be deficit in the other linguistic components also. The younger children had more generalized problems while the older ones had more specific types of disordered language. Some children have difficulty with comprehension but they can perform tasks that are primarily repetitive. Many will have better comprehension than production.

SPECIAL GROUPINGS OF CHILDREN

Because of our tendency to group on the basis of major criteria we have special classes for pupils who are mentally retarded, trainable retarded, emotionally disturbed, learning disabled, hearing impaired, and physically handicapped. Students are placed in these classes on the basis of their performance and school personnel provide a special curriculum for them. In smaller school districts these children may be in one or two special rooms because there are fewer children to be served. In other districts only the pupils with the most severe disabilities are in special classes, while all the others receive assistance through the resource rooms.

Many of these students have multiple handicaps. They may be both mentally retarded and hearing impaired, learning disabled and physically handicapped, emotionally disturbed and mentally retarded, or any similar combination. In addition, there are gradations of all of these—pupils may have mild, moderate, or severe degrees of the disabling condition. Many have communication problems. They need to be identified and receive instruction and therapy to fit their needs. In the following section we will identify the language deficits of several of these groups.

MENTAL RETARDATION

The American Association for the Mentally Retarded has defined mental retardation as a group of conditions characterized by inadequate social adjustment, reduced learning capacity, and a slow rate of maturation, present singly or in combination, due to a degree of intellectual functioning below average, and usually present from birth or soon after.

The child who is mentally retarded seems to follow a pattern of language development that is similar to that of normal children. This statement, however, does not imply that they use the linguistic structures either to the same extent or the same way as normal children. It does not mean that they "catch up over time," that is, that they reach the level of understanding and utilization of language expected of normal children by the chronological age of 12. The studies show that there are both qualitative and quantitative differences in their language use, compared to normal children.

According to studies of educable retarded children, a high percentage of them have deviations in articulation. In a group of almost 800 between 6 and 16 years of age in classes for the retarded in St. Louis County, Missouri, more than half had articulation deviations (Wilson, 1966). Types of errors were similar to those of normal children, with substitutions and omissions decreasing and distortions increasing among those with higher mental ages (MA). Number of errors was also associated with MA level. Children with MAs between 3 and 5½ years had an average of 17 errors, while those between 8½ and 12 had 10.

Some categories of phonemes were easier for the children to master than others. There tended to be fewer errors on nasals, plosives, glides, fricatives, affricates, and sibilants, in that order. The number of errors on the sibilants did not decrease, however, among those with the higher MAs. Evidently, this set of consonants presents some special problems also for the educable retarded.

Newfield and Schlanger (1968) studied the inflections of a group of mentally retarded children ranging in chronological age from 8 years 10 months to 12 years 1 month, with a mean mental age of about 6. They compared their scores with those of a normal group of 30 children with a mean chronological age of 6 years 10 months. The results, using lexical items to evaluate the plural, present progressive, past tense, third person singular verb, and possessive inflections are given in Table 3–15. Only two inflections, the present progressive *ing* and plurals requiring [z] and [s], were 90 percent correct. It would seem that these two were the only inflections that had been mastered at that level by the retarded. However, the normal children had command of almost all the items at that level and did not fall below the 80 percent correct level on any of the categories. In comparison, the retarded were severely deficient in most of the other inflections.

Naremore and Dever (1975) obtained spontaneous language samples from 30 educable mentally retarded and 30 normal children at mental age levels of 6, 7, 8, 9, and 10 years. The retarded ranged in chronological age from 8 to 12 years and the normal group from 6 to 10 years. The authors analyzed the verbal output in terms of the syntactic structures the children used. They found that they could discriminate the two groups by the number of subject and predicate elaborations and the number of relative and subordinate clauses. At the earlier mental ages the sentence elaboration was similar for the two groups, but by mental age 10 the normal children were integrating the information they gave in more mature sentence forms. The retarded children tended to use the coordinated sentence, with the conjunction *and* as the major connecting word. As a result the syntax seemed to be more typical of that of younger normal children.

Table 3–15. Data on Lexical Items from a Normal and a Retarded Sample

Class	Allomorph	Lexicon Words	Mean Percentage Correct	
			Normal	Retarded
Nouns	[-z]	dogs doors guns paws leafs, leaves	99	90
	[-əz]	watches garages noses dresses glasses	81	41
Noun subtotal mean			90	66
Verbs	[-ɪŋ]	running	100	97
	Vowel change plus final consonant change	ringed, rang	90	25
	Vowel change plus final consonant change	singed, sang		
	[-t]	kicked	100	50
	[-d]	played	100	17
	[-əd]	melted skated batted	82	23
	[-əz]	judges dances	87	18
Verb subtotal mean			90	32
Possessives	[-z]	dog's	100	60
	[-s]	chick's	90	47
	[-əz]	claus's	80	27
Possessive subtotal mean			90	44
Total means			90	48

Source: M. U. Newfield and B. Schlanger. The acquisition of English morphology by normal and educable mentally retarded children. *Journal of Speech and Hearing Research, 11,* 693–706 (1968).

Part of the Monroe study (1971) involved a group of children who were considered to be delayed in language development. Of the four mentally retarded children with CAs between 3 years 6 months and 4 years 10 months, none displayed knowledge of the concepts of plurality, time, or discrimination nor did any succeed on any of the tested inflections—plurals, future and past tense, and comparative and superlative forms of the adjectives—at either the comprehension or use level. Responses on the expressive level were primarily no reply, imitation of the experimenter, unintelligible response, or naming an object in the picture.

On tests to measure verbal expression, word meanings, word associations, and analogies, the educable retarded function either at the same level as their MAs or below. They have a limited vocabulary of both comprehension and use. Some of them will "talk" a great deal, but the content is inappropriate.

There is clinical support for these statements that the educable retarded pupils have more than their share of deficits in all facets of language. They seem to learn the language structure at a slower pace and use its forms inappropriately or in less complex ways than their normal counterparts.

The children who are labeled trainable have more severe language deficits than the educable. Some of them have not learned any oral language; some have mastered either a few signs or some minimal language. Others have attained enough language proficiency to be able to manage themselves at home or in community placement centers. About this group we can say that they have deficits in the same aspects of language as those who are educable, but their performance level is lower.

LEARNING DISABILITIES

The child who is considered learning disabled is usually identified by the end of the first grade. Although each school district sets its own standards for identifying these children, in general the children have the following characteristics: (1) they have normal intelligence as measured by standard tests; (2) they have difficulty learning school subjects; and (3) they are not able to function at capacity in the regular classroom. Depending upon the severity of their difficulties and the school's facilities, the children are either placed in a special classroom for the learning disabled or remain in the regular classroom and receive remedial instruction. The special instruction may be provided through a resource room teacher or a specialist, such as the teacher of remedial reading.

These children demonstrate a wide range of communication and language skills. Some have normal receptive and expressive language, at least while they are in the primary grades. Others show specific oral language problems. Teachers and speech clinicians have reported that many of them have immature articulation skills for their ages and social group. Some are slow in mastering morphologic endings. In a study of a group of children enrolled in classes for the learning disabled, Moran (1977) found that even the regular verb past tense endings had not reached a 90 percent level of correct production. The children studied were between the ages of 7 and 9, had normal intelligence, and had been placed in these classrooms because of their inability to learn in the regular classrooms. They had less than half of the irregular past tense inflections correct. A few did not have the present progressive form of the verb; others did not have the appropriate marker for future time. They use prepositions incorrectly, possibly as a part of their difficulties with concepts.

Teachers have noted that some of the children have syntactic and semantic deficits as well. They may use immature forms of question and negative sentence types. They have difficulty telling a story in the correct sequential order of events. Wiig and Semel (1973) reported that their ability to process and comprehend sentences that included some selected concepts was significantly lower than children of the same age and intelligence without a learning disability. Some examples of the questions asked by

Wiig and Semel are: Are parents older than their children? Bill was painted by George. Who painted? Does spring come before winter? Relationships such as these were difficult for them to fathom, and so they gave wrong answers.

Some learning disabled take twice as long as other children to complete tasks. Others require frequent repetition of directions before they can complete a task. Assignments that take 15 or 20 minutes for normal children require more than 60 minutes for some of them.

SOCIAL ENVIRONMENT

There has been considerable interest in the proficiency of language use by those in various socioeconomic groups for the past fifty years. Much of the early research pointed to differences in cultural strata, but only in recent years have researchers evaluated specific linguistic aspects of English. In this section we will present some highlights from the research literature.

Templin (1957) has reported on the acquisition of phonemes by children aged 3 to 8 from upper and lower socioeconomic groups. She found that the development of phonemic skills was faster among the upper than the lower socioeconomic group. Templin reported that for all categories of phonemes the upper group had scores for correct production that were higher than those in the low group. It took an additional year for the low group to master the phonemic system.

Sociolinguists have pointed out that morphologic rules take different forms in Black English from those in Standard English. One study of black children from low socioeconomic backgrounds in New York City reported how six such rules were utilized by pupils across preschool and four grade levels (Ramer and Rees, 1973). In the constructions of plurality, past tense, possessives (singular and plural), and a single act (today she *eat*), a zero marker is used in Black English; in the third person singular continuous action, the copular *be* is utilized (she *be* eating). The study showed that the pupils knew and used the rules of morphologic construction of both Black and Standard English. As the age of the groups increased, the pupils demonstrated fewer instances of Black English. However, not even the oldest group, those in eighth grade, used the Standard English forms completely. In other words, there was a mixture of the two dialects.

Gerber and Hertel (1970) gave the Illinois Test of Psycholinguistic Abilities (Kirk, 1968) and obtained a spontaneous speech sample from a group of normal preschool children from two cultural groups—one considered to be disadvantaged and the other nondisadvantaged. The test scores indicated that the disadvantaged children were significantly behind their advantaged counterparts on all but one subtest, the visual motor association test. On the total test the disadvantaged children were more than one year below the advantaged group. The former followed a pattern similar to those in the latter group, however It appeared that mastery of the linguistic skills was delayed, but not necessarily deficient. The authors reported that the disadvantaged seemed to understand and relate the meanings of symbols, but they were particularly weak in expressing their ideas. The length of their utterances was considerably below that of their advantaged counterparts, also. Thus, they showed their expressive language weakness not only in the tests, but in the length of their utterances.

Studies of black middle- and lower-class children indicate that the former have language skills that are superior to those in the latter group. Just as with white students the black middle-class group utilize more elaborate sentence structures, are more adept at story-telling and interpretation, and employ more general and abstract vocabulary than the lower-class group.

The Templin (1957) comparisons between the high and low socioeconomic groups of children on the syntactic and semantic aspects of the language show that in almost every instance the upper group had higher scores. On tests of meaning of words, length of utterances, and syntactic complexity, those whose fathers hold professional, managerial, or skilled status showed greater proficiency. However, the differences were significant in only 28 percent of the comparisons, with a high concentration in the grammatical complexity and vocabulary tests.

Bernstein (1962) reported that adolescents from working-class families in England used a restricted code for communication. In other words, the adolescents used minimal words to express their ideas. He hypothesized that the family structure itself inhibited the development of both elaborate syntactic structures and large vocabularies.

Because Bernstein's samples were small and were not randomly selected, some researchers, like Poole and Field (1971), were not willing to generalize from the Bernstein reports to other populations. To test the reliability of the reports' findings Poole and Field studied the verbal output of college freshmen at the University of New England in Australia. The first-year students were classified in four groups on the basis of father's occupation and level of education: (1) working class—skilled or semiskilled, (2) working class—unskilled, (3) middle class—rural, professional, and (4) middle class—urban, professional. A structured individual interview that tapped verbal planning from description to abstraction was utilized to obtain the language sample.

They reported that there were significant differences in the syntactic and semantic aspects between the students in the four socioeconomic groups. However, fewer differences were noted between students from the professional middle class who were urban and those who were rural. They pointed out also that only the brightest children from the working classes were admitted to the university and therefore the sample from the working class was a superior group. In spite of this factor the elaborated syntactic structures and the descriptive vocabulary differentiated the four social groups from one another.

CEREBRAL PALSY

Cerebral palsy has been described in many different ways. The following is a definition used by Perlstein (1952): "a condition characterized by weakness, paralysis, incoordination, or any other aberrations of motor functions due to pathology of the motor control centers of the brain." If the speech production mechanism is involved, we would expect deficits in the articulation of this population. When other areas of the brain are also damaged, we find deficiencies in the related structure of language.

When Irwin (1955) studied the vowel and consonants used by cerebral palsied children, he found that both the type and frequency were considerably below that of normal children. Mean vowel types ranged from 6 for 1- to 2-year-olds to about 9 for 7- to 8-year-olds. The mean consonant types ranged from 5 for 1- to 2-year-olds to about 11 for the 7- to 8-year-olds. In his total 7- to 8-year-old group an average of only 20 phonemic types was present. In comparison, normal children utilize an average of 20 types at 16 months.

Another way to look at the vowels and consonants is to consider their frequency of occurrence in connected speech. Irwin reported the mean frequency of vowels in his sample of cerebral palsied children from 1 to 8 years clustered around 50. Consonant frequency averaged about 100. In all, the frequency of phonemes, including both vowels and consonants, averaged about 150. Normal children of 30 months of age are using 150.

Another way to analyze their phonemes is to consider the initial, medial, and final positions. Irwin reported that the highest frequency of correct production occurred among the initial phonemes, then the medial, and then the final. Still another way to examine phonemes is to compare the order of acquisition by normal and cerebral palsied children. Byrne (1959) found that the phonemes were acquired in the same order for the two groups of children, but the proficiency with which they used the phonemes was considerably different. Only five phonemes, [m], [d], [w], [h], [b], were utilized by 75 percent of the children with cerebral palsy, who ranged in age from 2 to 7 years. We can compare that figure with what we know about normal children, 75 percent of whom have these phonemes and many more by age 3.

When we talked about types of errors at the phoneme level, we indicated that we could classify them as substitutions, omissions, distortions, or additions. With most children omissions are negligible. With Byrne's cerebral palsied sample there was almost an equal percentage of omission and substitution errors. Of all the errors which they demonstrated, approximately 15 percent were omissions and 16 percent were substitutions.

When Lencione (1966) studied the phoneme production of cerebral palsied pupils between the ages of 8 and 14 years, she also found that the production followed the pattern of normal children. In her 8-year-old group; 75 percent of them had achieved correct production of the nasals, plosives, [l], [h], [w], and [j] in the initial position. She found that even among her 14-year-olds, however, the 75 percent level of proficiency was not attained for five phonemes. Contrast this with the average 6-year-old who has mastered most or all his phonemes.

Because of the low proficiency in articulation, researchers have been discouraged from studying other aspects of the language of the cerebral palsied. We do have some information about their acquisition of first morphemes and beginning syntactic structures. The range in single words is somewhere between 15 and 27 months. The Byrne (1959) sample were all educable quadriplegics and their first words appeared at age 15 months. The Denhoff and Holden (1951) group included all types of cerebral palsied children and he considered them to be a random sample of this population. That group had a mean of 27 months for the appearance of first words. Hood and Perlstein (1956) indicated that children were about 21 months of age before they used their first words. They also reported a mean of 31 months for two-word presentences and Byrne reported 36 months. Denhoff and Holden reported that among those children who used three-word utterances some were 37 months of age, but many at that age had not reached that stage. Byrne reported a mean of 78 months for three-word utterances. There is probably less delay in the acquisition of the single morpheme, but more difficulty with two- and three-word syntactic units. We can compare these figures with normal children who for the most part have three-word presentences by 30 months of age.

Few studies of the semantic aspects of the language have been reported. Dunsdon (1952) reported that the vocabulary of the British population which he studied was delayed three to four years. Love (1964) felt that the educable cerebral palsied child whose speech is intelligible has no problem with semantics either in terms of comprehension or production. His sample, however, was a very select one. Many children are not intelligible and could not have been included in Love's study.

EMOTIONAL DISTURBANCE

Children whose primary problem is an emotional one have varied degrees of skill in language. Some may have no deficits, but others may have no language at all. The degree and type of emotional disturbance is a major factor in the development and use of normal language.

Much of our information about the language of these children has come from case studies and reports. Most of these deal with the psychotic child and his very serious deficits in communication. Shervanian (1967) summarized the characteristics as they have been reported in the literature. Some children use no language, only some animallike noises. Some are silent except for a rare perfectly formed and articulated sentence. Some have no words, but do combine some phonemes in syllables. Some have language, but the articulation is characterized by substitutions and omissions. There are pronomial reversals, reversals in word order, perseveration, echolalia, incomplete sentences, and irrelevant and bizarre outbursts that reveal a large vocabulary.

In a study of precommunicative psychotic children, Shervanian (1959) found that they had the vowels and nasals, but not the plosives, fricatives, [l], and [r]. There was a reduction of both types and frequency in their vowel and consonant production that was out of proportion to expectations in view of their ages.

Shapiro and his co-workers (1972) followed the language development of a schizophrenic boy over a four-year period. They obtained a 10-minute spontaneous language sample periodically from the time he was 2 years 10 months until he was 6 years 2 months. During this period 13 samples were analyzed to determine how many utterances of more than two words he used (excluding echolalia) and selected characteristics of those utterances. At 2 years 10 months he had only 7 utterances in the 10-minute period, and all of them were simple declarative sentences. A year later he used 36 utterances, but 19 of them were judged to be stereotyped utterances. Of the remaining 6 were simple declarative sentences, 4 were question or imperative sentences, and the rest were primarily incomplete phrases. At 4 years 9 months there was a drop in verbal output. There were only 11 utterances, 3 of which were stereotypes and only 2 were sentences. At age 6 years 2 months the number of utterances rose to 43, with 5 stereotyped comments, 26 incomplete phrases, and only 4 sentences.

This child, Freddi, showed some progress in language use over the four years, but at least for one year he showed marked regression. As we indicated above, he had 36 utterances at 3 years 10 months, but during that year the number slipped each time a recording was made. It reached 11 at 4 years 9 months. Shapiro reported that his mean length of utterance at 63 months was only 2.6. With that length of utterance, it is not possible to use many inflections, expanded noun phrases or verb phrases, or many transformations.

HEARING IMPAIRMENT

Just as with other groups of children with special problems, the hearing impaired show great variation in their mastery of language. Some deaf students have such excellent command of English that they have been awarded Woodrow Wilson and other fellowships for graduate study. Others, at the opposite end of the continuum, never achieve any facility with oral language, but have learned and use manual language.

Several recent reports focus on the rules that the deaf may be using in formulating sentences. In one study Sarachan-Deily and Love (1974) found that deaf students in two different residential programs probably have unstable or limited syntactic rules for the reconstruction of active, passive, negative, and passive-negative sentences. When they were asked to write down sentences of these types that were read to them, they tended to delete major sentence constituents and to use incorrect noun and verb inflections, incorrect word order, and inappropriate verb substitutions. As a result of these types of errors their written utterances were atypical of English syntax. The sentences they heard contained no more than eight words in each, so that we cannot say they could not hold them in memory. In addition, they all had been taught by either a strictly oral or an oral plus finger-spelling procedure.

Quigley, Wilbur, and Montanelli (1974) investigated the comprehension of question formation of deaf students aged 10 to 18 years. They asked the students yes-no, wh-, and tag questions and requested that they encircle the correct answers to the questions. They found that yes-no questions were easier for them to comprehend than wh- questions and both were easier than the tags. The deaf students scored 74 percent correct on yes-no's, 66 percent on the wh's, and 57 percent on the tags. The normal hearing children who were the control group and were 8 to 10 years of age achieved 90 to 100 percent on all three.

When the researchers studied the abilities of these deaf students to judge the grammaticality of question forms, they found less proficiency than for the answers to the question forms. The deaf made the correct judgments on the yes-no question types 66 percent of the time and on the wh- question types 58 percent of the time. The authors concluded that skill in making judgments about the grammaticality followed the comprehension of the question forms themselves. In neither the question of comprehension nor judgment of grammaticality, however, did these students come close to the performances of normal hearing children who were 8 to 10 years old. There was a gradual improvement in scores of the age groups of the deaf, but not even the 18-year-olds performed as well as the normal hearing sample.

Rules for the use of the conjunction *and* to conjoin nouns as subjects, nouns as objects, and verb phrases have also been explored by Wilbur, Quigley, and Montanelli (1975). They gave the deaf students written instructions like these:

> The girl chased the ball. The boy chased the ball.
> "Make one sentence from the two sentences."
> The girl ______________________________

The students had 24 such sets to reconstruct. Although the older deaf students completed the coordination tasks with more correct sentences than the younger ones, even they made mistakes. The deaf, even at age 18 years, did not achieve the proficiency of normal hearing 10-year-olds.

All of the studies on grammatical structures show that the deaf improve over time. If we can determine what inefficient rules they are using, we may be able to develop programs that will help them to master the language more easily and quickly.

DELAYED OR DEVIANT?

There is a difference between deviant language and delayed language development. The latter refers to the slow mastery of the linguistic structures that we see in many children. They are learning the grammar in an orderly fashion, but they are doing it at a slower pace than other children of the same age. For instance, they are using the correct inflections for regular plurals and regular past tense verbs, but they are overgeneralizing those endings to other nouns and verbs. They have the concept, but as yet they have not mastered some of the specific inflections. Also, they may still be using a simpler syntactic structure than other children of their age. They have the simple affirmative-declarative sentences with some transformations, but not the degree of embedding and coordination that they might be utilizing.

Those children whose language is deviant are in a different category. Some of them have syntactic structures that are different from those of children of their age group. They are different in terms of correctness, complexity, and variety. In many instances, even though the word order is correct, there are major omissions of either noun phrases or verb phrases. In addition to the syntactic errors there are morphological problems. This group may omit all of the inflections that are needed to express the many concepts. There is an unevenness in their mastery of all or several aspects of the structure of language. They show a peak of development well below their chronological ages. For instance, at age 5 they may still be using incorrect pronouns. They may not have learned the rule for contractions, and forms of the copula and auxiliaries are not appropriate.

We might summarize the differences between these two groups of children by saying that the truly delayed language group know the rules consistent with their level of development but have not learned to apply them correctly in all instances. The deviant group either do not have a set of rules or have a set and apply them in ways that are not correct. Their language differences are distinct.

There is a group of children whose expressive language falls somewhere between the two. We are not sure whether it is a question of delayed development or deviant use. This is the group who require more extensive testing and observation. Their language samples need to be analyzed more carefully in order to help us to determine into which group the children fall. In spite of very careful analyses, however, there will be some whose expressive language has characteristics of both delay and deviancy. These characteristics have implications for program planning.

SUMMARY

In Chapter 3 we have reviewed language acquisition of children and their language deficits. We do not have complete information about many aspects of both acquisition and deficiency and as a result there are gaps in our presentation.

Normal acquisition proceeds quickly during ages 2 to 4; there is growth in all aspects of language. By age 8 most children have acquired all the phonemes and by age 12 the morphologic and syntactic units. The semantic aspect continues to develop throughout life.

The deficits can be described in relation to the phonologic, morphologic, syntactic, and semantic aspects of English. Regardless of whether the language deficit is the primary problem or the secondary one, we can describe the language within the same framework.

With some children and adolescents there is a question whether or not the language is just delayed or is really deviant. In both instances it is different from the average for the age of the person. The degree of difference and the age of the individual must be considered in making a determination of normal, delayed, or deviant.

REFERENCES

Aram, D. M., and Nation, J. E. Patterns of language behavior in children with developmental language disorders. *Journal of Speech and Hearing Research*, *18*, 229–241 (1975).

Berko, J. The child's learning of English morphology. *Word*, *14*, 150–177 (1958).

Bernstein, B. Social class, linguistic codes, and grammatical elements. *Language and Speech*, *5*, 221–240 (1962).

Blasdell, R., and Jensen, P. Stress and word position as determinants of imitation in first-language learners. *Journal of Speech and Hearing Research*, *13*, 193–202 (1970).

Bloom, L. *One word at a time: The use of single word utterances before syntax*. The Hague: Mouton, 1974.

Brown, R. *A first language: The early stages*. Cambridge, Mass.: Harvard University Press, 1973.

Byrne, M. C. Speech and language development of athetoid and spastic children. *Journal of Speech and Hearing Disorders*, *24*, 231–240 (1959).

Carrow, E. *Test for auditory comprehension of language*. Austin, Tex. Learning Concepts, 1973.

Chen, H. P., and Irwin, O. C. Infant speech: Vowel and consonant types. *Journal of Speech Disorders*, *11*, 27–29 (1946).

Chomsky, C. *The acquisition of syntax in children from 5 to 10* (Research Monograph No. 57). Cambridge, Mass.: MIT Press, 1969.

Darley, F., and Winitz, H. Age of first words: Review of research. *Journal of Speech and Hearing Disorders*, *26*, 272–290 (1961).

Denhoff, E., and Holden, R. H. The developmental ladder in cerebral palsy. *The Crippled Child*, *29*, 4–5 (1951).

De Villiers, P. A., and De Villiers, J. G. Early judgments of semantic and syntactic acceptability by children. *Journal of Psycholinguistic Research*, *1*, 299–310 (1972).

Dundson, M. I. *The educability of cerebral palsied children*. London: Newness Educational Publishing, 1952.

Fraser, C., Bellugi, U., and Brown, R. Control of grammar in imitation, comprehension, and production. *Journal of Verbal Learning and Verbal Behavior, 2*, 121–135 (1963).

Gerber, S. E., and Hertel, C. G. Language deficiency of disadvantaged children. *Journal of Speech and Hearing Research, 12*, 270–280 (1970).

Gesell, A. *The first five years of life*. New York: Harper & Row, 1940.

Hood, P., and Perlstein, M. Infantile spastic hemiplegia: V. oral language and motor development. *Pediatrics, 17*, 58–63 (1956).

Horowitz, F. D. (Ed.). Visual attention, auditory stimulation, and language discrimination in young infants. *Monographs of the Society for Research in Child Development, 39*, Nos. 5–6 (Serial #158) (1974).

Hubbell, R., Byrne, M. C., and Stachowiak, J. Aspects of communication in families with young children. *Family Process, 13*, 215–224 (1974).

Ingram, D. Phonological rules in young children. *Journal of Child Language, 1*, 49–65 (1974).

Irwin, O. C. Infant speech: Consonantal sounds according to place of articulation. *Journal of Speech Disorders, 12*, 397–401 (1947a).

Irwin, O. C. Infant speech: Consonant sounds according to manner of articulation. *Journal of Speech Disorders, 12*, 402–404 (1947b).

Irwin, O. C. Phonetic equipment of spastic and athetoid children. *Journal of Speech and Hearing Disorders, 20*, 54–57 (1955).

Irwin, O. C., and Chen, H. P. Infant speech: Vowel and consonant frequency. *Journal of Speech Disorders, 11*, 123–125 (1946).

Kirk, S. *Illinois test of psycholinguistic abilities* (Rev. ed.). Champaign: University of Illinois Press, 1968.

Lee, L. *Northwestern syntax screening test*. Evanston, Ill.: Northwestern University Press, 1971.

Lencione, R. Speech and language problems in cerebral palsy. In W. Cruikshank (Ed.), *Cerebral Palsy*. Syracuse, N.Y.: Syracuse University Press, 1966.

Loban, W. D. *The language of elementary school children* (Research Report No. 1). Champaign, Ill.: National Council of Teachers of English, 1963.

Love, R. J. Oral language behavior of older cerebral palsied children. *Journal of Speech and Hearing Research, 7*, 349–359 (1964).

McCarthy, D. A. *Language development in children*. In L. Carmichael (Ed.), *Manual of child psychology*. New York: Wiley, 1954.

McNeill, D. *The acquisition of language. The study of developmental psycholinguistics*. New York: Harper & Row, 1970.

Metraux, R. W. Speech profiles of the pre-school child 18 to 54 months. *Journal of Speech and Hearing Disorders, 15*, 37–53 (1950).

Monroe, N. *Concept learning in the acquisition of inflectional endings*. Doctoral dissertation, University of Kansas, 1971.

Moran, M. and Byrne, M.C. Verb inflections of normal and learning disabled children. *Journal of Speech and Hearing Research, 20*, 529–542 (1977).

Naremore, R., and Dever, R. B. Language performance of educable mentally retarded and normal children at five age levels. *Journal of Speech and Hearing Research, 18*, 82–95 (1975).

Newfield, M. U., and Schlanger, B. The acquisition of English morphology by normal and educable mentally retarded children. *Journal of Speech and Hearing Research, 11*, 693–706 (1968).

O'Donnell, R. G., Griffin, W. J., and Norris, R. C. *Syntax of kindergarten and elementary school children: A transformational analysis* (Research Report No. 8). Champaign, Ill.: National Council of Teachers of English, 1967.

Perlstein, M. Infantile cerebral palsy: Classification and clinical correlations. *Journal of the American Medical Association, 149*, 30–41 (1952).

Poole, M. E., and Field, T. W. Social class and code elaboration in oral communication. *Journal of Speech and Hearing Research, 14*, 421–427 (1971).

Prather, E. M., Hedrick, D. L., and Kern, C. A. Articulation development in children aged two to four years. *Journal of Speech and Hearing Disorders, 40*, 179–191 (1975).

Quigley, S. P., Wilbur, R. B., and Montanelli, D. S. Question formation in the language of deaf students. *Journal of Speech and Hearing Research, 17*, 699–713 (1974).

Ramar, A. L., and Rees, N. S. Selected aspects of the development of English morphology in Black American children of low socioeconomic background. *Journal of Speech and Hearing Research, 16*, 569–577 (1973).

Sanders, L. S. The comprehension of certain syntactic structures of adults. *Journal of Speech and Hearing Research, 14*, 739–745 (1971).

Sarachan-Deily, A. B., and Love, R. J. Underlying grammatical rule structure in the deaf. *Journal of Speech and Hearing Research, 17*, 889–898 (1974).

Shapiro, T., et al. The speech of the schizophrenic child from two to six. *American Journal of Psychiatry, 128*, 92–97 (1972).

Sharf, D. J. Some relationships between measures of early language development. *Journal of Speech and Hearing Disorders, 37*, 64–74 (1972).

Shervanian, C. C. *The speech developmental level of precommunicative psychotic children*. Doctoral dissertation, University of Pittsburgh, 1959.

Shervanian, C. C. Speech, thought, and communication disorders in childhood psychoses: Theoretical implications. *Journal of Speech and Hearing Disorders, 32*, 303–313 (1967).

Solomon, M. Stem endings and the acquisition of inflections. *Language Learning, 22*, 43–50 (1972).

Templin, M. *Certain language skills in children*. Minneapolis: University of Minnesota Press, 1957.

Templin, M. C., and Darley, F. L. *The Templin-Darley Tests of Articulation*, Second Edition. Iowa City: University of Iowa, 1969.

Weir, R. *Language in the crib*. The Hague: Mouton, 1962.

Wiig, E. H., and Semel, E. M. Comprehension of linguistic concepts requiring logical operations by learning-disabled children. *Journal of Speech and Hearing Research, 16*, 627–636 (1973).

Wilbur, R. B., Quigley, S. P., and Montanelli, D. S. Conjoined structures in the language of deaf students. *Journal of Speech and Hearing Research, 18*, 319–335 (1975).

Wilson, F. B. Efficacy of speech therapy with educable mentally retarded children. *Journal of Speech and Hearing Research, 9*, 422–433 (1966).

Winitz, H., and Irwin, O. C., Syllabic and phonetic structure of infants' early words. *Journal of Speech and Hearing Research, 1*, 250–256 (1958).

Wyatt, G. *Language learning and communication disorders in children*. New York: Free Press, 1969.

Zonshin, J. *One-word utterances of Hebrew speaking children*. Masters Thesis, University of Tel Aviv, 1974.

THE PHYSICAL DETERMINANTS Chapter 4

The anatomical structures involved in the formulation of the language code and the production of speech include the nervous system, the respiratory system, the oral portion of the digestive tract, and the auditory sense receptors. All of these structures are involved in the biological adaptation of the individual through acts such as breathing, sucking, chewing, swallowing, and alertness to danger signals. Speech and language production requires the use of organs that, in the view of some writers, have more primary functions than speech. This opinion is the source of descriptions of speech as an "overlaid function." Jackson and Jackson (1937) point out that in addition to producing voice for speech, the larynx functions in emotional cries, in keeping foreign objects out of the lungs, in removing foreign objects from the lungs through coughing, as a regulator of oxygen-carbon dioxide exchange in breathing, and in fixing the chest for lifting heavy objects, in defecation, and in childbirth.

This concept of speech as an overlaid function clearly reveals the intimate connection of the speech mechanism with other more primary physiological activities. Often speech must cease when more primary physiological activities take place. Speech comes to a halt when deep, rapid breathing follows highly strenuous exercise.

Because of the overlaid nature of speech, many disorders of language and speech production and reception are determined by defective anatomical structures and defective physiological functions caused by disease and maldevelopment.

THE MEDICAL MODEL

The medical model of physical pathology is based on the assumption that the overt manifestations of pathology are symptoms of an underlying disease process. Since many diseases result in similar symptoms, a differential diagnosis must be made to determine the underlying disease. The diagnostic procedure includes the case history and an appropriate battery of laboratory tests. One by one the possible diseases are eliminated as causative factors until the illness has been diagnosed or labeled. If possible, the treatment is directed toward elimination of the underlying disease, since the symptoms will disappear once the disease has been brought under control.

The medical model has been applied to speech and hearing problems. The problems are viewed as symptoms of an underlying disease process. The term *disease* is broadly generalized to include factors such as specific diseases, biochemical inadequacy, structural damage, hereditary factors, embryological defects, and maturational defects. These are the physical factors which affect the structures and functions of speech and hearing.

These physical factors are problems which may be treated by physicians through medication, reconstructive surgery, or preventive medicine, and by other specialists, such as dentists and physical and occupational therapists, depending on the type and severity of the problem.

The speech pathologist views speech and hearing pathologies as behavior to be dealt with through the use of appropriate psychotherapeutic and educationally sound intervention programs. Having a physical problem of speech or hearing does not mean that the person is so psychologically different that the basic laws of behavior do not apply. In actual practice the medical model as such has limited application to speech and hearing problems, since most behavior is multiply determined. The person with a cleft palate may have a speech pathology, but there are factors of a psychological and social nature that influence his speech.

THE SPEECH MECHANISM

Language and speech are produced by the physiological activities of a number of anatomical structures. The structures include the brain for the conceptualization and formulation of the linguistic code; the central and peripheral nervous system for transmission of nerve impulses; the lungs for the creation of air pressure; the vocal folds for the generation of sound; the throat, nose, mouth, palate, tongue, jaws, and lips for the production of consonant and vowel sounds that combine into words and sentences; and the ears for the monitoring of speech. The process is illustrated in Figure 4–1, adapted from Carhart (1969).

The physical structures function in a highly organized and integrated fashion, with the various parts synchronized with one another in order to produce a meaningful sequence of accurate speech sounds, using an established linguistic code and employing proper levels of loudness, pitch, and a pleasing voice quality.

INTRODUCTION TO SOUND

In the communication act sounds are produced by the speaker, transmitted through the medium of air, and received by the listener. They are highly structured sounds that serve as the currency of exchange in speech communication. The physical attributes of the sounds have occupied the attention of a number of scientists from a

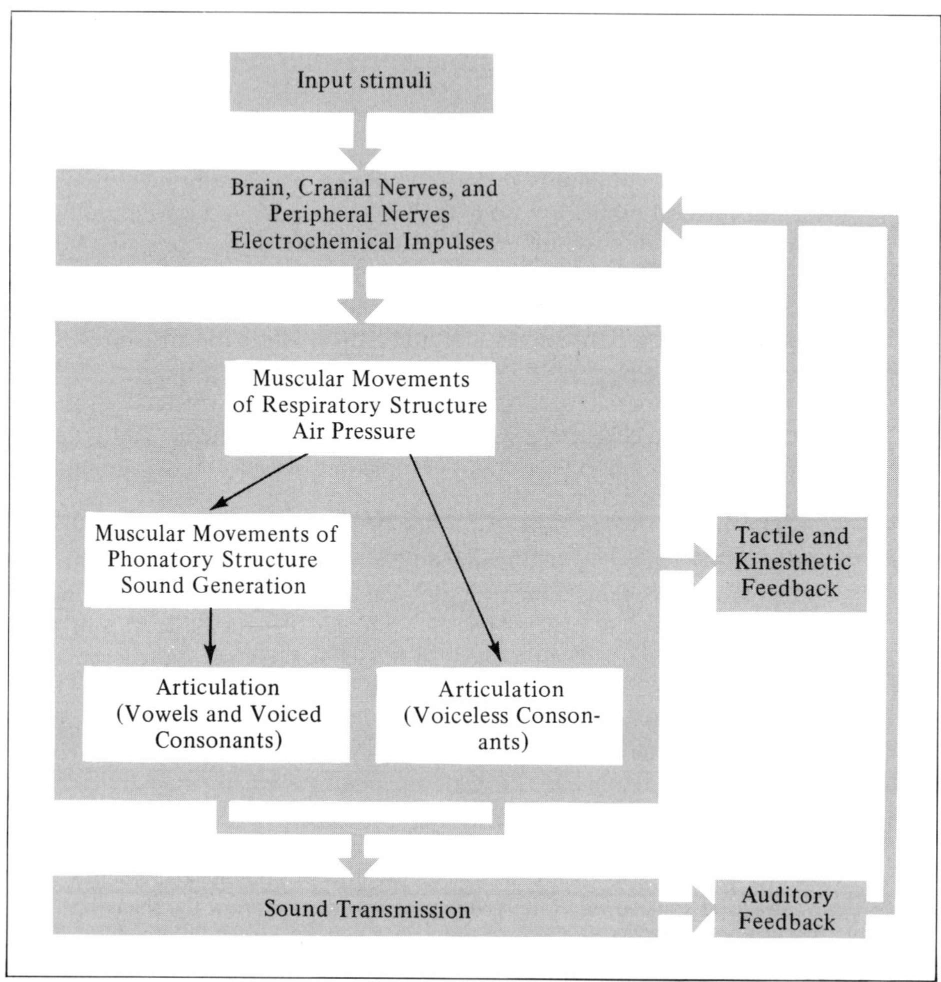

Figure 4–1. The speech act.

variety of disciplines. Physicists have analyzed and labeled their components. Engineers have devised instruments for measuring them and for transforming them into electrical energy for telephone and radio transmission. Speech and hearing scientists have especially been concerned with the production, transmission, and reception of these human sounds in both their normal and pathological forms. They have been joined in these efforts by experimental psychologists and psycholinguists. Our understanding of speech sound production, transmission, and reception will be greatly enhanced if we acquire a few nontechnical concepts of the physics of sound as they are applied to speech communication.

A sound wave motion begins with a source of energy which can initiate movement. The finger striking a piano key or plucking a string on a harp provides the energy for vibrating the strings to produce sound. The major source of energy for activating speech sound waves comes from a column of air. A column of air under the pressure of being forced out of the lungs causes the vocal folds, which are at the top of the column, to vibrate.

In addition to a source of energy, there must be something which can be forced to move back and forth or to vibrate from its rest position. Thus, the vibratory source must have properties of mass and elasticity. The strings of the piano or harp have these qualities. Once struck or plucked they vibrate, producing sound waves until all the energy which initiated the movement is expended. The vocal folds also have the characteristics of mass and elasticity, although they are certainly not like strings. Rather, they are like muscular lips at the end of an air column which is under pressure. The air blows the lips apart, and because they are elastic, they spring back together again, only to be blown apart again and again. The opening and closing movement causes the air to vibrate.

There must be a medium to carry and transmit the vibrations. The medium most used for sound is the air, although sound can travel through water and, as every apartment dweller knows, through plaster walls, concrete floors, and, for that matter, any medium that can be made to vibrate. When there is no medium, there can be no transmission of sound. A bell placed inside a glass dome can be heard to ring. When the air is removed and a vacuum created inside the dome, the bell can be seen vibrating, but no sound is heard, because there are no sound waves unless there is a medium.

Sound travels through a medium by means of movements of the molecules of the medium. Air is an elastic medium with many billions of molecules per cubic inch. A vibratory mass activates the molecules into an identical vibration. If we were able to observe the molecules greatly enlarged (Figure 4.2), we would see that when they are

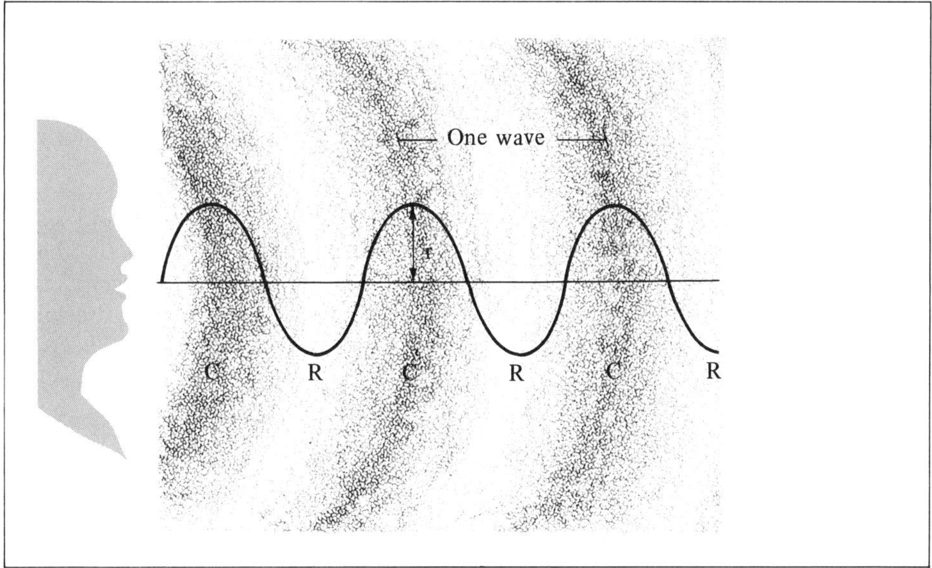

Figure 4–2. Schematic representation of sound wave being propagated through space. The dots represent molecules as they pile up in condensations (C) and spread apart in rarefaction (R). When sound is represented by a wave, condensation is at the crest and rarefaction at the trough of the wave.

disrupted by a vibration they move away. As they move, they strike one another and tend to pile up. This piling up is called a *condensation*. Being elastic, they "bounce" away after striking one another. This explosion is called a *rarefaction*. By means of successive condensations and rarefactions the sound is propagated in waves in a spherical manner away from its source until it strikes an object. Depending on the surface size and shape of the object, the sound will either be absorbed or reflected or will set the object into a vibration.

SOUND INTENSITY AND LOUDNESS

The force with which the molecules strike one another determines the distance molecules will travel when set into motion and the amount of energy the sound will contain. The magnitude of the sound energy is called sound pressure amplitude. This can be converted to a more useful measure called *intensity*. Research has shown that the measurements indicating the intensity of a sound approximate what the human ear perceives as the *loudness* of a sound.

The unit of measure for the intensity of a sound is a ratio called a decibel (dB). Since the decibel is a relative number, it must be stated in terms of an existing reference level. Most often .0002 dynes per centimeter square is used in speech and hearing research. This figure is roughly equivalent to the smallest pressure vibration sufficient to produce an audible sound wave. Thus 0 dB with the reference level of .0002 dynes per cm^2 is the smallest audible sound wave. In contrast 130 dB intensity is the strongest sound we can hear without feeling pain. Other dB intensity values are as follows (Denes and Pinson, 1973):

1. An average whisper produces an intensity of 20 dB 4 feet from the speaker.
2. The level of night noises in a city is about 40 dB.
3. Normal conversation at a distance of 3 feet is usually at an intensity of 60 to 70 dB.
4. A pneumatic drill 10 feet away makes a 90 dB noise.

SOUND FREQUENCY AND PITCH

The *pitch* or the ear's perception of the highness or lowness of a sound is determined by the number of cycles of condensations and rarefactions per second. This is illustrated in Figure 4–3. The number of cycles per second is called the *frequency* of a sound. The unit of measure is the Hertz (Hz). Thus, if a sound wave contains 500 vibratory cycles per second, it would be described as having a frequency of 500 Hz. A sound which contains only one frequency is called a *pure tone*. Pure tones do not occur in nature. They are generated electronically or somewhat less accurately through tuning forks.

Speech and hearing scientists depict sounds in three ways: as a wave, as a graph, or as a spectrograph. Figure 4–3*a* shows a 500 Hz pure tone as a wave. A variety of electronic and mechanical instruments are capable of producing an illustration of this type. For our purposes, the significant parts of this illustration include the horizontal axis which is marked time in seconds. Each cycle of the wave occupies $^1/_{500}$ of a second since this is a sound of 500 Hz. The vertical axis is amplitude, revealing the intensity of the sound. Figure 4–3*b* takes the same 500 Hz sound and depicts it as a bar graph.

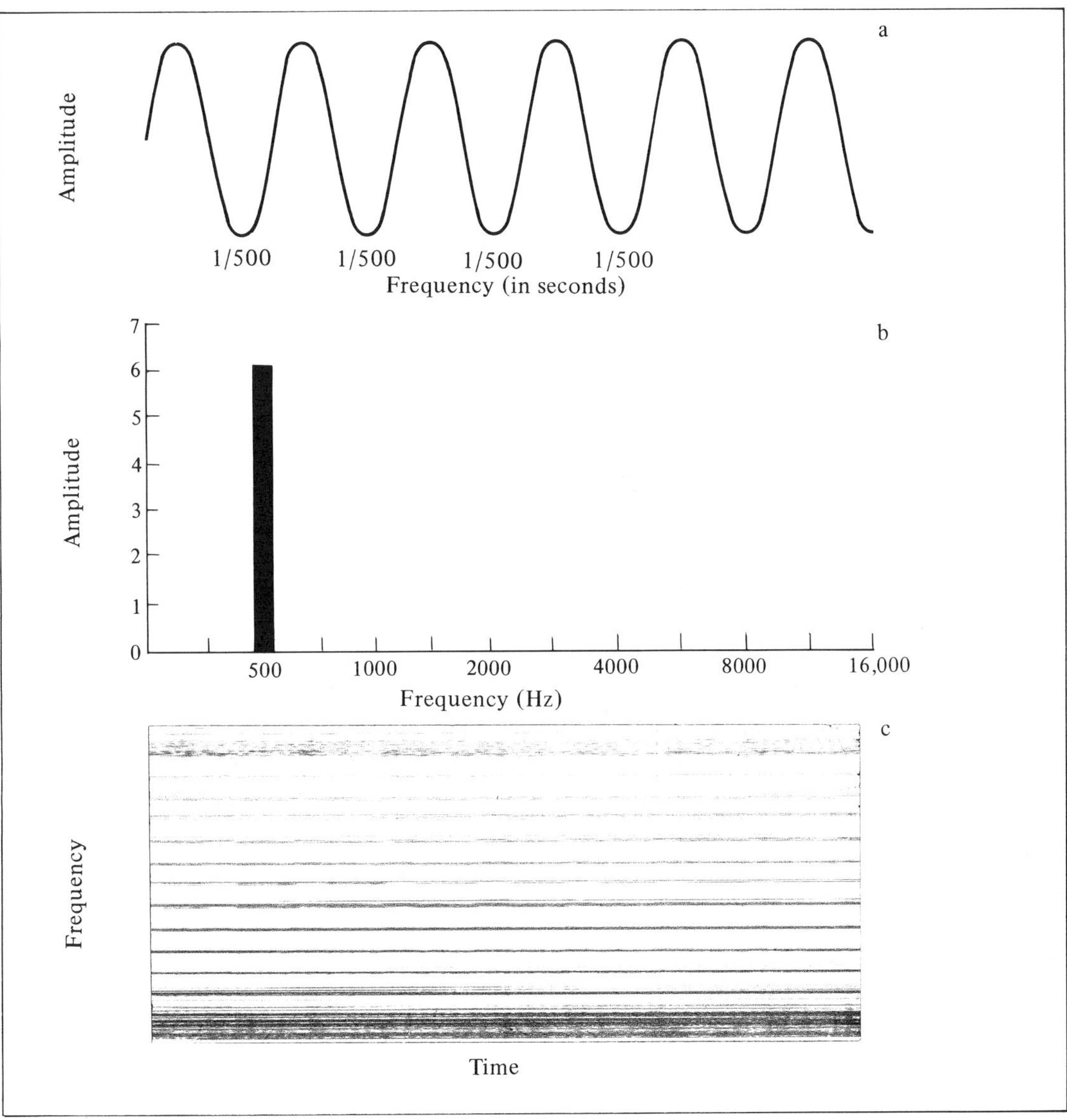

Figure 4–3. Three Methods of Representing a 500 Hz Pure Tone. (*a*) The tone is depicted as a wave. Each cycle is $^{1}/_{500}$ of a second. Time is indicated on the horizontal axis. The vertical axis is the amplitude of the wave or the intensity of the sound. (*b*) The tone is represented as a bar graph. Only the frequency 500 Hz is depicted. Amplitude is indicated by the height of the bar. (*c*) The tone is represented as a sound spectrogram. Frequency is indicated on the vertical axis, time on the horizontal, and amplitude by the darkness of the ink.

The horizontal axis in the bar graph represents frequency and the vertical axis represents intensity (amplitude) in dB. Figure 4–3*c* once again takes the 500 Hz sound and uses an electronic instrument, the sound spectrometer to analyze and create a spectrograph of the sound. The horizontal axis represents time, the vertical axis represents frequency and the darkness of the ink is an indicator of the intensity. Figure 4–4 gives a schematic picture of the sound spectrograph.

A sound which contains more than one frequency is called a *complex tone*. Vowel sounds are complex sounds. The lowest frequency of a sound is called the fundamental. The other frequencies are called overtones or partials. They are an integer number of the fundamental. Those overtones in a vowel which show energy peaks are called formants. Figure 4–5 shows a complex tone, actually the vowel [ɑ] as a wave, its spectra with its formant clearly visible, and a sound spectrogram.

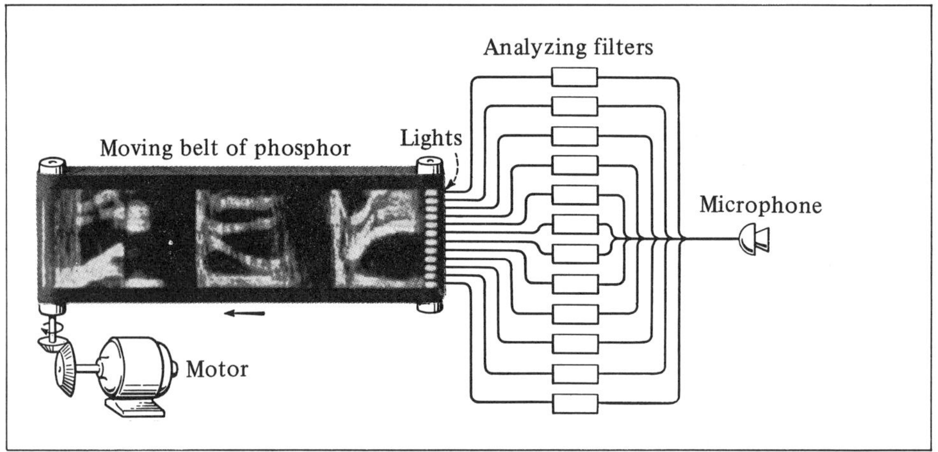

Figure 4–4. Schematic view of the sound spectrograph. From *The Speech Chain*, copyright © 1963 by Bell Telephone Laboratories, Inc. Reprinted by permission of Doubleday & Company, Inc.

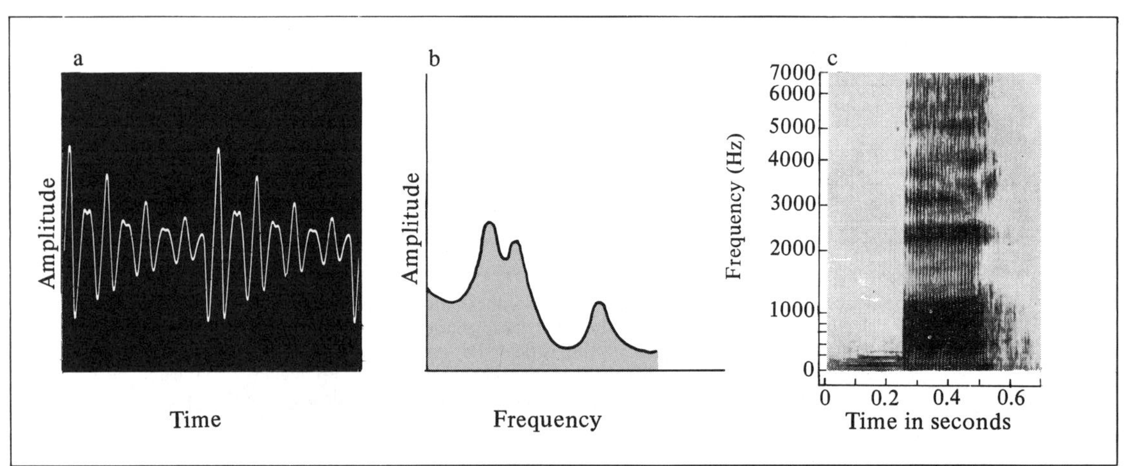

Figure 4–5. The vowel [ɑ]: (*a*) the waveshape of [ɑ], (*b*) the spectra of [ɑ], (*c*) the sound spectrogram of [ɑ]. From *The Speech Chain*, copyright © 1963 by Bell Telephone Laboratories, Inc. Reprinted by permission of Doubleday & Company, Inc.

SOUND WAVE COMPLEXITY AND QUALITY

The pattern of fundamental and overtones in a sound is called the *wave complexity*. The human ear perceives the wave complexity as the *quality* of a sound. There is no symbol for the wave complexity, since it is not a discrete unit. It is a pattern that is composed of the frequency and intensity of the fundamental and each overtone. If it is not possible to ascribe a fundamental to a sound because of very rapid changes, we perceive it as *noise*.

SOUND TIME AND DURATION

Sound continues over a period of time until its energy has been dissipated. The human ear perceives the length of time as the *duration*. This is measured in milliseconds.

THE NERVOUS SYSTEM

NEUROLOGICAL STRUCTURES UNDERLYING THE RECEPTION, CENTRAL PROCESSING, AND EXPRESSION OF SPEECH AND LANGUAGE

The nervous system underlies all the processes of language and speech. It is highly complex, both in its structure and function. While a great deal is known about the anatomical components, knowledge of the details of functioning is in large measure conjectural and hypothetical (Carhart, 1969). We will introduce you to some of the more widely held views of the system.

The nervous system consists of (1) the central nervous system—the brain and spinal cord and (2) the peripheral nervous system—the sensory nerves which link the sensory receptors to the central nervous system and the motor nerves which link the central nervous system to the muscles and glands.

The functions of the nervous system during speech and language production are: (1) afferent nerves carry sensory information to the brain, (2) central processing of information is carried out in the brain, and (3) efferent nerves transmit activating information from the brain to the muscles and glands.

More specifically, sensory stimuli are received by the senses. The sensory information is coded and transmitted along afferent nerves to the brain. The receptors important in speech include organs of hearing, vision, touch, and kinesthesis (the sense of movement and position of parts of the body in space). Central processing includes: perception (mental awareness of a sensory stimulus), memory, concept formation, thought, and language formulation. It is through these and other central processes that we give meaning to what we hear, mediate the information, formulate a response, and implement the response. Efferent nerves relay the directions to activate and coordinate muscles and glands of the organs of breathing, voice, and articulation to produce speech.

NEURON. The entire nervous system is based on a highly specialized form of living cell called the *neuron*. The brain alone is organized with well over 10 billion neurons. There is considerable understanding of how these cells transmit nerve impulses.

A schematic view of the neuron is shown in Figure 4–6. The neuron consists of (1) a cell body with its nucleus, (2) dendrites which appear to branch out from the cell body and serve as contact receptors of impulses from adjacent cells, (3) an axon—a nerve fiber which extends from the cell body and ends in the axon terminal. Axons range in length from a few thousandths of an inch to 3 feet.

The function of the neuron is to transmit electrochemical nerve impulses. Nerve impulses received by dendrites travel to the cell body and then along the axon to its terminal which connects to the next dendrite. The point of juncture between terminal and dendrite where neurons connect is called a synapse. Afferent neurons carry nerve impulses from the senses to the central nervous system and efferent or motor neurons carry nerve impulses to the muscles and glands from the central nervous system. There are also neurons which carry impulses between different points of the central nervous system.

Nerves themselves consist of bundles of axons and serve as pathways for impulses. Some axons are covered with a fatty fibrous myelin sheath which is thought to facilitate the conduction of nerve impulses.

Central Nervous System. The central nervous system with brain and spinal cord are shown in a schematic drawing, Figure 4–7. The important subdivisions and their arrangements are illustrated. The central nervous system appears to follow a hierarchical organization, with the spinal cord controlling simple automatic reflex behavior such as the knee jerk and higher units responsible for more voluntary actions. The brain stem, cerebellum, hypothalamus, and thalamus each share increasingly more complex regulatory mechanisms and coordinating activities over the lower structures. The

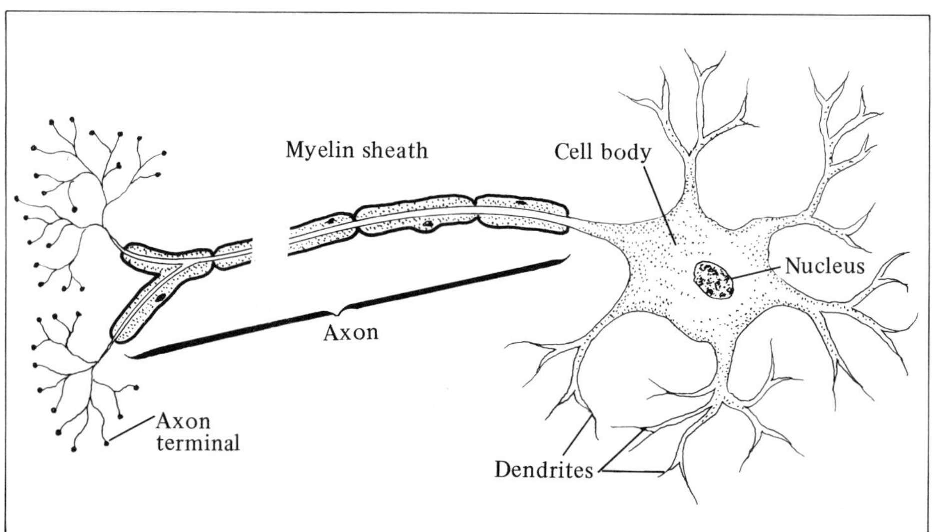

Figure 4–6. Schematic view of the neuron.

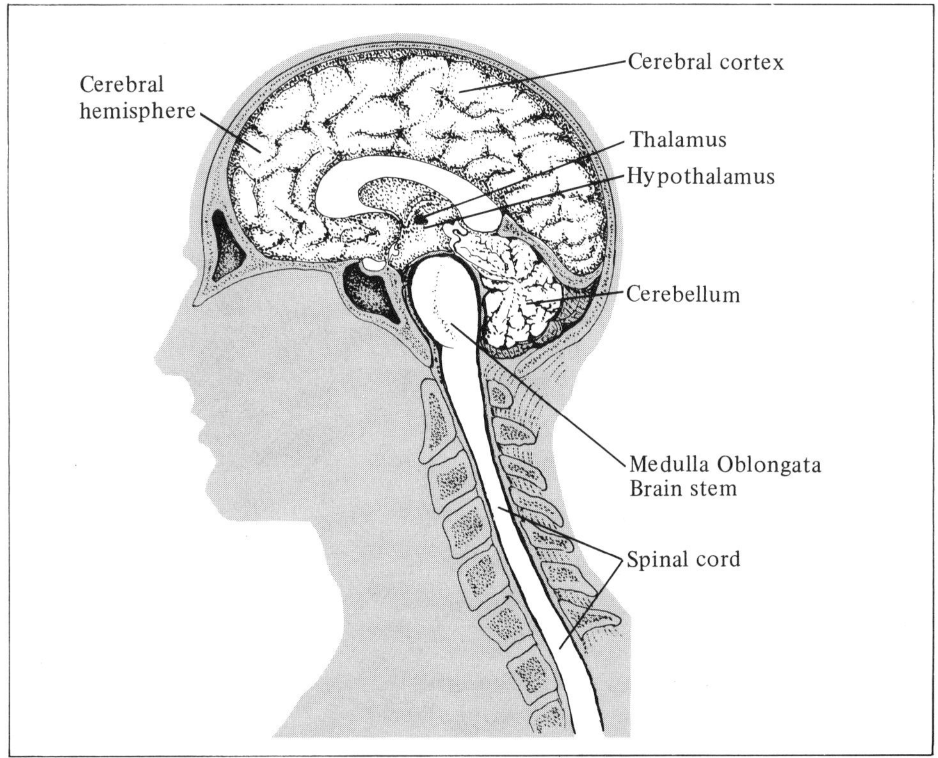

Figure 4–7. Central nervous system.

highest level of adaptive control is the cerebrum which differentiates man from all other animals in its symbolic and rational control of behavior.

CEREBRUM. The cerebrum with its right and left hemisphere makes up the largest part of the brain. Its surface, the cerebral cortex, is a highly wrinkled, thick layer of nerve cells which form an unbelievably complex network.

It is in the cortex that the specialized sensory and motor areas are located. Figure 4–8 shows these supposed localizations on the cortical surface. With the exception of the sense of smell, sensory reception of impulses from the left half of the body is found on the right side of the cortex and vice versa. This type of opposite side brain control is true for the motor areas as well. Brain damage in the motor areas of the right hemisphere produces paralysis in the left half of the body.

The human brain has yet another type of specialization. In most people the left hemisphere of the brain is dominant in the control of speech, language, and skilled movements of the right hand, while the right hemisphere controls activities such as form perception and spatial organization. Recent studies show that some control of speech reception is found in the right hemisphere and some control of spatial reception is in the left hemisphere, but such controls are basically in the dominant hemisphere (Sperry, 1968).

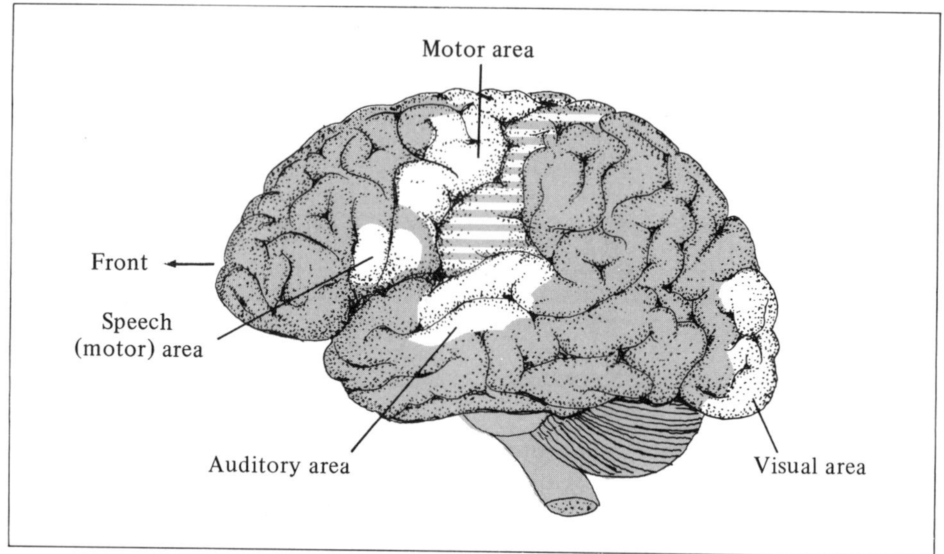

Figure 4–8. Sensory and motor areas of the brain.

About 5 percent of the population have a left-handed preference; they perform most of their skilled movements with that hand. However, control over speech and language remains in the left hemisphere. Only 5 to 10 percent of left-handed people have right hemisphere dominance (Hebb, 1972). When brain injury occurs in the left hemisphere prior to age 10, it is thought that the right hemisphere compensates by developing dominant control over language and speech.

The functions of the cerebral cortex include control over all the higher complex mental processes including perception, consciousness, memory, reasoning, problem solving, learning, and language. How this takes place and what neural activity relates to the various mental processes is still not known.

THALAMUS. The thalamus is located under and is surrounded by the cerebrum. It functions as the major relay station for transmitting sensory impulses to the cortex from most of the sense receptors, including those of hearing. Another role it may play in communication is transmitting impulses from the motor speech area of the cortex.

HYPOTHALAMUS. The hypothalamus is a small structure located beneath the thalamus. It may have some control over motor functions, but its major function is homeostatic regulation of body temperature, water, metabolism, endocrine balance, appetite, and sleep. Through its influence over endocrine glands, it affects the muscular functions of speech, especially when strong emotions are involved.

CEREBELLUM. The cerebellum is attached to the rear of the brain stem under the cerebrum. Its major functions include coordination of muscular actions, maintenance of muscle tone, and balance. Since speech involves a fairly precise coordination of a large number of muscles of the voice and articulation mechanisms, the cerebellum's role in oral communication is an important one. Cerebellar dysfunctions result in certain types of clumsy, imprecise dysarthric speech.

BRAIN STEM AND SPINAL CORD. The brain stem is an upward extension and enlargement of the spinal cord. It contains the medulla which in addition to controlling heartbeat and swallowing has reflex control over breathing. Most of the nerve fibers and bundles from the higher centers of the brain have pathways down through the brain stem to other parts of the body. These include sensory and motor pathways important to speech. Many cranial nerves which are part of the peripheral nervous system connect with the central nervous system at the level of the brain stem.

The spinal cord is a downward continuation of the brain stem. It is encased in the vertebral column. It serves as the primary reflex pathway, carrying impulses to and from the brain. Spinal nerves which enter and leave the spinal cord through the vertebra have a role in this process. They innervate muscles of the chest and abdomen, some of which are involved in breathing, as well as organs and glands of the body.

CRANIAL NERVES. We have noted that the cranial nerves, most of which have sensory and motor fibers, are connected at the level of the brain stem. Seven of the nerves are of interest to us here because they innervate sensory receptors, muscles, and glands important for speech and hearing. Table 4–1 lists these cranial nerves and their functions.

NEUROLOGICAL DISORDERS AND SPEECH AND LANGUAGE

Any disorder in neurological structures and functions can have a profound effect on all aspects of speech and language. The nature of the effect and the degree of severity

Table 4–1. Cranial Nerves Important for Speech and Hearing

Number	Name	Function
5th	Trigeminal	Controls movements of jaw; carries sensory fibers from the lips and face
7th	Facial	Carries motor fibers to face and lips
8th	Auditory	Carries sensory fibers from the inner ear
9th	Glossopharyngeal	Carries sensory fibers from the tongue and pharynx; carries a few motor fibers to the pharynx, velum, and posterior root of the tongue
10th	Vagus	Carries motor fibers to the larynx; carries a few motor fibers to the muscles of the pharynx, velum, and posterior root of the tongue
11th	Accessory	Carries motor fibers to certain muscles used in inhalation and to muscles of the pharynx, velum, and posterior root of the tongue
12th	Hypoglossal	Carries motor fibers to the intrinsic and a portion of the extrinsic muscles of the tongue and to muscles involved in forced inhalation

Note: Cranial nerves are usually referred to by both number and name. There are 12 pairs.

vary. Problems of neurological dysfunction can range from a massive destruction of the cerebral cortex, as in a severe cardiovascular accident, causing widespread defects in all symbolic receptive, mediational, and expressive language functions, to a very mild articulation problem during rapid speech caused by a peripheral nerve paralysis of the lip.

Depending on the site of the neurological damage and the degree of severity the symptoms may be in any component of the linguistic code, paralinguistic structures, or the mechanism for speech production, namely, respiration, phonation, articulation, resonance, or hearing.

Breakdowns in the brain may result in aphasia, dysarthria, apraxia of speech, and learning disabilities, while those in the spinal cord or peripheral nervous system are the dyarthrias.

Aphasia. Aphasia, according to Darley (1964), is a disorder of the capacity to deal with symbolic language. Aphasia affects all aspects of the language function. These include the symbolic processes associated with reception and comprehension, central processing and formulation, and the expression of meaningful morphologic, syntactic, and semantic functions. Specifically, it adversely affects the use of words, competence in and performance of morphologic and syntactic rules, and denotative and connotative aspects of meaning. It is to be differentiated from loss of intelligence, emotional disturbance, hearing loss, and motor dysfunctions, although these may be present to some degree in the aphasic.

Causes of adult aphasia according to Schuell (1969) are found in cerebrovascular accidents or strokes. These occur when the blood vessels supplying nutrition and oxygen to the brain are blocked because of thrombosis or embolisms or when the blood vessels rupture because of weakness in the walls of the vessel, high blood pressure, or trauma. Other causes include brain tumors, head injuries as in war or automobile accidents, infectious diseases, and toxins.

In classifying aphasia according to type, we must keep in mind that we are dealing with a symptom complex, that is, a grouping of symptoms that frequently occur

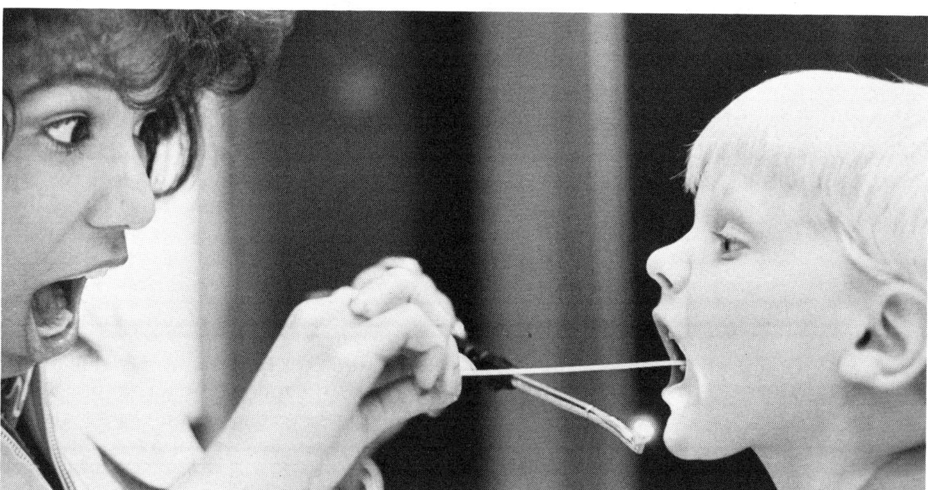

together. The descriptive terms are behavioral and are not to be interpreted as implying a localization in some specific area of the brain. The two types of aphasia are expressive and receptive.

Predominantly expressive aphasia is a disturbance in the ability to express ideas symbolically. It represents a disorder in the use of the linguistic code, not in the physical production of speech. It includes language symptoms in a number of areas. The patient may have difficulty in remembering specific words when he speaks. He may block on a word, substitute a synonym, or use circumlocutions. There is hesitancy, blocking, and frustration in talking, and sentences, are short, lacking in auxiliary words, and agrammatical.

There are dysfunctions in the prosodic features, with abnormal intonations and stress patterns. The speech may lack vocal variety and color (Berry and Eisenson, 1956).

Predominantly receptive aphasia is a difficulty in the ability to comprehend and understand spoken or written words (Weisenberg and McBride, 1935). Often coupled with the difficulty in comprehension is the inability to monitor and control verbalization, resulting in expressive problems as well. In extreme cases the individual may "talk" in a free-flowing jabber of incomprehensible nonsense words, since he cannot monitor his own speech to keep it orderly. Such individuals may talk with proper rate of speech, with copious streams of words accurately articulated, but with incomprehensible content.

Another aphasic disturbance is agnosia, the inability to discern configurations of objects or pictures, even though the sense organ is not significantly defective.

Dysarthria. Dysarthria is a speech disorder that may affect the processes of respiration, phonation, articulation, resonance, and prosody. It is caused by weakness, paralysis, or incoordination of the neuromusculature due to a lesion of the central or peripheral nervous system. Research of Darley, Aronson, and Brown (1969a, 1969b), has greatly clarified this speech problem as it occurs in adult patients with neurological disorders. The clinical neurological diseases include pseudobulbar palsy, amyotrophic lateral sclerosis, bulbar palsy, cerebellar disease, Parkinson's disease, dysarthria, and choreoathetosis. Each of these diseases affects specific parts of the motor nerve tracts from the cerebellum to the spinal cord. Darley and his associates were able to classify the resulting breathing, voice, and articulation problems into five discernible symptom types. Their speech typology was accurate enough to be useful in diagnosing the disease.

Cerebral palsy, which usually has its origins in brain injury in childhood, results in a dysarthria of respiration, voice production, articulation, and paralinguistic attributes. The identification and speech and language symptomatology have been discussed in Chapter 3.

Apraxia of Speech. Apraxia of speech is a disorder in articulation caused by brain damage. Unlike dysarthria, in which there is a neuromuscular weakness, paralysis, or incoordination which affects articulation as well as other willed and reflex responses, apraxia of speech is characterized by impairment "of the capacity to program the positioning of the speech musculature and sequencing of muscle movements for volitional production of phonemes and sequencing of phonemes" (Darley, 1964; Johns and Darley, 1970). The person with apraxia is capable of producing the muscular movements involved in articulation production, but may fail when attempting to combine those movements in articulation of meaningful phonemes or when sequencing the articulatory movements in morphemes.

Martin (1974) takes exception to the term apraxia of speech. As defined above it appears to be most closely associated with speech production. Martin argues that the problem falls in the realm of aphasia, since it is an impairment in the processing of the linguistic unit, the phoneme, clearly an aspect of language.

Special Learning Disabilities. In following the lead of the National Advisory Committee on Handicapped Children (1968), we have grouped together under the label children with special learning disabilities all those who have been variously referred to as having perceptual handicaps, brain injury, minimal brain dysfunction, and developmental aphasia. These children manifest disturbances in the psychoneurological processes which underly the receptive and expressive aspects of language and of cognition, including listening, thinking, talking, reading, writing, spelling, and arithmetic. Excluded from this group are children with learning problems due primarily to visual, hearing, or motor handicaps, emotional disturbance, mental retardation, or environmental disadvantagement.

THE RESPIRATORY SYSTEM

THE PROCESS OF RESPIRATION

Breathing for life purposes is so natural and effortless a process that the normal person hardly thinks about it. Yet he completes, on the average, 14 cycles of breathing every minute of his entire life. A respiratory cycle has two phases: inhalation, the act of bringing necessary oxygen gases into the lungs, and exhalation, the act of expelling carbon dioxide gases from the lungs. The oxygen is carried by the blood to the cells of the body in exchange for the carbon dioxide, which is a waste gas. If breathing is arrested for a prolonged period, as in drowning, despite eventual resuscitation, the neurological organs such as the brain begin to break down from anoxia (oxygen deprivation), causing irreversible brain damage.

A study of Figure 4–9 will be helpful in understanding the respiratory structures and the mechanics of breathing. The body is divided into two cavities by the diaphragm, a hemidome-shaped tendinous muscle. The upper cavity is the thorax or rib cage which contains the lungs and the heart. The lower or abdominal cavity contains the stomach and viscera.

Inhalation occurs when certain muscles attached to the chest contract, thereby lifting the thorax in an upward and outward direction. This action increases the volume of the chest in its front-to-back and side-to-side dimensions. At the same time, contraction of the muscles of the diaphragm cause it to move downward to a flattened position, thus increasing the vertical dimensions of the rib cage. The lungs inside the rib cage, being spongy masses, expand to fill the enlarged space. This overall increase

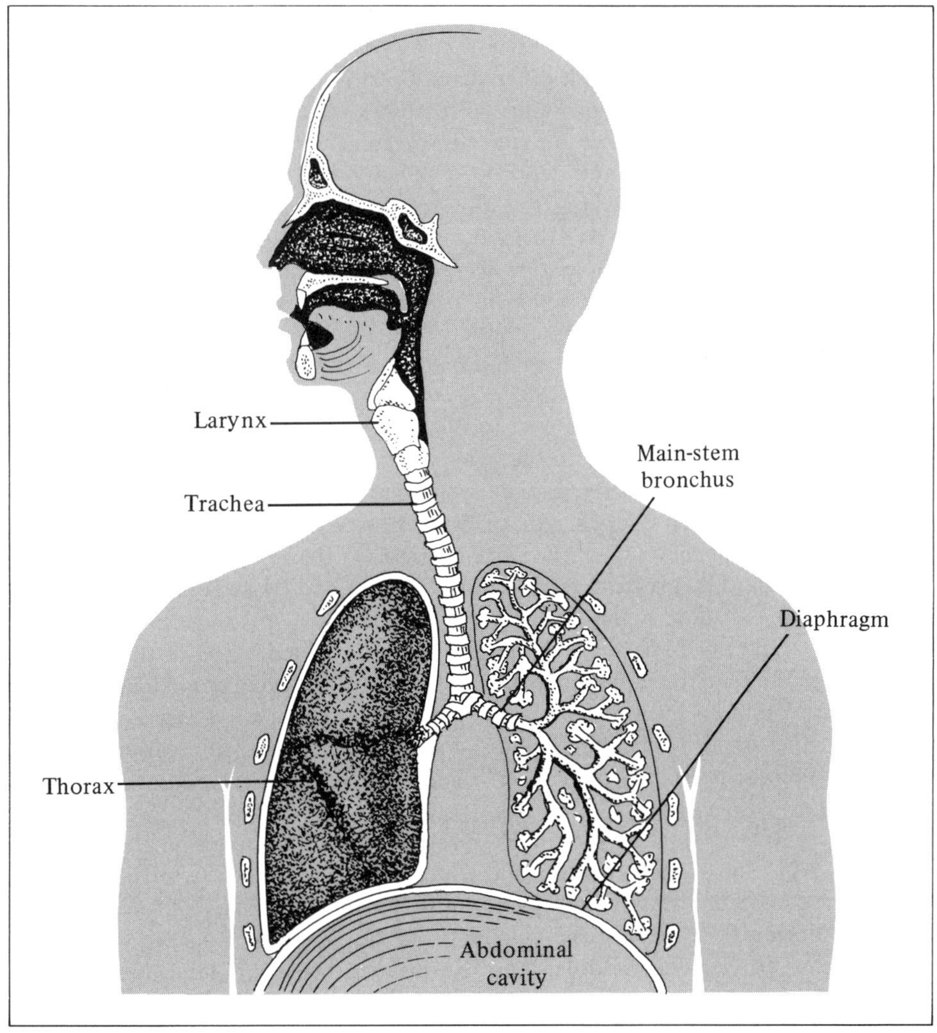

Figure 4–9. Respiratory mechanism.

in the volume of the thorax creates a negative pressure or partial vacuum inside the lungs. Since the air pressure outside the lungs is greater than inside, air travels through the respiratory pathway, inflating the lungs, until there is an equal pressure outside and inside the lungs.

The process is reversed for active exhalation. The volume of the thorax is decreased when contraction of abdominal muscles pulls the rib cage in a downward and inward direction and indirectly causes the diaphragm to return to its dome shape. The decrease in the volume of the thorax places pressure on the lungs, forcing air out through the respiratory tract.

The primary purpose of breathing is for life purposes, but this in no way minimizes the importance of breathing for a second major process—speech production. Our breathing provides the source of energy for speech.

Breathing for speech differs from breathing for life purposes during rest in several ways. Examination of Figure 4–10 shows the differences found in the two curves of breathing. The curve for quiet respiration is rhythmic and smooth, with approximately equal time and depth for inhalation and exhalation. In contrast, the curve for respiration for speaking reveals a more rapid and deeper inhalation and a greatly prolonged and uneven exhalation. Thus the pattern of respiration for speech purposes is modified by a comparative decrease in time of inhalation, increase in time of exhalation, increase in volume of air inhaled, and unevenness of exhalation. All of these factors are related to the production of the linguistic structure. A rapid and deeper inhalation allows for fewer interruptions in the flow of words for intake of air and greater volume of air permits more words to be uttered on one exhalation. Syllable and word stress within the utterance are possible because of the available air. Usually, inhalation takes place in the pauses between thought units.

The function of respiration in speech is to provide energy for producing the vowel and consonant sounds. Air pressure causes the vocal folds to vibrate and produce voice. The loudness of the voice increases as the air pressure increases. Air pressure is increased by greater air flow from the lungs and by increasing the degree of resistance to the air flow at the vocal folds.

Untrained speakers, wishing to produce a loud voice, as in shouting at a football game, tend to employ increased air flow. If kept up over too long a period of time, the pressure on the vocal folds can produce temporary hoarseness or laryngitis. On the other hand, trained speakers, such as actors, wishing to project their voices, tend to increase resistance at the vocal folds with no apparent ill effects.

Respiration at Birth. Respiration must be initiated in the newborn quickly to avoid anoxia. Much of the fluid which fills the lungs before birth is squeezed out by the presure of the mother's pelvic muscles and vaginal walls on the neonate's thorax during the course of the delivery. The physician then suspends the newborn by his feet to drain out residual fluid. Respiration begins spontaneously or with a stimulus from the physician. Unless the infant is defective or has been asphyxiated or drugged,

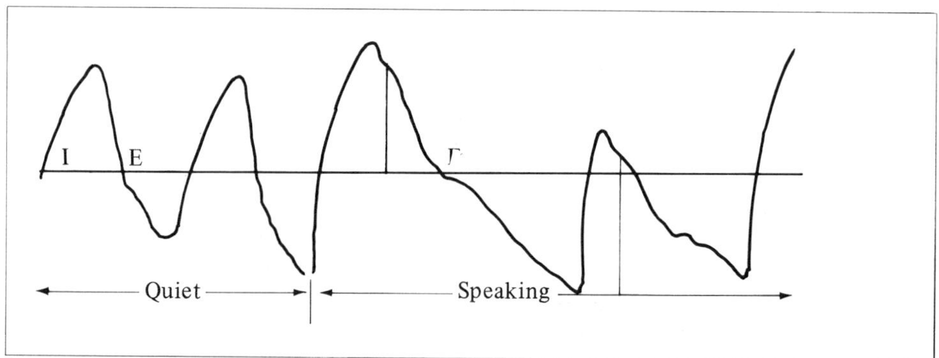

Figure 4–10. Two curves of breathing. (Adapted from Luchsinger, R. and Arnold, G. E. *Voice-Speech-Language*, Belmont, Cal.: Wadsworth Pub., 1965. Reprinted by permission of the publisher.

initial respirations are shallow, irregular, and rapid. Some fluid still remains in the lungs.

Lung capacity at birth is limited, proportionally less than that of the adult, but postnatal development of the lungs is rapid. Respiratory rate during the first day ranges from 28 to 78 cycles per minute, with the average about 46 cycles, in contrast to the adult average of 14 cycles per minute.

Severe respiratory distress in the neonate may be indicative of anoxia and it has been found to be one of the factors predictive of later language problems.

Respiration in the Aging. Changes in respiration accompany the process of decline during aging. When groups of both sexes under 40 years and above 65 years were compared, Ptacek et al. (1966) found significant differences in the respiratory abilities of the older group. These in time influenced certain speech abilities. They were inferior in vital capacity (the maximum amount of air which can be expelled following maximum inhalation), maximum vowel duration (the length of time a vowel can be prolonged), maximum intraoral pressure (maximum pressure built up in the mouth), and maximum vowel intensity (maximum loudness of the vowel measured in dB).

These respiratory limitations in the aging are attributable to a reduction in the power of respiratory muscles and a loss of elasticity of the lungs themselves. In conversational speech these limitations would have significant influence only in extreme cases. They do, nevertheless, carry social and psychological significance.

RESPIRATORY DISORDERS

Respiratory disorders may affect speech in a number of ways depending on the type of disorder and degree of severity. Lesions of the lungs, such as found in emphysema, bronchial asthma, or cardiac and vascular diseases, reduce the air capacity of the lungs (Luchsinger and Arnold, 1965). In these cases, where there is a shallowness of breathing with a sharp limitation on the volume of air inhaled, there is a consequent limitation on the air available for sustained exhalation for speech. This necessitates frequent pauses for inhalation, causing a reduction in the length of phrases which can be spoken on each breath group and an interruption of phrases in places not related to the language structure or meaning. In addition to reduction of lung capacity there is also a diminution in expiratory strength. When there is inadequate air pressure, the voice may be weak, lacking the necessary loudness to be easily audible.

Dysarthrias of the breathing mechanism are found in such diseases as cerebral palsy, Parkinson's Disease, and multiple sclerosis. These diseases may result in reduced muscular control of the air flow, which may have an adverse effect on vocal loudness and steadiness of tone. Darley, Aronson, and Brown (1969a, 1969b) found that over 80 percent of dysarthric patients with multiple sclerosis had an impaired control of loudness.

PHONATION

Phonation is the process of producing voice by means of the vibrations of the vocal folds. The vocal folds are located in a structure called the larynx, popularly called the

Adam's apple. The larynx is tube shaped and open at both ends (Figure 4–11). The lower opening is continuous with the trachea or windpipe and the upper opening empties into the pharynx or throat.

The framework of the larynx is made up of cartilages held together by ligaments and muscles. The vocal folds themselves are embedded inside the laryngeal tube. They consist of two bands of muscles covered with mucous membrane and edged medially by a ligament. The vocal folds function in a valvelike fashion. When they are open, they form a somewhat triangular-shaped slit. This space between the vocal folds is called the glottis. The glottis is open during breathing to allow air to enter and leave the lungs. Closing of the glottis occurs during acts which require fixation of the rib cage such as lifting heavy objects, defecation, and childbirth.

To initiate phonation for speech production, the glottis is approximated or closed through the synergic action of a number of laryngeal muscles. This is the closed phase. The flow of expiratory air from the lungs builds up subglottal air pressure. When the air pressure becomes great enough, the folds are blown apart to begin the open phase. The air, which was under pressure, is released into the throat and mouth. With the reduction of air pressure the elastic reaction of the contracted vocal fold muscles causes them to approximate again, only to be blown apart again once the air pressure has

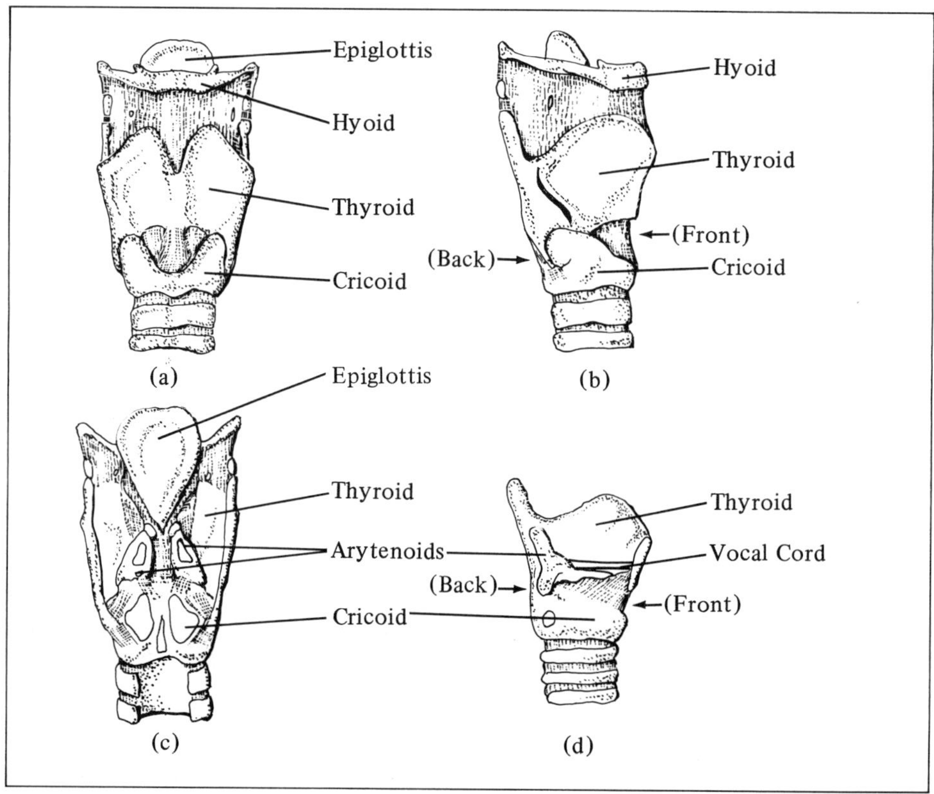

Figure 4–11. Various views of the larynx: (*a*) front, (*b*) side, (*c*) back, (*d*) cut-away side.

increased. The rapid action of opening and closing of the vocal folds many times per second creates an air turbulence that produces a sound somewhat like a Bronx cheer. This is the phonatory sound employed in speech production.

Inspection of the vocal folds by means of a dental mirror is called an indirect laryngoscopic examination. This procedure is used in making diagnoses of laryngeal pathology. Diagnoses of this type are done by laryngologists, physicians who have received specialized training in diagnosing and treating diseases of the larynx. Some speech pathologists with specialized training also do laryngoscopic examinations to observe the structures of the larynx and vibratory patterns of the vocal folds.

A modification of indirect laryngoscopic procedure with a high-speed camera to record the oscillations is used for research into the normal and abnormal aspects of vocal fold vibration. Figure 4–12 shows the camera setup. This type of research has been used extensively by the Bell Telephone Laboratories and Dr. G. Paul Moore at the University of Florida.

PHONATORY PITCH. The pitch as well as certain aspects of the loudness and quality of the voice are determined by the vocal fold structures and patterns of phonation.

The fundamental pitch and pitch variations in the voice are determined by the interrelation of three factors: the length of the vocal folds, the mass or thickness of the vocal folds, and the tension in the vocal folds. Variations in these three factors determine the number of vibrations of the vocal folds per second and it is the rapidity of the vibrations which we perceive as the pitch or highness or lowness in the voice.

Assuming the air pressure from the lungs remains constant, physicists calculate that increasing the length, increasing the mass or thickness, and decreasing the tension

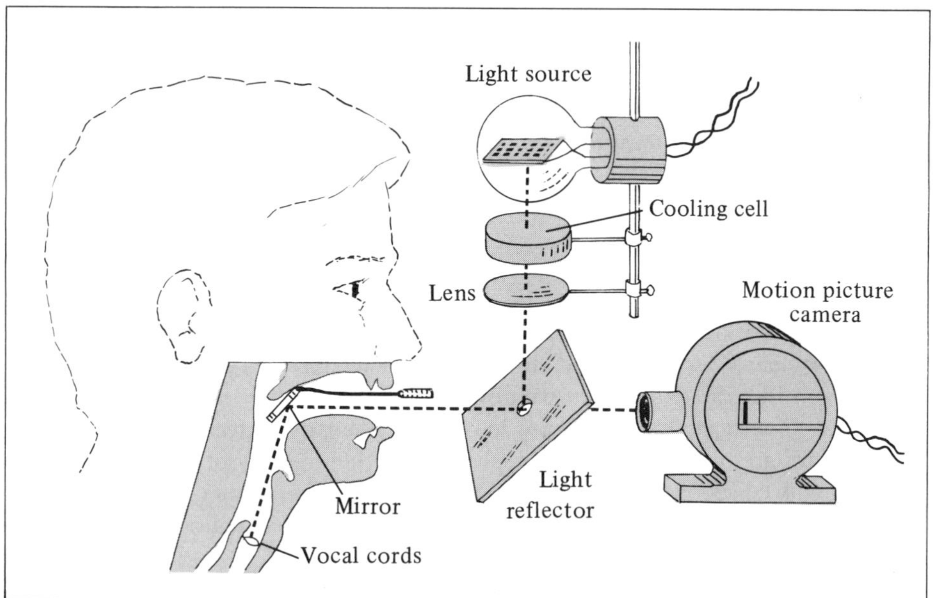

Figure 4–12. High-speed photographic equipment shown in position for recording vocal fold movements.

of the vocal folds brings about a lowering of pitch. Conversely, decreasing the length, decreasing the mass or thickness, and increasing the tension of the vocal folds brings about a raising of the pitch. High-speed motion pictures show that as the pitch becomes higher, the vocal folds do become thinner (decrease in mass) and more tense, but they also show that the vocal cords lengthen, contrary to the finding that higher pitch results from decreased length. It appears that because of the structure of the vocal folds, in order to decrease mass and increase tension, the folds must be stretched and they become longer. The major factors in vocal pitch rise are, therefore, decreased mass and increased tension, the combination of which compensate for the increased length.

The habitual pitch with which we produce an utterance belongs to the category of paralinguistic structures. It does not influence the meaning if a phrase is spoken by a man with a low pitch or a woman with a higher pitch or a child with a still higher pitch. However, it does carry some social and psychological significance if the vocal pitch is too high or too low for the age and sex of the speaker or if pitch changes are so slight as to produce impressions of monotony.

Pitch changes, such as the rapid upward pitch to end an interrogative sentence or the faded downward pitch to end a declarative sentence, do carry meaning and are a part of the prosodic elements of language. Disturbances of this type adversely affect communication of meaning.

Phonatory Loudness. The loudness of the voice is determined by the degree of air flow from the lungs. As the expiratory air pressures increase, there is an increase in the magnitude of the excursions of the vocal folds and thus an increase in the vocal loudness. In trained speakers the loudness of the voice can also be increased by the duration of the closed phase of the vocal folds during their cycle of vibration. When prolonged use of the voice at high intensities is required, this less vigorous vibration of the vocal folds reduces the possibility of damage to the folds.

The habitual loudness level of the voice is a paralinguistic structure. It does not carry linguistic meaning. Voices that are inappropriate to a situation by being too loud or soft or those lacking in variety of loudness so as to be monotones in the extreme may be socially or psychologically significant.

Phonatory Voice Quality. The quality of voice which ultimately emerges in speech is a result of two types of influences. The first influence comes from the pattern of vibration during phonation and the second from the modification of that voice in resonance as it is passed through the pharyngeal, oral, and nasal cavities. We will consider the latter when we discuss resonance.

Phonatory quality is a product of the vibratory patterns of the vocal folds which in turn are, to a great extent, dependent on the integrity of muscles, nerves, and tendinous edges of the vocal folds. Normal efficient vibratory patterns of the vocal folds create sounds that are musical in nature, that is, they consist of a fundamental, which is the lowest tone produced, plus a rich series of periodic overtones. High-speed motion pictures of the vocal folds in normal phonation show a rhythmic, sequential, wavelike movement of the vocal folds.

Timcke, Von Leden, and Moore (1958, 1959, 1960) studied the vocal fold movements of individuals with a variety of structural deviations, including cases of unilateral laryngeal paralysis, growths on the vocal folds, and edema or swelling of the vocal folds. They found many abnormal patterns of vibrations, including asynchronous and asymmetrical vibrations.

When the vibratory patterns of the vocal folds are abnormal, the vocal quality will also be abnormal. Instead of, or in addition to, musical tones being produced, varying degrees of noise will be the result of this type of vibration. These are considered breakdowns of phonatory quality. We hear the results in voices that are described as husky or hoarse.

Other breakdowns include breathiness and aphonia. When the vocal folds vibrate in such a way that they do not approximate completely, some air is allowed to escape without vibration. The vocal quality is said to be "breathy." If no vibration of the vocal folds occurs and the individual speaks only on expelled breath, the condition is called aphonia.

Phonatory Duration. The duration or length of a vowel sound is controlled by respiratory and phonatory factors. In English vowel sound duration is used in some dialects to convey phonemic meaning. In some cases syllable stress is indicated by an increase in vowel duration coupled with a slight increase in loudness. The clipping or prolonging of vowels may have regional significance or it may be a matter of individual differences.

Age and Sex Differences. Phonatory changes occur throughout the life cycle. Most are of a gradual nature, although some changes, such as those at puberty, are comparatively rapid. The processes of growth and development account for phonatory changes in the child and degeneration and decline for the aging. Most research has centered around pitch level changes rather than quality changes, probably because quality changes present a more difficult problem of measurement.

Pitch changes from birth through puberty are accounted for on the basis of the growth of the laryngeal structures. As the mass of the vocal folds increases with the growth of the child, there is a gradual lowering of the normal pitch of the voice. The male vocal pitch is slightly lower than that of the female. During puberty there is a spurt in the laryngeal growth, because of secretion of hormonal sex glands. At the conclusion of this period the larynx achieves adult size, and the pitch level has lowered in both sexes with male pitch at approximately one octave below middle C (256 Hz) and the female two-thirds of an octave higher. The rapid increase in size of the larynx during puberty may cause occasional "voice breaks," especially in males, when with uncertainty he moves from the habitually higher voice to the new lower voice. Huskiness and weakness of the voice may also be heard in this so-called mutational voice. These are usually temporary symptoms of rapid laryngeal growth.

Hollien and Shipp (1972) report that a slight lowering of pitch continues in the male until middle age when a gradual rise in pitch level begins. In females Hollien and McGlone (1963) found little change in the pitch level throughout adult life.

In a study of adults over 65 years of age Ptacek et al. (1966) found the range of the voice (the lowest to the highest pitch an individual can produce) had significantly narrowed, especially for the higher frequencies. The researchers felt that this difference and other "peculiarities of senile voice" can be explained by degenerative changes which have been found in histological studies of the laryngeal muscles of the aged. The muscles lose much of their elasticity and the cartilages of the larynx become more rigid and bonelike with calcification.

PATHOLOGIES OF VOICE

The physical determinants of voice pathologies fall into three categories: (1) structural inadequacies in the larynx itself, (2) damage or maldevelopment in the central or peripheral nerves which innervate the structures of the larynx, and (3) inadequacies in the hearing mechanism necessary for monitoring feedback control of voice production.

Structural Defects in the Larynx. Structural defects in the larynx are related to congenital maldevelopment of the larynx and vocal folds, endocrine problems, diseases, growths, traumatic injuries, or surgical alterations. The most frequent causes of defects are diseases and growths on the larynx and surgical alterations of the structure. The resulting voice symptoms are usually breathiness, huskiness, or hoarseness. Hoarseness is so common a symptom of laryngeal disease that Jackson and Jackson (1937), authors of one of the standard texts on laryngology, report that it is a symptom in more than 60 diseases in adults and 35 in children.

Vocal nodules and polyps are benign growths usually on the edges of one or both vocal folds. They are thought by most laryngologists to be caused by improper and excessive use of the voice. Prolonged use of a pitch that is unsuited for the vocal structure or use of excessive loudness over too long a period of time have been cited as causes. Along with vocal misuse or abuse Luchsinger and Arnold (1965) note that we must consider predisposing factors most often of a constitutional nature including personality, precipitating factors such as "a derangement of internal physiology," possibly endocrine imbalance, and aggravating factors including excessive drinking and smoking.

Vocal nodules have been found in all ages of the populace including young children. In children they are sometimes called screamer's nodes and in singers called singer's nodes. In a study on hoarseness in children Silverman and Zimmer (1975) reported that out of a group of 38 children, judged to have chronic hoarseness, 10 were examined by an otolaryngologist. Nine of those examined were found to have bilateral vocal nodules. Nodules have been known to disappear *spontaneously* and after vocal rest or voice therapy. Some are removed surgically.

The following is a case study that can be duplicated in many clinics. After his first week as a teacher Claude's voice became extremely hoarse. He consulted a laryngologist who diagnosed bilateral vocal nodules on the anterior third of his vocal folds with the probable cause vocal abuse. He referred him to a speech pathologist for voice therapy with the added suggestion that he seek a new occupation.

As is so often the case with a new teacher, Claude had been assigned to one of the most difficult third grades in the inner city. Sociologists have referred to this as an "ordeal by fire" to initiate new teachers into the system. It had indeed been extremely trying for him because he could not cope with the new situation. His own background was middle class and his training and student teaching had been geared to the suburban schools. Despite his desire to succeed, his approach to the children made any teaching well nigh impossible. In his effort to bring order and discipline to the classroom, he resorted to shouting. Teachers in adjacent classrooms who had a few more months experience tried to impart to him their quickly learned disciplinary methods, but it was too difficult for him to adjust to all of these demands in so short a period of time. As he lost control of the class, he would become more anxious and shout louder. At the end of each day his throat was sore and his voice became progressively more hoarse.

Hoarseness is among the earliest symptoms of malignant laryngeal growths. In most cases it appears well before any symptoms of discomfort or pain. Early diagnosis is of extreme importance from a life-saving point of view and also for laryngeal conservation. If detected early, surgical excision may be conservatively done with only a portion of the laryngeal structures removed rather than a laryngectomy which is total surgical removal of the larynx.

Ellen H., a 40-year-old businesswoman, is an example of what can happen. She gradually became aware that she was experiencing intermittent periods of vocal hoarseness. She mentioned this to her family doctor who referred her to a laryngologist. After a number of visits the physician was unable to determine the cause of the hoarseness. Four weeks later the hoarseness became noticeably worse. And this time the family physician referred Ellen to a large diagnostic facility in another state where a malignant growth was discovered on the under surface of the left vocal fold. The left vocal fold was removed surgically.

Following the surgery Ellen was aphonic. She could speak only in a hoarse whisper. This condition lasted until she consulted a speech pathologist. Therapy helped her to produce a hoarse but acceptable voice which allowed her to return to work.

When cancerous growths require a total laryngectomy, voice can no longer be produced in the usual manner. Most often the patient is taught to speak with esophageal voice. Air brought in through the mouth is captured in the upper part of the esophagus. When the air is forced out, muscular constrictions in the area produce a pseudo-glottis which creates voice. The voice is low pitched, monotonous, and hoarse, but despite its inadequacies it makes speech possible. In some cases where the patient cannot learn alaryngeal speech or there are other contraindications to teaching it, a mechanical vibrator is placed against the neck to create the sounds for speech. This device is called an artificial larynx.

DYSARTHRIAS OF THE LARYNX. Dysarthrias of the larynx may be produced by peripheral nervous system or central nervous system damage or disease. Paralysis of laryngeal nerves following thyroidectomy is the most frequent cause of peripheral nerve dysarthria. Other causes include diseases, such as diphtheria, and accidental injury to the larynx. Strokes, tumors, and degenerative diseases are the major sources of dysarthrias of central origin (Luchsinger and Arnold, 1965).

The vocal symptoms of dysarthria include aphonia, vocal weakness, breathiness, huskiness, hoarseness, and pitch disorders. Thus, pitch, loudness, and quality disorders result depending on the location and severity of the disease. In dysarthrias stemming from central degenerative diseases. Darley, Aronson, and Brown (1969a, 1969b) have shown that the clustering of vocal symptoms is characteristic of specific types of diseases and may have diagnostic value.

Hearing Loss and Voice. Hearing losses may cause voice problems because of the inaccuracy of the auditory monitoring feedback control. The type of voice problem is related to the type and degree of hearing loss. Those with conductive hearing losses—obstructions in the outer or middle ear, but with normal inner ear functioning—monitor their speech through bone conduction. What to them sounds like an adequately loud voice for conversation is, in fact, too soft. When they are told to speak louder, they invariably are convinced that they are shouting. In contrast, those with sensorineural hearing losses—a defect in the inner ear—tend to speak in a voice that is too loud. When they adjust their voices to the loudness which to them is conversation level, the impression of the listener is that they are shouting. In addition to the loudness problems, where the loss is severe, the pitch of the voice may be too high and the prosodic features of intonation and stress may be lost, giving the voice a monotonous quality.

ARTICULATION AND THE VOCAL TRACT

ARTICULATORY STRUCTURES

Articulation refers to the process of forming vowel and consonant sounds through movements of the speech mechanism. The structures of articulation are illustrated in Figure 4–13, which is a view of the vocal tract. They include the vocal folds, throat, mouth, tongue, teeth, lips, palate, and nose. When there is air flow from the lungs, specific movements of these structures modify the shape of the vocal tract and initiate vibrations. We have learned to identify the resultant articulation sounds as vowels or consonants. For our purposes vowel sounds are produced with the vocal tract vibrating free of obstructions, whereas consonant sounds are made with the vocal tract partially or completely obstructed. The discussion which follows will clarify these definitions.

There are three cavities in the vocal tract: the oral or mouth, the nasal or nose, and the pharyngeal or throat. Figure 4–13 shows their location and interconnections. The oral cavity contains the tongue and teeth. It is bounded by the lips in the front, the cheeks on the sides, and the pharynx in the back. The floor of the oral cavity is formed by the dorsum or top part of the tongue and the roof is formed by the palate. The palate is divided into two parts. The hard palate is a bony structure in the front section the roof. The gum ridge or alveolar process, which is part of this bony section, is a rounded protuberance slightly behind the teeth. The soft palate or velum forms the posterior portion of the roof of the mouth.

The nasal cavity extends from the nostrils in the front to the pharynx in the back. It contains many other bony structures which reduce the cavity size considerably. The pharynx, or throat, extends from the upper part of the larynx to connect with the oral and nasal cavities above. The opening between the pharynx and the nasal cavity is called the velopharyngeal opening.

The velopharynx remains open when the velum hangs down in a relaxed state. When certain muscles of the velum and the pharynx contract, the velum moves up to make a sphincterlike contact with the pharyngeal wall, thus closing off the nasal cavity from the pharyngeal and oral cavities. This process is called velopharyngeal closure.

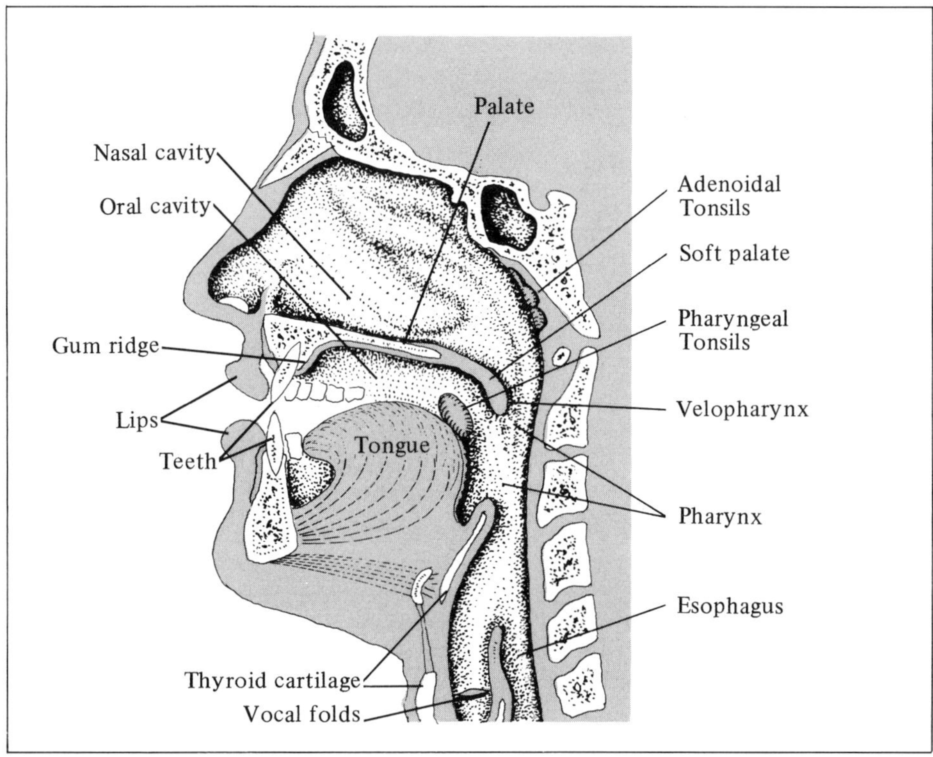

Figure 4–13. Structures of articulation.

Consonant Sounds

Consonant sounds may be classified in several ways. Table 2–2 lists the place of articulation and the manner of articulation including whether voiced or unvoiced. We have already dealt with these from a phonemic point of view in Chapter 2. Here we will be concerned with the physiological articulatory movements involved in speech production of English.

The terms used to describe place of articulation are labial for lip, bilabial for both lips, dental for teeth, alveolar for gum ridge, palatal for the roof of the mouth, velar for the back part of the palate, and glottal for the vocal folds.

An examination of our classification by place shows that it is not totally foolproof, but it is functionally useful. One example of sounds by the place of articulation should suffice. Bilabial sounds involve the use of both lips. Sounds made in this manner include [p] as in *p*en, [b] as in *b*in, [m] as in *m*e, and [w] as in *w*ing.

The classification by place is useful, but not complete in differentiating between sounds. We need additional information in terms of the manner of articulation. This refers to the kind of articulatory movements involved in producing the sounds.

Plosives. Plosives are sounds produced by an occlusion of air by the articulators with a build-up of intraoral air pressure followed by a sudden explosive release. This class of sounds includes [p] as in *p*in, [b] as in *b*in, [t] as in *t*o, [d] as in *d*o, [k] as in *k*eg, and [g] as in *g*o. The sounds [p], [t], and [k] are further classified as unvoiced sounds because they are made without vibration of the vocal folds; [b], [d], and [g] are called voiced sounds because they are made with vocal fold vibration.

Fricatives. Fricatives are sounds produced by constriction of articulators to allow a narrow opening through which air is forced under pressure. The result is a hissing, frictionlike noise. The [s] sound as in *s*ee is a fricative. The sound is produced when air is forced through a narrowly grooved tongue, which is in contact with the alveolar ridge. The stream of air cuts across the edges of the front teeth to create friction. If we add voicing in the form of vocal fold vibration, we produce the [z] sound as in *z*oo.

Affricates. The affricates, [tʃ] as in *ch*ew and [dʒ] as in *j*ust, combine the characteristics of the plosive with the fricative sounds. The sound begins with complete obstruction of the air pathway and a buildup of intraoral air pressure, followed by an explosive release blended immediately into a frictionlike sound by forcing air through a constriction. The production of affricates is similar except that [tʃ] is unvoiced and [dʒ] is voiced.

Nasals. The three nasal sounds are [m] as in *m*e, [n] as in *n*o, and [ŋ] as in ri*ng*. They are all voiced sounds made with oral obstruction and the velopharynx open, thus allowing for nasal resonance. These are the only sounds on which nasalization is legitimately allowed in English. They owe their differentiating qualities to the place of articulatory obstruction in the oral resonator. Bilabial obstruction produces the [m] sound; lingual-alveolar obstruction produces the [n] sound, and velar obstruction produces the [ŋ] sound.

Liquids. The liquid sounds [l] and [r], both voiced, are produced in several ways, resulting in allophonic variations. We shall describe one variant of each. The [r] as in *r*ed may be produced by raising the sides of the tongue, barely touching the molar teeth, and curling the tongue tip upward. The [l] as in *l*ie is made by raising the tongue tip to the alveolar arch and allowing the sound to travel over both sides of the tongue.

Semivowels. Two sounds are classified as semivowels: [w] as in *w*ing and [j] as in *y*ellow. They are made with vocal fold vibration, no interruption of the air stream, and a limited constriction of the vocal tract—characteristics they share with vowel sounds. Yet, in their production there is more constriction than is found in vowels and somewhat less than in the production of other consonant sounds. Hence, the name semivowel is descriptive.

VOWELS

The production of vowel sounds requires the vibration of the vocal folds, the molding and sometimes the tension of the tongue and in some cases the shaping of the lips to produce a characteristic resonance phenomenon which we acoustically recognize as a vowel. In all English vowels there is velopharyngeal closure during production to exclude nasalization. Some languages, such as French, nasalize certain vowels, and some slight nasalization usually occurs in English. Vowel sounds are determined by three factors: (1) the position of the tongue in the mouth; (2) the amount of tension in the tongue, and (3) the shaping of the lips. Manipulation of these three variables creates all variety of vowels. Vowels may be classified according to the three factors, although classification is usually based on the position of the highest part of the main body of the tongue. By this means we may describe the relative position required for each of the vowels. This is done schematically in the vowel diagram in Figure 4–14. It has been superimposed on a cross-sectional view of the vocal tract.

In producing a vowel the highest point of the main body of the tongue may be in the front, central, or back part of the mouth and may be high, mid, or low in the mouth. According to this descriptive system the vowel [i] as in h*e* is classed as a high, front vowel, since the main body of the tongue is forward in the mouth and the highest part of the tongue is high in the mouth. Other front vowels in descending order relative to the height of the tongue are: [ɪ] as in h*i*m, [e] as in ch*a*otic, [ɛ] as in m*e*t, and [æ] as in c*a*t.

In the production of English front vowels the lips are retracted, whereas most back vowels require rounding of the lips. Contrast the lip retraction on the front vowels with the lip rounding on the back vowels [u] as in f*oo*d, [ʊ] an in p*u*t, and [o] as in *o*bey.

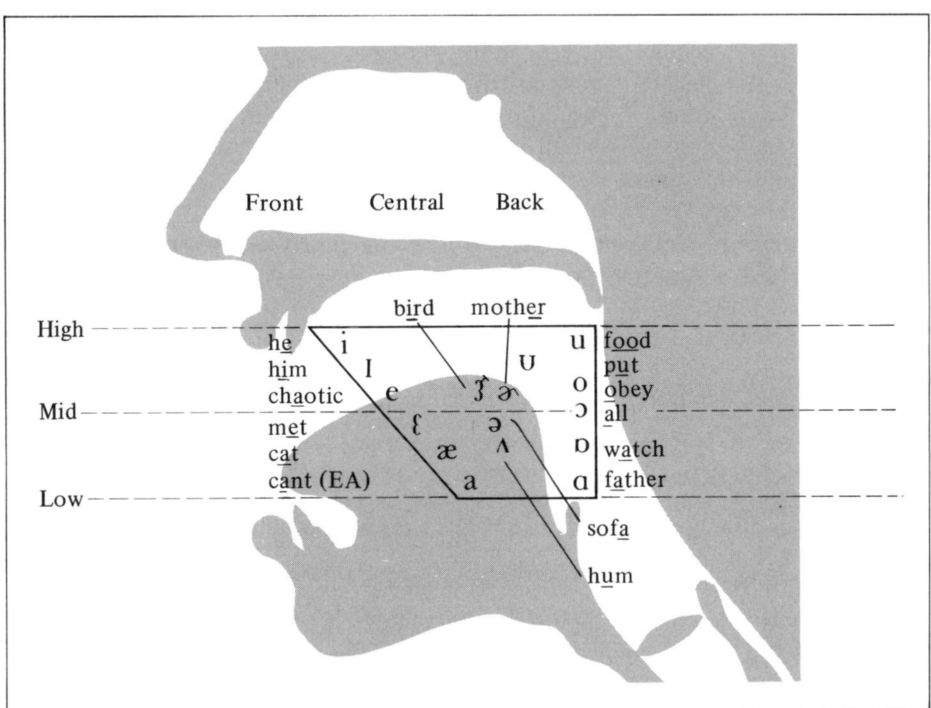

Figure 4–14. Vowel diagram based on position of the tongue. (Adapted from Perkins, W. H. *Speech Pathology An applied behavioral science*. St. Louis: C. V. Mosby Co., 1971 (diagram only; not key).

Muscular tension is a third factor used in classifying vowels. The major differentiating factor between [i] and [ɪ] is not tongue position; they are made in similar positions. Rather it is the degree of muscular tension in their production which differentiates the two; the [i] is tense and [ɪ] is lax. Therefore a description of [i] as in h*e* would be that of a high, front, tense vowel, with lips retracted, and that of [ɪ] as in h*i*m would be a high, front, lax vowel with lips retracted. For reference, Table 2–1 lists the vowels of English and key words.

ALLOPHONE ARTICULATION AND ASSIMILATION

We have described articulation in a somewhat static fashion that might mislead the student to conclude that there is only one position for producing a correct sound. For example, we may describe the lingual-alveolar plosive [t] as contact of tongue tip with the alveolar ridge, buildup of air pressure, and then release of pressure with an explosive noise. What is not revealed in this description is that speech sound production is influenced by context. Both the sounds that precede and follow a given speech sound influence its production. This is true not only for the sounds within words, but also within the context of phrases. The context of a sound determines the type of physiological movements necessary for its production.

If you experiment by producing the following series of [t] sounds, you will become aware of the contextual determinant of sounds. Listen to the [t] sounds as you produce the words *tick*, *hit that*, *button*, and *mantle*. The [t] in *tick* is followed by a front vowel. It requires the tongue tip to be moved to and touch the alveolar ridge. The explosive release is followed by a slight aspiration as the tongue moves toward the vowel position. To produce the [t] sound in *hit* in the phrase *hit that* the tongue anticipates the [ð] sound in *that* by assuming an alveolar-interdental contact. The explosion is almost interdental and there is no aspiration. The [t] in *button* is in fact a nasal explosive in anticipation of the [n] which follows the [t]. The [t] in *mantle* is exploded laterally on both sides of the tongue in anticipation of the [l] sound.

Linguists refer to the different productions of [t] as allophones. A careful study of these physiological productions shows that they require very different movements, yet we perceive them as belonging to the same phoneme. Alterations in phoneme production according to sound context are called assimilation or coarticulation. Speech scientists are interested in coarticulation in terms of phonetic theory.

SELF-MONITORING OR FEEDBACK IN ARTICULATION

Our discussion of articulation has centered around the structures and movements involved in producing speech sounds. There is another facet to this study which, although less obvious, is of extreme importance, namely, the monitoring or feedback of information during the production of speech. We have all caught ourselves unintentionally mispronouncing a word. It usually surprises us and we may go back and correct our error. This is a single example of the self-monitoring or feedback of information. In speech production the most utilized sensory receptors are aural, tactile, and kinesthetic.

We use our hearing to monitor aspects of loudness of voice, appropriateness of pitch and intonation, as well as precision of articulation. Our reaction time is rapid enough to correct most errors of vowel and consonants in process except for those of short duration such as plosives (Daniloff, 1973). Rousey and Holzman (1967) point out that perception of our voice and speech is influenced by personality factors which may introduce defensive distortions of their own.

Tactile and kinesthetic sensory receptors give additional clues as to the accuracy of the movements of articulation, but it should be noted that the parts of the oral mechanism are not equally endowed with tactile and kinesthetic nerve endings so there are limitations on the information. For example, Locke (1968) says that tactile feedback in tongue tip sounds such as [t] and [d] is much greater than in palatal sounds such as [k] and [g]. The struggle of a person with new dentures as his tongue searches for the right tactile surface for producing a correct [s] should convince us of the need for this feedback for accurate speech.

DEVELOPMENT AND DECLINE OF ARTICULATION

One might look at the development of articulatory skill in children as two processes. The first process is the development of articulation of speech sounds through the infant's production of noncrying sounds, cooing and babbling, and later through echolalic vocalizations. The child passes through stages of development of phonetic sounds that closely parallel his motor development and integrative behavior. The second process is learning articulation of phonemic sounds which are part of a linguistic structure. Thus the first process is the development of the physical capability of producing the sounds and the second is the development of the ability to use those sounds.

One might view the development of phonetic speech sounds in the child as a "learning how-to-learn" process. The child practices the various sounds and intonations as a means of facilitating later speech development.

> The development of the complex, language-directed articular movement arises during infancy when children initially move their articulators in an exploratory non-language way, during crying, babbling, feeding, or breathing. At birth the respiratory system and much of the vocal tract are coordinated at a reflex level, to produce distress and pleasure cries. This coordination includes the diaphragm, intercostal muscles, larynx, tongue, jaw, lips, etc. The latter structures produce the open tract for vowel-like cries, and the rapid lip and tongue movements which create consonant-like noises. Conscious language-directed articulation develops from this initial repertoire or substructure of early vocal tract behaviors" (Daniloff, 1973).

We reported in Chapter 3 that Irwin studied these early speech sounds in infancy. He shows that the sounds develop in an orderly and predictable fashion. McCarthy (1954) thinks that the earliest sounds are intimately connected with physiological movements of breathing and sucking. Lingual-alveolar sounds appear to be added to the sound repertoire as the introduction of more solid foods requires chewing.

Articulation once learned remains relatively stable thoughout life. Any decline in articulation skill results from presbycusis, a hearing loss which accompanies decline, and from deterioration in the muscular and motor nerve control. A reduction in the reaction time (Jarvik, 1975) and in the rapidity of reciprocal muscular movements, including those of speech are aspects of the aging process.

PHYSICAL DETERMINANTS OF PATHOLOGIES OF ARTICULATION

The physical determinants of articulatory breakdowns fall into three different groups. (1) There may be structural inadequacies in the vocal folds, tongue, lips, teeth, palate or resonating cavities. These make the necessary articulatory movements difficult or impossible. Most structural defects of this type are of a developmental nature, although some result from traumatic accidents, surgical intervention, or disease. (2) Damage or maldevelopment of the central or peripheral motor nerves which innervate the speech mechanism accounts for the second group of breakdowns. With one exception they are called dysarthrias. (3) Inadequacies of the sensory receptors required for monitoring feedback information, such as deafness or hearing loss, comprise the third group.

Structural Inadequacies and Articulatory Pathologies. Articulation deficits may be caused by inadequacies in the oral structures if they interfere with the (1) buildup of intraoral air pressure, (2) direction of the stream of air, or (3) proper tongue, lip, jaw, or palatal movements discussed under manner of articulation. Missing front teeth and malocclusions (deviations in the relationship of the upper and lower teeth when the jaws are closed) are the most common problems of this type, but there are, in addition, problems of cleft palate, maldevelopment of the tongue, and surgical removal of structures in treating malignant growths.

Missing front teeth or large spaces between the teeth may cause a distortion of the [s] and [z] sounds (Snow, 1961; Bankson and Byrne, 1962). In malocclusions such as overbite, where the upper front teeth overlap the lower front teeth to a considerable extent and where there may be an accompanying protrusion of the upper teeth and underdevelopment of the lower jaw, there may be substitution of a [θ] for [s] and [ð] for [z]. Underbite, in which the lower jaw juts out beyond the upper jaw causing the lower front teeth to be forward of the upper teeth, may contribute to defects of the [s] and [z]. If severe, labial and labiodental sounds may be affected.

Now that we have mentioned the possibilities for structural deviations and articulation defects it is important to note that in cases where the structures are not too seriously impaired most children and adults manage to produce sounds correctly using compensatory movements. They may plug up openings between the teeth with the tongue to prevent the generation of additional distorting sounds. Often one can observe the compensatory movements of the jaw in cases of malocclusion. The speech literature has a number of cases illustrative of individuals who have achieved intelligible speech despite gross tongue and oral deformities (Weinberg et al., 1969) and surgical removal of the entire tongue. Compensatory movements of the cheeks and other structures are substituted for the missing parts. In these cases, of course, there are errors of articulation, but the speech is intelligible.

Among some of the most serious structural inadequacies which may have a detrimental influence on the functions of articulation are the clefts of the lip and of the palate. These include deformities of the bones and muscular tissue of the oral and surrounding regions including the nose, lips, upper jaw, palate, velum, and pharynx. There are five types: (1) cleft of the upper lip, (2) cleft which include the lip, palate, and velum, (3) cleft of the hard palate and velum, (4) cleft of the velum, and (5) insufficient palate (Koepp-Baker, 1971).

These clefts are the result of embryological maldevelopment during the critical period for fusion of the lips and palate, between the sixth to twelfth weeks of development. Hereditary factors are most frequently cited to account for the failure of development. However, clefts have been created in offspring of experimental animals through dietary deficiencies in the pregnant animal and the use of a wide variety of drugs. The possibility of multiple causation cannot be discounted.

Before generalizing about the relationship of cleft lip and palate to articulation, we must take into account the factors which would influence this relationship. Foremost, of course, is a consideration of the structural integrity of the parts. Is the upper lip cleft? Is it a unilateral cleft (one side only) or bilateral cleft (both sides)? Is some of the muscular or other tissue missing through lack of development? Has the surgical repair been successful or is there scar tissue and displacement of muscles making the lip nonfunctional or only partly functional? Has tissue loss made the repair functionally inadequate? Similar questions would be asked about the alveolar arch, the hard palate, and the velum.

A second factor to consider is whether the surgery was done before or after the child learned speech. Early articulation habits learned with inadequate structures might continue after structural repair. Additionally, surgical repair may produce structures which are adequate at the time of the repair, but because of growth in the facial and oral areas, become inadequate later, making proper function impossible.

Of particular importance is the malformation of the oral structures. The teeth may be missing, misplaced anywhere in the palate, or nonaligned. The nasal and oral facial contours may be deviant, especially the size, shape, and relationship of the upper to lower jaw, thus creating cosmetic problems and serious malocclusions. Because of structural inadequacies in the palatal and pharyngeal areas, these children are more prone to ear infections which increase the probability of their developing mild to moderate hearing losses.

Depending on the degree of success in surgical repair of the lip and palate, or prosthetic treatment of the palate as well as the other factors cited, the articulation skills of individuals with cleft palate range from normal to nearly unintelligible. There are both wide variability in articulation skills among cleft palate individuals and inconsistency in articulation skill within the individual (Moll, 1968). This finding means that the following generalizations about the articulation of individuals with cleft palate must be interpreted with caution.

The most frequent problem of articulation centers around the nasalization of vowel and consonant sounds as a result of inadequate closure of the velopharynx. Inadequate closure also contributes to the weakness or distortion of plosive sounds. Plosives require a buildup of air pressure in the oral cavity, but with incomplete closure the air escapes through the nose making proper articulation of [p], [b], [t], [d], [k], and [g] impossible.

Fricative sounds may also be absent or distorted in cleft palate speech. These sounds require an air stream directed through the mouth. Air escaping through the nose reduces the oral pressure and direction, thus distorting [s], [z], [ʃ], [ʒ], [f], and [v]. In extreme cases a snorting nasal fricative sound may be substituted for other fricatives. Because of their articulatory similarities to plosives and fricatives, all of the affricates are likewise distorted. Semivowels and glides are less affected than the other consonants and the nasal sounds are considered normal.

Apraxia of Speech. Brain damage can also cause articulation deficits that are due not to weakness, paralysis, or incoordination in the muscles per se, but rather to the central formulation of the positions and movement of the articulators and the sequencing of the positions and movements in the articulation of phonemes. This is called apraxia of speech. These same muscles and movements may remain unimpaired in reflex and automatic acts such as in chewing, sucking, and swallowing. This contrasts with the more commonly occurring dysarthrias in which the muscles and their coordination are impaired in both willed and nonvolitional movements.

Rosenbeck et al. (1973) described some speech and language conditions under which apraxia of speech is more likely to occur. They found that there are more errors on fricatives, affricates, and clusters of two or more consonants, especially at the beginning of a word, than on vowels, nasals, or plosive sounds. Errors also occur if the sequencing of successive phonemes in the word requires longer excursions of the articulators. For example, the articulators must travel greater distances in producing the word *scream* [skrim] than in the word *tinny* [tɪnɪ] and the consonant cluster of [skr] in the initial position is more difficult than the consonant followed by a vowel, as in [ti]. Apraxic errors increase with greater word length and rarity of the words.

Hearing Loss and Articulation. The self-monitoring of speech is adversely affected by hearing loss. The type of hearing loss, the severity, and the time of onset must be taken into account. Children who are born with or develop severe or profound hearing losses prior to age 3 years do not hear others sufficiently well and cannot monitor their own speech to produce articulated sounds in the usual way. They must be taught to speak using visual, tactile, and kinesthetic cues. Many are able to develop intelligible speech, albeit with a number of articulation problems. Vowels are nasalized, substituted, and distorted by being prolonged into diphthongs. Consonant sounds are nasalized, substituted, and distorted; voiceless consonants may be voiced. Consonant clusters are distorted (Hudgins, 1934; Hudgins and Numbers, 1942). These articulation problems are not surprising when we consider the laborious means by which the sounds and words are learned and maintained by the deaf.

Children and adults who become deaf after language has been well-established retain their speech for a time and then gradually show a decline in speech skills. Knowledge of morphological, syntactic, and semantic forms remains stable, but articulation and voice deteriorate. In some cases the speech cannot be distinguished from those who were born deaf. Following is an example of an adult who had normal hearing and then lost it.

Jerry was a war veteran who became profoundly deaf in both ears following exposure to an accidental explosion of ammunition. Two years after discharge from the service his speech had deteriorated to typically deaf speech with monotonous nasal quality. His speech is barely intelligible despite speech conservation therapy. He has rejected oral communication because of frustrations he experiences when he tries to talk. He prefers to substitute written for oral communication. His writing indicates complete control of all aspects of language structure.

Among the hard-of-hearing those with moderate hearing losses may show some slight articulation errors, especially if they have high frequency sensorineural losses. The group who have moderately severe hearing losses with high frequency deficits show multiple articulation errors. Those consonant sounds that are weak in volume and contain many high frequencies tend to be distorted, omitted, or substituted. The sounds distorted or omitted include [s], [z], [ʃ], [ʒ], and [tʃ].

RESONANCE: THE MODIFICATION OF THE PHONATORY SOUNDS

During phonation, the vocal folds produce voice. It is a complex musical sound having a fundamental frequency, which we recognize as the pitch of the voice, and a rich series of periodic overtones, which contribute to the quality of the tone. However, this is not the voice which is ultimately emitted. The sound originating during phonation goes through the dual processes of modification, namely, resonance and damping.

The structures involved in the modification are the three major cavities of the speech mechanism: the pharyngeal, oral, and nasal cavities. These are shown schematically in Figure 4–15. Two or more of these cavities are coupled to modify the voice

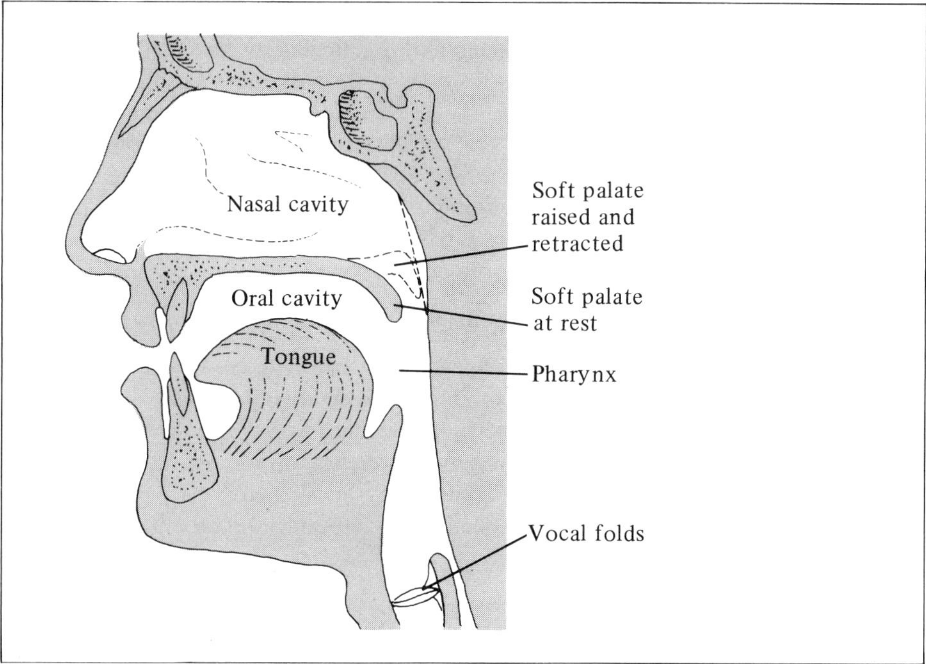

Figure 4–15. Resonating cavities

produced by the vocal folds by selectively resonating or increasing the loudness of certain overtones or by damping or reducing the energy contained in others. Resonance, of course, does not create new energy; it is a process which redistributes the existing energy. Nor does damping destroy energy; it transforms sound energy into another form.

Cavities will resonate overtones to which they are tuned. If you hold a vibrating tuning fork over a series of different size tubes, you will find one tube which makes the sound swell a great deal. This swelling of the tone is the process of resonance and the tube creating the greatest resonance would be most nearly tuned to the frequency emitted by the tuning fork.

The cavities of the speech mechanism may be likened to tubes which are tuned to a range of frequencies. Factors which influence the resonance include the size of the tube, the size of the opening, and the hardness of the walls. Larger tubes resonate lower overtones and smaller tubes resonate higher overtones. Small openings resonate lower overtones than do wide openings. Hard walls resonate and soft walls dampen sounds (Pronovost, no date).

When considering cavity resonance of the vocal tract, we are dealing with a complex phenomenon since the tract is capable of a wide variety of alterations. The size, shape and number of cavities, size and number of openings, coupling of the cavities and degree of hardness of the walls contribute to the changes. Some of these alterations in resonating cavities are required for proper articulation; some are acceptable individual differences in voice production. Serious deviations in resonance may result in articulation errors and voice quality disorders.

Resonance in Consonant and Vowel Articulation. Resonance is an essential aspect of articulation. It is resonance that creates the characteristic vowel and nasal consonant sounds. In our discussion of articulation we noted that vowel sounds are articulated by producing constrictions of the tongue in certain parts of the mouth and by varying lip position. Each of these articulatory tongue and lip positions alters the resonating characteristics of the vocal tract. They produce two or three important peaks of energy in the overtones or formants by which we acoustically recognize the vowel. Figure 4–16 shows the tongue position and resultant patterns of formants. The nasal consonants are produced when the phonatory sound has been resonated by passing through the coupled resonators.

Resonance and Voice Quality. In addition to the linguistic function of phoneme production where speech sound differentiation is conveyed primarily through the formants, resonance also contributes to the paralinguistic vocal attribute of voice quality. It influences the pattern of overtones beyond those necessary for distinguishing between phonemes and it contributes to the uniqueness of individual voices.

We have already identified phonatory vocal quality, a paralinguistic attribute, as the pattern of overtones produced by the vibratory mode of the vocal folds. Improper phonating results in the phonatory quality disorders of breathiness, huskiness, and hoarseness.

The resonance component of voice quality can contribute greatly to the esthetic aspects of speech. Voice improvement teachers have devised methods of increasing the resonance of lower overtones by relaxing the walls of the pharyngeal cavity and by

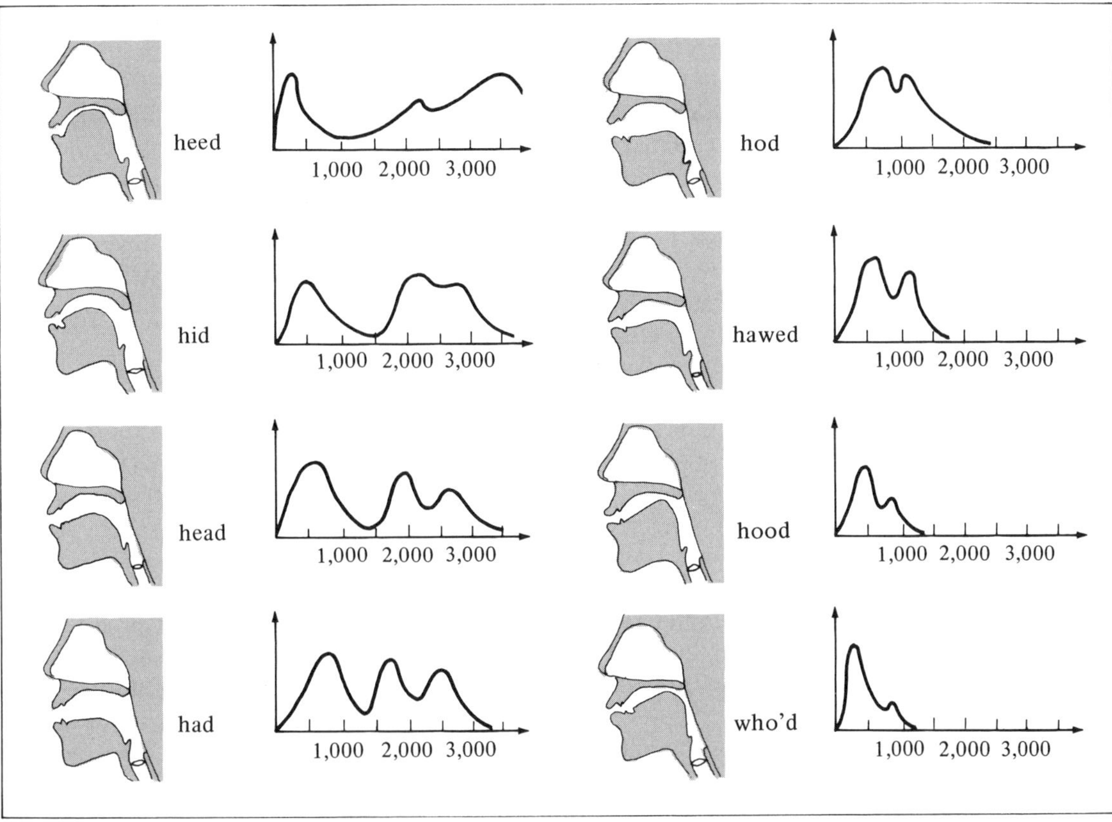

Figure 4–16. Tongue position and formants. (P. Ladefoged. *Elements of acoustic phonetics.* Chicago: University of Chicago Press, 1962.) Reprinted by permission.

increasing its size through muscle contractions, thus widening the pharynx (Anderson, 1961). These manipulations of the resonators are done indirectly through the use of auditory and other monitoring feedback of the voice.

PHYSICAL DETERMINANTS OF RESONANCE QUALITY PATHOLOGIES. Nasality and denasality are voice quality defects of resonance that are often physically determined. These disorders are caused by structural inadequacies or defects, neurological disorders, and monitoring-feedback problems as in hearing loss and deafness.

Nasality is a disorder in which nasal resonance is incorrectly added to sounds that should be articulated without nasal resonance. In the mildest form of nasality nasalization occurs as a coarticulation factor when a vowel preceding or following a nasal sound becomes nasalized through anticipation of the nasal consonant or by assimilation following the nasal sound. In the word *can* [kæn] the vowel [æ] becomes nasalized in anticipation of the articulation of the [n]; or in the word *knock* [nɑk] the [ɑ] becomes nasalized through assimilation as the articulators move from the [n] to the [ɑ] position. In the more serious form nasality occurs when sound enters the nasal cavity during the production of nonnasal sounds. All of the vowel and consonant sounds become nasalized.

We noted that the nasal cavity is partially separated from the oral cavity by the hard palate and the velum. Complete separation of the nasal cavity from the oral cavity requires velopharyngeal closure. Separation of the two cavities may be impossible because of a cleft in the hard palate or the velum, either congenital or acquired through disease or surgery, or because of insufficient length of the velum. In these cases all the sounds become severely nasalized and air pressure during the production of unvoiced sounds also enters the nose creating a snorting type nasal resonant emission. These problems of nasality coupled with the articulation disturbances discussed earlier make the speech of the person with cleft palate nearly unintelligible.

Neuromuscular disturbances of the speech mechanism which we have identified as the dysarthrias can affect the velopharyngeal closure through weakness or paralysis of the musculature or a lack of coordination with other speech movements. Nasality results from this lack of velopharyngeal control. Darley, Aronson, and Brown (1969a, 1969b) have found nasality one of the characteristics of spastic and flaccid dysarthria types and nasal emissions characteristic of the flaccid dysarthria types. The speech of deaf individuals who have lost or never acquired the auditory monitoring ability frequently show extreme nasalization of all vowel sounds.

Denasality occurs when the nasal resonance which is required for proper production of the sounds [m], [n], [ŋ] is either missing, reduced, or distorted. If the adenoidal tonsils, which are found in the nasal pharynx, are greatly enlarged, they may block off the nose from the mouth and prevent proper velopharyngeal opening, giving a typical adenoidal "cold in the nose" sound to the voice. A distorted [b] is substituted for the [m], [d] for [n], and [g] for [ŋ].

Enlarged adenoids may not only prevent nasal resonance, but also impede proper breathing through the nose and ventilation of the middle ear. The adenoids produce, in addition to the speech problem, a health hazard as well. Surgical removal of hypertrophic adenoids has been known to produce nasality (Lawson et al., 1972). Velopharyngeal movements are unnecessary when the adenoids block the opening. Following removal, the habitual patterns of inactivity are retained producing nasality where there formerly was denasality. In some cases it has been discovered that enlarged tonsils masked what was revealed after surgery to be a velum of insufficient length to make a proper closure, or a submucous cleft of the palate.

Another type of denasality is produced when the anterior part of the nose is partially or completely obstructed by a severe deviation of the septum, growths in the nose such as polyps, or by swelling of the mucous membrane lining of the nose caused by infections and allergies. These cause a diminution and distortion of the nasal resonance with a characteristic "boggy" or muffled quality.

HEARING

STRUCTURE OF THE AUDITORY SENSE ORGAN

The ear is the sensory organ for hearing. Its most important structures are imbedded in the temporal bone of the skull (Figure 4–17). The ear can be divided into three parts: the outer, middle, and inner ear.

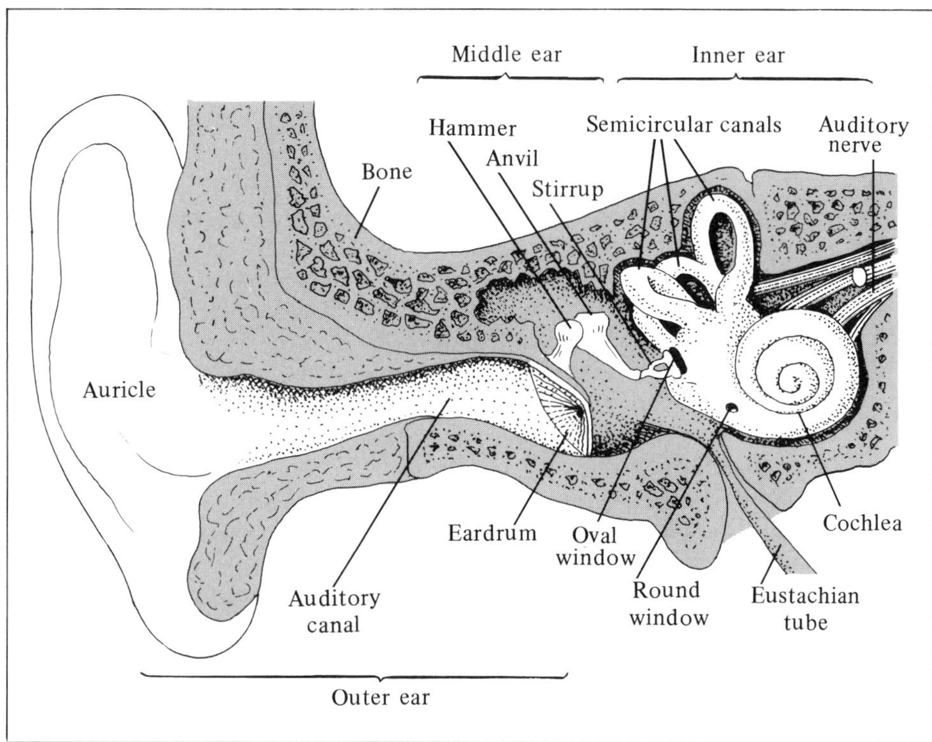

Figure 4–17. The ear.

THE OUTER EAR. Attached to the side of the head is the auricle, a cartilaginous shell-like structure covered with skin which leads to an opening, the external auditory canal. This canal is approximately ¾ inch in length in adults and contains glands which secrete a waxlike substance to keep the skin moist. At the end of the canal is the eardrum dividing the outer from the middle ear. Sound waves are captured by the auricle, condensed and lead through the canal to the eardrum causing the latter to vibrate.

THE MIDDLE EAR. The middle ear is an air-filled space in the temporal bone. It is bounded on the outermost side by the inner surface of the eardrum. Attached to the eardrum is the hammer, the first of three bones in the middle ear which are connected by ligaments and articulate with one another. The second bone is the anvil, which in turn is connected with the stirrup. The foot plate of the stirrup is attached to the oval window which connects to the inner ear.

The three bones or ossicles serve as a bridge to conduct and magnify mechanical movements from the eardrum to the oval window. Attached to the handle of the hammer is the tensor muscle which when contracted may have some influence on the responsiveness of the eardrum. Of more importance is the stapedius muscle, attached to the stirrup. It contracts in response to loud sounds as part of the acoustic reflex. Some writers think it may help to protect the inner ear from sudden loud sounds. On the inner wall below the oval window is the round window, another opening covered by a membrane which connects the middle ear with the inner ear.

The eustachian tube connects the middle ear with the nasopharynx. It is a ventilating pathway through which air travels to the middle ear to allow equalization of the air pressure on both sides of the eardrum. Acts such as swallowing, yawning, and chewing open the eustachian tube to admit air to the middle ear.

The transmission of mechanical movements over the ossicular bridge may be analyzed from two points of view: (1) impedance, the structure's resistance to conduction of sound energy and (2) admittance, the facility with which the sound energy is conducted. The terms are, of course, correlated; as impedance goes up, admittance goes down and vice versa (Greenberg, 1975). Any increase in stiffness in the movement of the ossicular bridge increases its impedance and decreases its admittance and may reduce hearing.

The Inner Ear. The inner ear is a more complex structure. It is composed of the cochlea which contains the sensory nerve endings for hearing and the vestibular apparatus which contains the nerve endings for balance. Because of their proximity, former developmental connection, and the fact that they are innervated by the eighth cranial nerve, it is not unusual for disturbances of balance and dizziness to accompany certain kinds of inner ear hearing losses.

The cochlea is shaped like a snail shell with two and a half turns. The widest turn at the bottom is called the basilar end and the opposite tip is called the apical end. Figure 4–18 contains schematic drawings of the cochlea somewhat unwound for easier visualization and in cross section. There are three ducts to the cochlea. The uppermost is the vestibular duct which forms the vestibule or entrance into the cochlea. It starts at the oval window and ends at the apical end of the cochlea. The lowermost duct is the tympanic duct which is continuous with the vestibular duct, beginning at the apical end of the cochlea and ending at the basilar end with the round window. Both the vestibular and tympanic ducts are filled with perilymph fluid. The middle duct is called the cochlear duct and it is filled with endolymph fluid. The roof of the cochlear duct, which separates it from the vestibular duct, is Reisner's membrane; its floor, which separates it from the tympanic duct, is formed in part by the basilar membrane and in part by a bony shelf which extends from the inner core of the cochlea. Seated on and running the full length of the basilar membrane, is the organ of Corti, which contains thousands of sensory nerve endings for hearing. The organ of Corti consists of hairs imbedded in a membrane called the tectorial membrane. Each hair is attached to a neural fiber which is rooted in a nerve cell. The nerves travel through the bony shelf to the inner core of the cochlea, where they form the auditory branch of the eighth cranial nerve. The eighth cranial nerve is attached to the brain stem from which its connections are made with the cortex of the cerebrum.

The function of the cochlea in hearing is to transform movements resulting from sound stimulation into electrochemical nerve impulses which are carried to the brain. This action occurs when the pumping and turning movements of the stirrup against the oval window set the perilymph fluid into motion. Since there is little compression in fluids, every inward movement of the oval window is accompanied by a bulging outward of the round window and vice versa. The resulting wave motion causes movements of the membranes of the cochlear duct, which in turn sets off wave

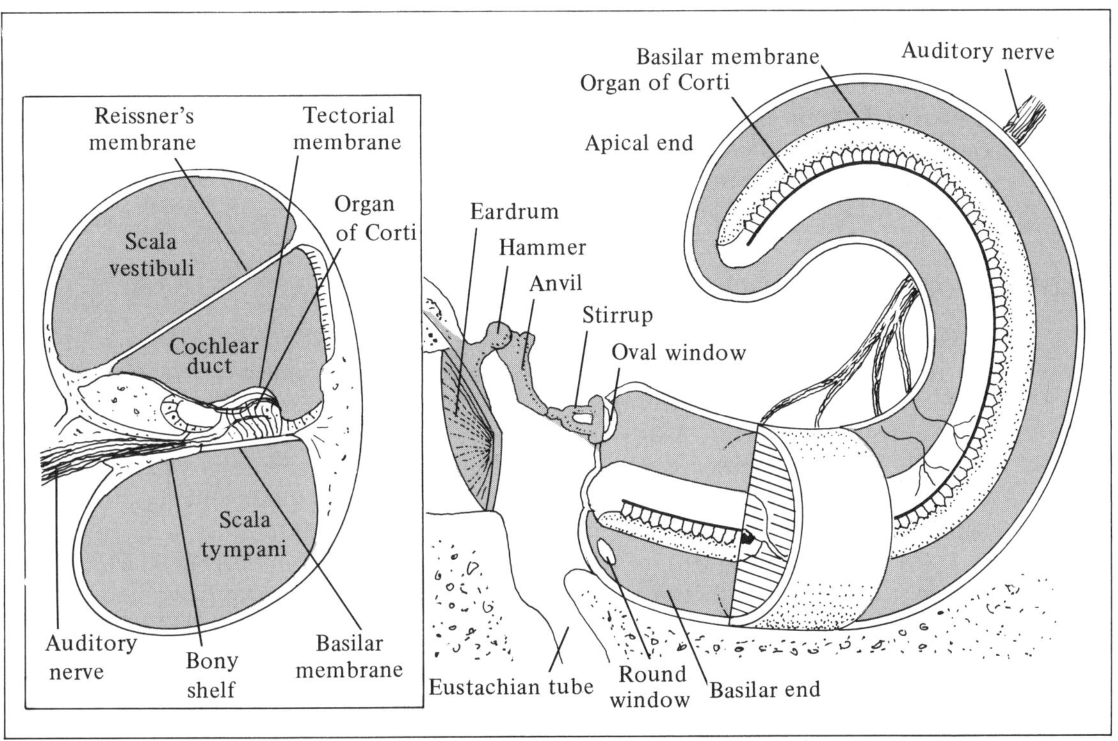

Figure 4–18. Schematic view of the cochlea with cross-sectional view of the organ of Corti.

motions of the endolymph fluid. Hairs of the organ of Corti are excited by the waves and in turn stimulate nerve cells to which they are attached. These electrochemical impulses are carried by the eighth cranial nerve to the brain for interpretation.

The means by which the ear analyzes the sounds into loudness and pitch is not fully understood. It is thought that loudness is determined by the number of hairs, hence nerves, excited by the waves and also by the stimulation of some selected hairs that require greater wave action for excitation of nerves. Even more conjecture is necessary to attempt to describe pitch perception. It is thought that different pitches stimulate different areas along the basilar membrane; high pitches excite the basilar portion and low pitches excite the apical portion of the cochlea. More complex interpretations of sound take place in the auditory cortex about which even less is known.

AIR AND BONE CONDUCTION OF SOUND

In our discussion of the auditory structure we described the pathway of sound reception for hearing. Sound, in its various transformations, is captured by the outer ear, transmitted across the middle ear, and received by the inner ear. This is called hearing by air conduction.

There is another pathway for sound reception. Since the inner ear is imbedded in the temporal bone of the skull, sound can cause the bones of the skull to vibrate, which in turn produces movements in the fluid of the inner ear and excites the nerve endings of the organ of Corti. The outer and middle ear are bypassed in this process and sound goes directly to the inner ear. This type of sound reception is called hearing by bone conduction. It should be noted that sounds have to be considerably louder to be heard by bone conduction and we are not aware of hearing by this means unless there is some pathological obstruction in the outer or middle ear.

THE MEASUREMENT OF HEARING

Pure-Tone Audiometry. The most frequently employed instrument for testing hearing is the pure-tone audiometer. This is an electronic instrument which generates pure tones at known frequencies and at a wide range of intensities. The frequencies most often tested are 125, 250, 500, 750, 1000, 1500, 2000, 3000, 4000, 6000, and 8000 Hz. The intensities are calibrated in degrees from a reference point of 0 dB, called the hearing threshold level (HTL). This reference point for each frequency has been adopted by the International Standards Organization (ISO).

Essentially, the purpose of the test is to determine the intensity level at which the subject can just detect the sound of the test frequencies, that is, to determine the subject's threshold of hearing for that frequency in relation to the HTL. Four thresholds of hearing are measured: hearing by air conduction for each ear and by bone conduction for each ear. Earphones are used to test hearing by air conduction; a small vibrator placed on the mastoid process of the temporal bone behind each ear is used to test hearing by bone conduction.

The Audiogram. A graphic representation of an individual's threshold of hearing for each ear by air and bone conduction is called an audiogram (Figure 4–19). The chart for the audiogram lists frequencies from 125 to 8000 Hz on the horizontal axis and indicates the intensity of sound from −10 dB to 110 dB on the vertical axis. Air conduction thresholds are shown by the symbols O for the right ear and X for the left; bone conduction thresholds are shown by the symbols > for the right ear and < for the left.

Reading the threshold curves on an audiogram gives information as to the type and degree of hearing loss. In the audiogram in Figure 4–19 the bone conduction curves are normal for both ears, but the air conduction curves show a hearing loss that is about the same for both ears. A bone conduction curve closer to normal than an air conduction curve indicates that some pathology in the outer or middle ear is obstructing the conduction of sound. The audiogram shows a bilateral, conductive hearing loss of moderate severity.

The audiogram in Figure 4–20 shows normal hearing in the bone and air conduction curves of the right ear. Both bone and air conduction curves show an equal loss in the left ear. This indicates that the sound is being conducted normally to the left ear, but a pathology exists in the sensorineural parts of the inner ear or beyond. The conclusion from the audiogram is unilateral, sensorineural hearing loss of the left ear of moderate degree.

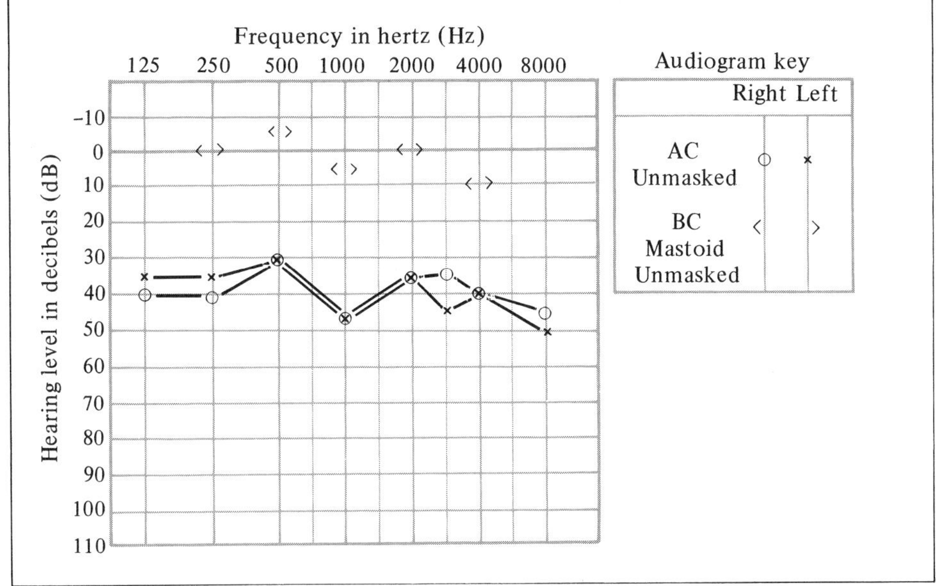

Figure 4–19. Audiogram showing a bilateral conductive hearing loss.

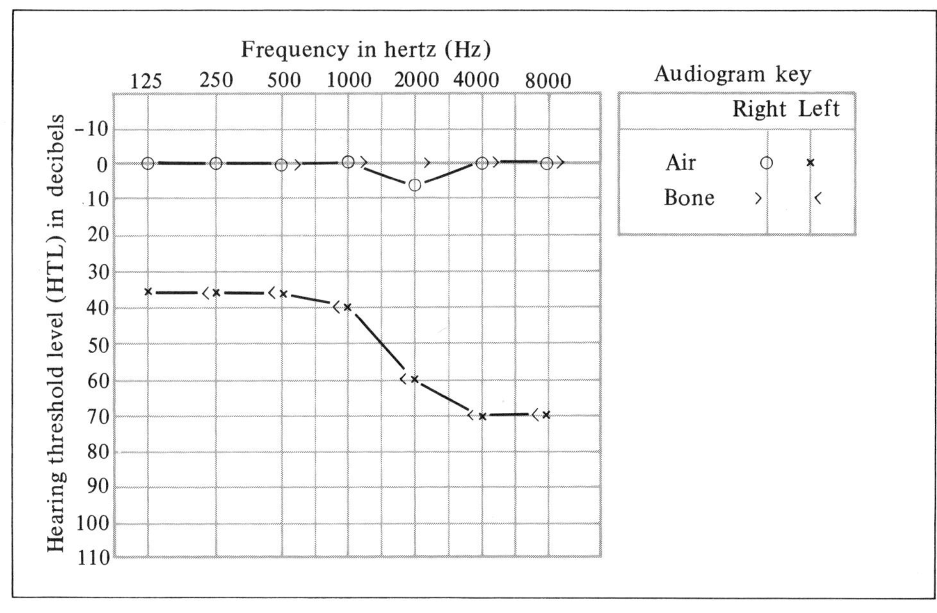

Figure 4–20. Audiogram showing a unilateral sensorineural hearing

Mixed impairments are also possible with the audiogram showing losses in both bone and air conduction.

Speech Audiometry. Proper assessment of hearing loss requires information in addition to what can be obtained from pure-tone audiometry. Pure tones are abstract sounds which do not exist in nature. An individual's response to more meaningful sounds throws light on the functional use of his hearing. Speech audiometry gives a measure of a person's sensitivity to speech.

One measure of the individual's degree of sensitivity to speech and thus an indication of hearing loss for speech is called the speech reception threshold (SRT). This is approximately the level at which the individual can just understand speech.

Another assessment in speech audiometry is the person's ability to discriminate speech when it is presented at a loudness level well above his speech reception threshold. Using established word lists as tests the percent of correct responses is called the person's speech discrimination score.

Impedance Audiometry. Recent developments in impedance audiometry and admittance audiometry have been extremely helpful in discovering and differentiating pathologies of the middle ear as well as the location of sensorineural lesions. Basically, it is a measure of the amount of energy flow through the middle ear. We shall not describe the technique which, until recently, involved cumbersome instruments and was time consuming. New instrumentation and methodology has simplified the administration and increased the test efficiency. When it was used to screen the hearing of 539 elementary school children, the impedance technique detected 94 percent of the hearing disorders, whereas a screening technique based on a modification of the pure-tone audiometer detected only 24 percent (Cooper et al., 1975).

DEVELOPMENT AND DECLINE OF HEARING

The prenatal and neonatal development of hearing has been studied by Eisenberg (1970a, 1970b). She reported that responses to sound appear during the fifth month of fetal life by which time the middle and inner ear have developed to their adult size. In the sixth month the fetus gives autonomic responses to pure tones, although noise bands are more effective in eliciting responses. Remarkably complex auditory differentiation of coding, intensity, and frequency is demonstrated during the seventh month.

On the basis of these findings on the prenatal development of hearing, it is not surprising to learn that after a series of studies on the newborn Eisenberg concluded that "it seems likely that auditory sensitivity at birth approximates 'normal' adult threshold values."

Decline in hearing due to changes in the inner ear is attributable to the process of aging. Hearing losses begin at about age 55 to 60 years and become progressively more noticeable with each decade of life. The highest frequencies are affected first and there is a gradual spread so the loss includes frequencies from 2000 to 8000 Hz (O'Neill and Oyer, 1966). In addition to a decline in auditory acuity there is an accompanying decrease in auditory discrimination of speech particularly for those over 60 years

(Blumenfeld et al., 1969). The speech discrimination problem is particularly vexing, since increasing the loudness of the speech through hearing aids offers little help.

TYPES OF HEARING LOSS

Hearing losses result from pathologies which interfere with the proper functioning of the ear. Pathologies may occur in the outer, middle, or inner ear. Conductive losses originate in the outer or middle ear and sensorineural losses from the inner ear. Hearing losses attributable to eighth nerve damage are called retrocochlear; losses attributable to breakdowns in the brain are called central hearing losses. Figure 4–21 shows the type of loss, location and audiometric air and bone channel.

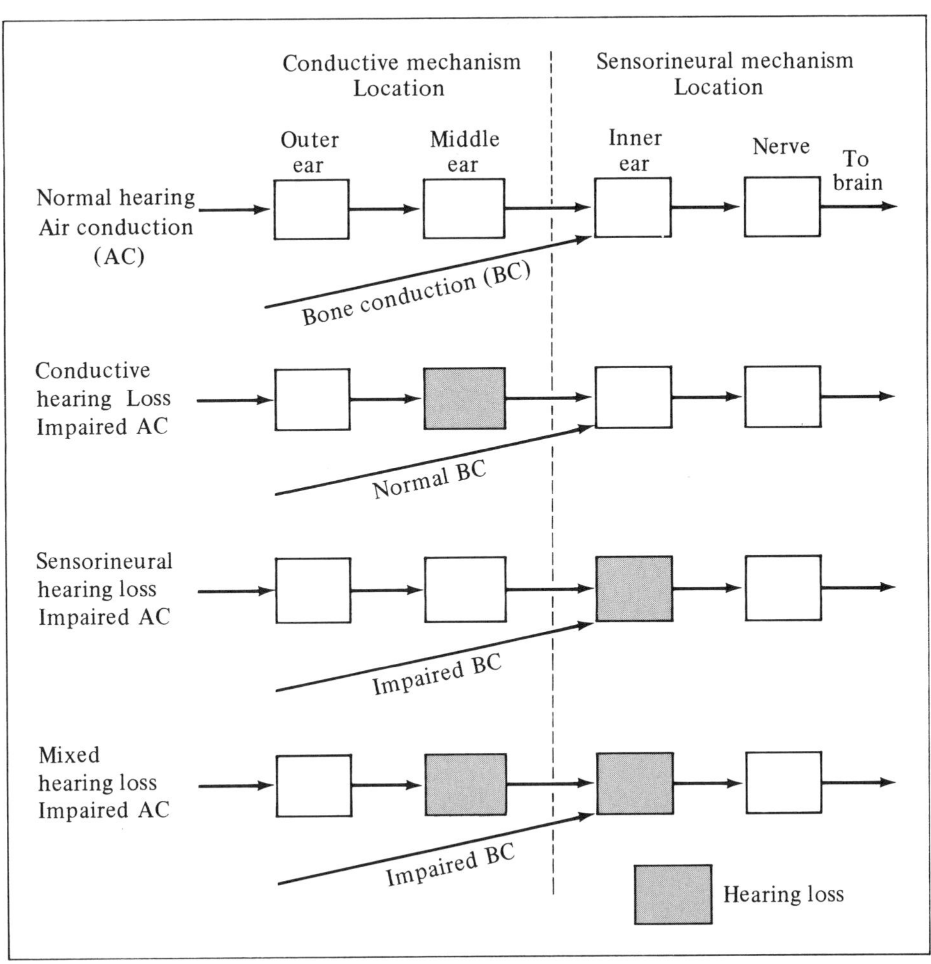

Figure 4–21. Type, location, and channel of hearing losses. (F. N. Martin. *Introduction to audiolosy.* © 1975, p. 5. Reprinted by permission of Prentice-Hall, Inc. Englewood Cliffs, New Jersey.

Outer Ear Hearing Loss. Outer ear conductive losses may be temporary. For example, impacted ear wax lodged against the eardrum may prevent proper vibration of the drum. Otologists sometimes discover small objects that have been inserted into the ear by children. More permanent outer ear conductive losses are those due to congenital atresia where the ear canal itself has not formed during embryological development. In some cases this lack of development may include structures of the middle and inner ear as well.

Middle Ear Hearing Loss. Children are especially prone to middle ear infections. Otitis media, an inflammation of the middle ear, may develop as a result of colds, allergies, measles, mumps, or sinusitis. The middle ear may become filled with pus, causing pain and impeding the conduction of sound through the middle ear. Repeated infections, especially if not treated medically, may leave adhesions which permanently impede energy flow across the middle ear.

Another cause of otitis media is a malfunctioning eustachian tube. The tube ventilates the middle ear in order to keep an equal balance of air pressure on both sides of the eardrum. If the tube becomes obstructed by enlarged adenoidal tonsils, infections of the throat, or serious allergic conditions, the air in the middle ear becomes absorbed, the eardrum is distended, and finally the ear fills with fluid which cannot drain. Medical attention is necessary to avoid permanent hearing loss. Children with clefts of the palate are especially prone to middle ear infections and conductive hearing losses because of maldevelopment in the palatal region which interferes with proper eustachian tube opening for ventilation and drainage.

Otosclerosis is a hereditary disease which causes abnormal bony growth to develop around the stirrup's footplate, fixing it more or less and impeding its vibratory action. The hearing loss associated with this condition usually appears in the late teens, although it could begin earlier, and it becomes progressively more serious. It appears initially as a conductive hearing loss, but a sensorineural component develops in the later stages if the results of the disease process are not dealt with surgically.

Warren S. was a 38-year-old businessman who consulted an otologist at the insistence of his friends who were concerned about his hearing. Warren already knew he had a hearing loss, but his symptoms seemed exaggerated in recent months. He spoke in a loud voice that seemed inappropriate to the situation, although it did go along with his highly assertive, aggressive personality. One problem was that he seemed inattentive at times. This was subsequently attributed to the finding that he was missing large segments of the conversation, despite his excellent speech-reading ability which he had learned on his own. His articulation and language structure had suffered no deterioration. His neighbors had frequently complained to the building management about his excessively loud television and hi-fi.

Warren had been reluctant to see an otologist because he felt he knew the diagnosis. He had been treated by specialists since childhood for ear, nose, and throat infections and allergies. He had a continuous problem of tinnitus, a ringing in the ears. Doctors had told him years before that his hearing loss was the result of early otitis media and acoustic trauma. He had worked his way through college as an inspector in a canning factory where loud noise levels were constant. Much to his surprise, audiological and otological examination showed that the major source of his hearing loss was from the hereditary disease of otosclerosis. The diagnosis was mixed hearing loss. An inner ear sensorineural component had developed from the otosclerosis.

SENSORINEURAL HEARING LOSS. Sensorineural losses result from a wide variety of conditions ranging from prenatal damage to decline in old age. Prenatal sensorineural damage has been found in cases where there was maternal illness during pregnancy. Illnesses include rubella, kernicterus, viral infections, and meningitis. Other prenatal causes include blood incompatibility between mother and fetus, the so-called rh factor. Certain drugs taken during pregnancy also are known to produce damage in the fetus (Konigsmark, 1972). Cerebral palsied children of the athetoid type have been found to have a higher than average incidence of sensorineural hearing losses.

Sensorineural hearing losses can also result from childhood diseases including measles, mumps, influenza, scarlet fever, and meningitis (Jensema, 1975). The inner ear damage may stem from accompanying high temperatures, direct bacterial infections, or the toxins of the bacteria. Frequently the vestibular mechanism is also impaired.

Some industrial chemicals and a number of drugs have a toxic and ultimately destructive effect on the inner ear, leading to permanent sensory hearing losses. The drugs include quinine and members of the mycin family, particularly dihydrostreptomycin, streptomycin, and neomycin. Physicians who prescribe extended use of these drugs that have detrimental side effects do so primarily as a life-saving attempt.

Another cause is acoustic trauma, that is, the continuous or sudden exposure to loud noise, due to a noisy environment such as factories or the sudden explosion of bombs or gunfire. The noise may affect one frequency (4000 Hz is particularly susceptible) or the entire range of frequencies. These types of hearing losses are found more frequently among men than among women because men are more likely to work in noisy environments and to be exposed to gunfire, either in war or hunting. Some recent studies have shown that acoustic trauma may now be affecting a totally different group—the young of both sexes. Jerger and Jerger (1970) studied the noise level at a rock concert. They found noise levels ranged from 104 dB to approximately 120 dB with peaks as high as 130 dB. Keeping in mind that "Hammering on a steel plate two feet away produces a level of 115 dB, a sound almost at the threshold of feeling" (Denes and Pinson, 1973), it is no wonder that Jerger and Jerger concluded that "Performances of contemporary rock and roll music pose a serious threat to hearing."

Traumatic head injuries, such as those sustained in automobile and other accidents, can cause fractures of the temporal bone, damaging the structures of the inner ear, the ossicles, or the eardrum. Depending on the site of injuries the losses may be conductive, sensorineural, or both.

Among the profoundly deaf those with hereditary causes constitute the largest group. Konigsmark (1972) notes that there are 60 types of hereditary hearing losses. There are three general types of hereditary auditory defects: (1) embryological maldevelopment of the inner ear or the auditory nerve pathway, the most frequent type in children in schools for the deaf, (2) degenerative diseases of the sensorineural mechanism which can start any time in life following normal hearing, and (3) inner ear otosclerosis. There is no known medical treatment for these defects.

Presbycusis is a name given to a decline in the inner ear and neural functioning which attends the process of aging. The extent of the hearing loss varies among people and cultures, just as with other types of deterioration in the aged.

CLASSIFICATION OF HEARING LOSSES

Hearing plays the dominant role in three functions: (1) learning speech and language; (2) self-monitoring of speech, and (3) sensory reception of the speech of others. Loss in hearing will have adverse effects on all these functions. We have discussed the monitoring-feedback of one's own speech under articulation and voice. Before proceeding to discuss the other influences, though, we need some terminology concerning the severity and age of onset of hearing loss.

No completely satisfactory definition of severity of hearing loss exists because social and psychological factors account for large differences in the auditory functioning of individuals with the same degree of hearing loss. Keeping that caution in mind, the severity of hearing loss is sometimes calculated from the audiogram by taking an average of three frequencies: 500, 1000, and 2000 Hz in each ear, choosing the better ear's average, and making generalizations from that number. The rationale for choosing this index is based on the finding that this number is close to the speech reception threshold, a functional measure of the ability to perceive speech. However, it should be noted that all frequencies are important for speech.

Utilizing this index number the following scale of hearing impairment has been developed (Goodman, 1966):

Group I	minus 10 to 26 dB	Normal limits
Group II	27 to 40 dB	Mild hearing loss
Group III	41 to 55 dB	Moderate hearing loss
Group IV	56 to 70 dB	Moderately severe hearing loss
Group V	71 to 90 dB	Severe hearing loss
Group VI	over 91 dB	Profound hearing loss

Those individuals who are able to hear, although defectively, with or without a hearing aid, are identified as the hard-of-hearing. This includes the groups II through IV, although some of the more severe in group IV may fall into the next category—the deaf. The deaf are identified as those who are unable to use hearing for the ordinary purposes of life. The majority in group V and all in group VI fall into this category.

Age of onset of deafness is of extreme importance since it determines the extent to which language was learned prior to the deafness. Most children who become deaf after age 3 retain certain language and speech patterns. The deafmute, according to Beasley (1940), is "an individual who was born deaf or acquired deafness sufficiently early in life to prevent him from learning speech through the usual means" and the person totally deaf for speech is defined as one who "cannot hear speech under any circumstances, but acquired the hearing defect after learning to speak by ordinary means."

Using a threshold of hearing as a reference level, weak conversational speech would be 35 dB and loud conversational speech would be 65 dB; the average conversational speech is at approximately 50 dB (Newby, 1972). This may be helpful in assessing the

Table 4–2. Relationship Between Hearing Level and Speech Reception

Hearing Level (1964 ISO Reference)	Speech Reception
−10 to 26 dB	Normal
27 to 40 dB	Slight loss, difficulty in hearing faint or distant speech
41 to 55 dB	Understands conversational speech at a distance of 3 to 5 feet; difficulty in a classroom if voices are soft or out of line of vision; needs hearing aid
56 to 70 dB	Understands only very loud conversation; great difficulty in group and classroom discussion; needs hearing aid
71 to 90 dB	May hear a loud voice at 1 foot from the ear; may identify environmental noises; may distinguish vowels, but not consonants; benefits from hearing aid
over 90 dB	May hear some loud sounds, but does not rely on hearing as primary channel for communication

Source: Adapted from A. C. Goodman. Reference zero levels for pure-tone audiometers. Maico Audiological Library Series, Vol. IV, 1966.

impact of hearing loss on communication. To follow a weak conversation, for example, would require hearing of at least 25 to 30 dB. Table 4–2 presents a general summary of the relationship between hearing level and speech reception.

While there is no absolute rule, Huizing (1953) feels that 70 dB is a critical level for the natural development of speech and language in children. Children with greater losses need highly specialized speech and language training.

STUTTERING VIEWED AS A PHYSICAL PATHOLOGY

When parents observe the obvious struggle behaviors which accompany stuttering, they, as well as the stutterer himself, are convinced that there must be some physiological deficit which would account for the stuttering. They suspect that the cause must be in the nervous system or the more visible parts of the speech mechanism. In the latter the organ usually suspected of malfunctioning is the tongue. Undoubtedly for a combination of functional and symbolic reasons this explanation is well-known to psychoanalysts.

Van Riper (1958), who has collected some fascinating tidbits on the history of stuttering, describes the partial glossectomies of some stutterers. The surgical removal of the tongue was intended to cure the errant organ. It should be noted that these operations were performed prior to the development of general anesthesias and asceptic techniques. Of course, a certain number of stutterers must have been "cured," but all too permanently!

Let us not condemn these early practitioners too harshly in their attempts to eliminate stuttering. In our own time the same type of logic was used by surgeons who performed lobotomies on psychotic patients. The results indicate the same degree of success as in the cases of glossectomies on stuttering.

In applying the medical model to stuttering hundreds of research studies have been conducted to determine whether stuttering is a symptom of some underlying neurological or physiological deficit within the stutterer. Studies have been conducted in the neurological area to determine if there are brain wave differences or interferences of the nervous impulses from the brain which coordinate muscular activity of the speech mechanism. There have been many studies of the biochemistry of the stutterer to determine differences in the blood sugar levels. Others have examined respiratory changes during stuttering and still others have looked at the effect on stuttering behavior of drugs ranging from coffee to tranquilizers to LSD.

The findings from these studies are somewhat difficult to interpret. Studies have found breathing disturbances during stuttering, differences in blood sugar level, blocked or poorly timed nerve impulses to the paired speech musculature, and brain wave differences, but because two conditions are found to occur at the same time or are found to be correlated, it does not follow that they are necessarily causally related. There are a number of possible explanations. The differences may cause the stuttering or the stuttering may cause the differences. Both the stuttering and the differences may stem from a common factor which has yet to be identified. Also, the research itself may be faulty; the differences may be due to chance factors or have low significance.

Much of the past research does not fit the rigors of present-day research methodology. Many of the studies were pilot or exploratory research with few subjects and many did not employ control groups.

A large number of research studies were directed toward discovering physical determinants of stuttering during the 1920 to the mid-1940 period. The results were largely negative or ambiguous. Each new area under investigation stimulated interest and then failed to sustain its original promise. Hill (1944a, 1944b) summarized and interpreted the biochemical and physiological studies in 1944. The literature was brought up to date and reinterpreted by Perkins with essentially the same conclusions (1970). A few studies have appeared since that time.

SUMMARY

We have viewed the physical determinants of speech and language in terms of its structures, functions, and disorders. The structures include the nervous system, the respiratory system, the oral portion of the digestive tract, and the ear. The functions include neurological innervation and processing, breathing, phonation, articulation, resonance, and hearing. These are considered overlaid functions on the foundation of more basic physiological activities. The pathologies of speech are examined in the light of the medical model.

REFERENCES

Anderson, V. *Training the speaking voice*. New York: Oxford University Press, 1961.

Bankson, N. W., and Byrne, M. C. The relationship between missing teeth and selected consonant sounds. *Journal of Speech and Hearing Disorders*, *27*, 341–348 (1962).

Beasley, W. C. The general problem of deafness in the population. *Laryngoscope*, *50*, 856–905 (1940).

Berry, M., and Eisenson, J. *Speech disorders*. New York: Appleton, 1956.

Blumenfeld, W., Gruber, V., Bergman, M., and Millner, E. Speech discrimination in an aging population. *Journal of Speech and Hearing Research, 12*, 210–217 (1969).

Carhart, R. (Ed.). *Human communication and its disorders–An overview*. Bethesda, Md.: National Institute of Neurological Diseases and Strokes, Department of Health, Education, and Welfare, 1969.

Cooper, J. C., Jr., Gates, G. A., Owen, J. H., and Dickson, H. D. An abbreviated impedance bridge technique for school screening. *Journal of Speech and Hearing Disorders, 40*, 260–269 (1975).

Daniloff, R. G. Normal articulation processes. In F. Minifie, T. Hixon, and F. Williams (Eds.), *Normal aspects of speech, hearing, and language*. Englewood Cliffs, N.J.: Prentice-Hall, 1973.

Darley, F. L. *Diagnosis and appraisal of communication disorders*. Englewood Cliffs, N.J.: Prentice-Hall, 1964.

Darley, F. L., Aronson, A., and Brown, J. Clusters of deviant dimensions in the dysarthrias. *Journal of Speech and Hearing Research, 12*, 462–496 (1969a).

Darley, F. L., Aronson, A., and Brown, J. Differential diagnostic patterns of dysarthria. *Journal of Speech and Hearing Research, 12*, 246–269 (1969b).

Denes, P. B., and Pinson, E. N. *The speech chain*. Garden City, New York: Anchor Press, Doubleday, 1973.

Eisenberg, R. B. The organization of auditory behavior. *Journal of Speech and Hearing Research, 13*, 453–471 (1970a).

Eisenberg, R. B. The development of hearing in man: An assessment of current status. *Asha, 12*, 119–123 (1970b).

Goodman, A. C. Reference zero levels for pure-tone audiometers. *Maico Audiological Library Series*, 4 (1966).

Greenberg, H. J. Fundamentals of acoustic impedance or admittance measurement. *Asha, 17*, 729–732 (1975).

Hebb, D. O. *Textbook of psychology*. Philadelphia: Saunders, 1972.

Hill, H. Stuttering. I. A clinical review and evaluation of biochemical investigations. *Journal of Speech Disorders, 9*, 245–261 (1944a).

Hill, H. Stuttering. II. A review and integration of physiological data. *Journal of Speech Disorders, 9*, 289–324 (1944b).

Hollien, H., and McGlone, R. E. Vocal pitch characteristics of aged women. *Journal of Speech and Hearing Research, 6*, 164–170 (1963).

Hollien, H., and Shipp, T. Speaking fundamental frequency and chronological age in males. *Journal of Speech and Hearing Research, 15*, 155–159 (1972).

Hudgins, C. V. A comparative study of the speech coordinations of deaf and normal subjects. *Journal of Genetic Psychology, 44*, 1–48 (1934).

Hudgins, C. V., and Numbers, F. C. An investigation of the intelligibility of the speech of the deaf. *Genetic Psychology Monographs, 25*, 289–392 (1942).

Huizing, H. Assessment and evaluation of hearing anomalies in young children. In *Proceedings of the International Course in Paedo-audiology*. Groningen Verenigde Brukkerijen Hoitsema N.V., 88–97, 1953.

Jackson, C., and Jackson, C. L. *The larynx and its diseases*. Philadelphia: Saunders, 1937.

Jarvik, L. F. Thoughts on the psychology of aging. *American Psychologist, 30*, 576–583 (1975).

Jensema, C. Children in educational programs for the hearing impaired whose impairment was caused by mumps. *Journal of Speech and Hearing Disorders, 40*, 164–169 (1975).

Jerger, J., and Jerger, S. Temporary threshold shift in rock and roll musicians. *Journal of Speech and Hearing Research, 13*, 221–224 (1970).

Johns, D. F., and Darley, F. L. Phonemic variability in apraxia of speech. *Journal of Speech and Hearing Research, 13,* 556–583 (1970).

Koepp-Baker, H. Speech problems of the person with cleft palate and cleft lip. In L. E. Travis (Ed.), *Handbook of speech pathology.* New York: Appleton, 1971.

Konigsmark, B. W. Genetic hearing loss with no associated abnormalities: A review. *Journal of Speech and Hearing Disorders,* 37, 89–99 (1972).

Ladefoged, P. *Elements of acoustic phonetics.* Chicago: Univ. of Chicago Press, 1962.

Lawson, L. I., et al. Effects of adenoidectomy on the speech of children with potential velopharyngeal dysfunction. *Journal of Speech and Hearing Disorders, 37,* 390–402 (1972).

Locke, J. L. Questionable assumptions underlying articulation research. *Journal of Speech and Hearing Disorders, 33,* 112–116 (1968).

Luchsinger, R., and Arnold, G. E. *Voice–speech–language. Clinical communicology: Its physiology and pathology.* Belmont, Calif.: Wadsworth, 1965.

Martin, A. D. Some objections to the term apraxia of speech. *Journal of Speech and Hearing Disorders, 39,* 53–64 (1974).

Martin, F. N. *Introduction to Audiology.* Englewood Cliffs, N.J.: Prentice Hall Inc., 1975.

McCarthy, D. A. Language development in children. In L. Carmichael (Ed.), *Manual of child psychology.* New York: Wiley, 1954.

Moll, K. L. Speech characteristics of individuals with cleft lip and palate. In D. C. Spriestersbach and D. Sherman (Eds.), *Cleft palate and communication.* New York: Academic, 1968.

National Advisory Committee on Handicapped Children. *Special education for handicapped children. First report.* Washington, D.C.: Department of Health, Education, and Welfare, 1968.

Newby, H. *Audiology.* New York: Appleton, 1972.

O'Neill, J. J., and Oyer, H. J. *Applied audiometry.* New York: Dodd, Mead, 1966.

Perkins, W. Physiological studies. In J. G. Sheehan (Ed.), *Stuttering: Research and therapy.* New York: Harper & Row, 1970.

Pronovost, W. *The mechanism of speech.* Boston: Boston U., Mimeographed paper, no date.

Ptacek, P. H., Sander, E. K., Maloney, W. H., and Jackson, C. C. R. Phonatory and related changes with advanced age. *Journal of Speech and Hearing Research, 9,* 353–360 (1966).

Rosenbeck, J. C., et al. A treatment for apraxia of speech in adults. *Journal of Speech and Hearing Disorders, 38,* 462–472 (1973).

Rousey, C., and Holzman, P. Recognition of one's own voice. *Journal of Personality and Social Psychology, 6,* 464–466 (1967).

Schuell, H. Aphasia in adults. In R. Carhart (Ed.), *Human communication and Its Disorders. An Overview.* Bethesda, Md.: National Institute of Neurological Diseases and Strokes, Department of Health, Education, and Welfare, 1969.

Silverman, E., and Zimmer, C. H. Incidence of chronic hoarseness among school-age children. *Journal of Speech and Hearing Disorders, 40,* 211–215 (1975).

Snow, K. Articulation proficiency in relation to certain dental abnormalities. *Journal of Speech and Hearing Disorders, 26,* 209–212 (1961).

Sperry, R. W. Hemisphere deconnection and unity in conscious awareness. *American Psychologist, 23,* 723–733 (1968).

Timcke, R., Von Leden, H., and Moore, P. Laryngeal vibrations: Measurements of the glottic wave. *Archives of Otolaryngology, 68,* 1–19 (1958).

Timcke, R., Von Leden, H., and Moore, P. Laryngeal vibrations: Measurements of the glottic wave. *Archives of Otolaryngology,* 69, 438–444 (1959).

Timcke, R., Von Leden, H., and Moore, P. Laryngeal vibrations: Measurements of the glottic wave. *Archives of Otolaryngology*, *71*, 16–35 (1960).

Van Riper, C. Experiments in stuttering therapy. In J. Eisenson (Ed.), *Stuttering: A symposium*. New York: Harper & Row, 1958.

Weinberg, B., et al. Severe hypoplasia of the tongue. *Journal of Speech and Hearing Disorders*, *34*, 157–168 (1969).

Weisenberg, T., and McBride, K. F. *Aphasia*. New York: Oxford University Press, 1935.

THE PSYCHOLOGICAL DETERMINANTS Chapter 5

As the student of communicative disorders will soon discover, speech pathologists do not speak from a unified theoretical point of view. Our divergent approaches to the problems become most evident when we deal with the psychological determinants. A vast store of experimental and clinical information has accrued on all aspects of the psychological processes of both normal and deviant speech and hearing. However, no single theory or explanatory concept exists that can organize these data into a unified whole. No single theory has sufficient generality to be applied to all aspects of the problem.

At the present time a multiple approach to the psychological determinants is necessary. We must take into account the determinants of: (1) learning, (2) cognition or intellectual processes, and (3) personality and emotions.

We will consider the learning determinants from a behavioristic approach, with a special emphasis on operant conditioning. Much of the recent literature on stuttering and articulation explains these as learned phenomena following patterns of acquisition, maintenance, and extinction. Programs of therapeutic intervention in articulation, stuttering, voice, and language have emphasized learning principles. Work with the mentally retarded and the emotionally disturbed on their multiple problems has utilized this approach.

The cognitive or intellectual determinants will emphasize the theoretical approaches of Jean Piaget, although other points of view will be discussed. Cognitive explanations of mental retardation, learning disabilities, deafness, and autism have been particularly revealing.

The psychoanalytic theory is especially rich in explanatory concepts of emotional and personality determinants. Application of these principles has been made to problems of articulation, stuttering, and autism. We will present a modified neo-Freudian approach, with an emphasis on ego psychology.

Both the behavioristic learning theorists and the psychoanalytic theorists look at psychopathology in terms of their own orientations. We will discuss both the behavioral model of psychopathology and the psychodynamic medical model of psychopathology.

BEHAVIORISM AND LEARNING

Behaviorism is a psychological approach to the study of the individual. It deals exclusively with observable and measurable behavioral responses, in contrast to those psychological theories which are concerned with things that cannot be seen, those that are hypothetically within the "mind" of the individual, such as remembering, thinking, problem solving, libido, death instinct, and so forth. Leaders in the behaviorist movement include J. B. Watson, its founder, and B. F. Skinner.

Behaviorists are interested in determining the relationships that exist between behavioral responses and the conditions that elicit such responses. Operant conditioning, one of a number of learning theories that have evolved from a study of the relationships, has had considerable impact on the field of communicative disorders. B. F. Skinner developed and popularized this system, but its origins can be traced back to the respondent or classical conditioning theory of I. Pavlov.

A review of classical conditioning will serve as a brief introduction to operant conditioning. *Respondent behavior* is defined as an innate reflex behavior that exists without prior learning, such as the sucking response in infants and the knee jerk. When students are examining the oral structures, they try to avoid triggering the gag reflex when they use a tongue depressor. Audiologists utilize the acoustic reflex in impedance testing. Respondent behavior needs a stimulus to set it off. The sucking response appears after stimulation of the oral zone, the knee jerk is a response to a hammer blow to the tendon, and the acoustic reflex is a response to a sound.

Operant behavior is not a reflex behavior. It is a voluntary act which appears gradually and includes almost everything a person does: sitting, writing, answering a phone, talking. An action is taken to which there is a reaction and that reaction, in turn, affects future performance of the action. Lovaas (1966) has said: "Operant behaviors are a function of their consequences, and as a result of their consequences can be either strengthened or weakened."

RESPONDENT BEHAVIOR IN CLASSICAL CONDITIONING

Most discussions of respondent behavior begin with an illustration of Pavlov's dog experiment. We, however, will use the example of a person in an applied situation, the audiological clinic. Let us assume that the audiologist is testing the hearing of a child. If the child is too young to be able to cooperate and indicate responses in the typical audiometric test, he might use a galvanic skin response procedure, called GSR audiometry (O'Neill and Oyer, 1966), which is based on Pavlovian principles and makes use of a respondent behavior, the sweat gland reflex that is activated by an electric shock. This response is indicated on a galvanometer as change in the electrical resistance of the skin, the GSR.

The GSR is not voluntary and therefore does not require the child's cooperation. If the shock can be paired with an auditory stimulus, then her response to the auditory stimulus can be recorded by changes in the GSR. Earphones are placed on the child and electrodes are attached to her foot and leg. The electric shock is minimal, just strong enough for her to be aware of its presence. Before conditioning, when the audiologist presents to the child a 1000 Hz tone at 60 dB (a stimulus), there is no response. In the process of conditioning, the same auditory stimulus is followed by a shock (*unconditioned stimulus*), which shows up on our equipment as a GSR (*unconditioned response*). Thus we have the following.

Stimulus (tone) → no response
Unconditioned stimulus (shock) → unconditioned response (GSR)

During the conditioning the tone is paired with the shock several times, in order to strengthen the response. This is called *reinforcement*. At times the presentation of stimuli is varied by omitting the shock and presenting only the tone. This type of *intermittent reinforcement* tends to strengthen the conditioning. As conditioning proceeds we have this situation.

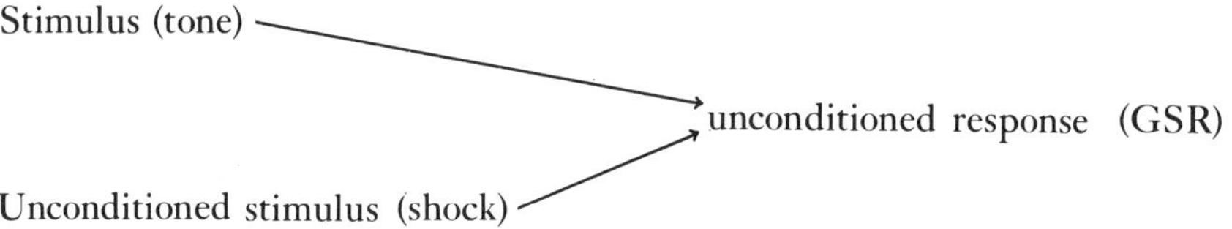

When the audiologist feels that the child has associated the tone and the shock sufficiently, he presents the tone without the shock. When the tone elicits a GSR, we say that the tone has become a conditioned stimulus which elicits a conditioned response. The child has been conditioned and we have the following.

Conditioned stimulus (tone) → conditioned response (GSR)

The audiologist can now begin the test of hearing. He reduces the loudness level of the tone until he gets a GSR response close to the child's threshold. If he is satisfied that he has a threshold for 1000 Hz, he is ready to test hearing at 500 Hz. He presents the new tone at 40 dB and the child responds with the GSR. Although this is a different stimulus from the 1000 Hz 60 dB tone with which she was conditioned, she responds. This is called *stimulus generalization*, a term applied when, after conditioning, similar stimuli produce the same response.

After many presentations of the tone without the shock, the GSR becomes weaker and finally the tone does not elicit a response. When a conditioned stimulus is repeated without the reinforcement, conditioning is weakened. This has been labeled *experimental extinction*. If the audiologist allows the child to rest and then resumes testing by presenting a tone without the shock, the child will again respond with a GSR. This is called *spontaneous recovery*.

OPERANT BEHAVIOR IN OPERANT CONDITIONING

Many of the principles of respondent behavior apply to operant behavior. The following experiment will illustrate the point.

There are a number of studies that report that infants confined to institutions vocalize less than their counterparts who grow up in homes (Brodbeck and Irwin, 1946). There are speculations that deficiency in vocal play may contribute to a child's delayed speech development. Rheingold, Gewertz, and Ross (1959) asked the question: can we increase vocalizations through conditioning?

During three periods on each of two days an experimenter stood next to an infant while the infant's vocalizations were being recorded. A count of the number of vocalizations was obtained and a mean or average of these was calculated. This average is called the *baseline*. On the third and fourth days the experimenter reinforced each vocalization immediately by smiling, saying *tsk*, and touching the infant's abdomen. The frequency of vocalization increased relative to the baseline obtained before conditioning.

On the last two days of the experiment the experimenter provided no reinforcement for the infant's vocalizations. The frequency of the vocalizations decreased to the level of the first two days. Extinction had taken place.

In operant conditioning the experimenter starts with a behavior he wishes to strengthen or increase in frequency of occurrence. He then focuses his attention on the consequences for that behavior, that is, actions or events which immediately follow the behavior, become associated with it, and therefore have an effect on it. The experimenter, or behavior modifier, can provide *positive reinforcers* or stimuli, to increase the frequency of the behavior; *negative reinforcers*, to strengthen responses which lead to the removal of those negative reinforcers and to weaken behaviors that elicit those negative reinforcers; or *neutral* stimuli, which have no effect.

Positive reinforcers are pleasure-producing stimuli. They may be *primary* or *secondary*, that is, learned or unlearned. For example, food, water, and sex are among the unlearned stimuli that act as positive reinforcement of behavior provided the individual has a heightened hunger, thirst, or sexual need. Learned, or secondary, positive reinforcers include approving gestures such as smiles, verbal praise, tokens, and money. Normal social development is based on the acquisition of many different, socially determined secondary reinforcers.

Negative reinforcers are unpleasant or aversive stimuli. Pain is the primary negative reinforcement and socially determined expressions of degrees of disapproval are secondary.

Reinforcement may also be direct or indirect. The withholding of a positive stimulus will have negative effects on behavior and the elimination of a negative stimulus will have positive effects. For example, in an experimental situation if we remove an unpleasant stimulus as soon as we see a desired response, the removal has the effect of reinforcing the desired behavior. Removal of an electric shock has the effect of reinforcing the behavior that immediately preceded it. Use of aversive stimuli is frowned upon by some researchers because it may have adverse side effects.

SHAPING

How can the experimenter elicit behavior that does not occur spontaneously? A behavior must occur before it can be reinforced. The experimenter may have to wait a long time before a desired behavior can be reinforced and complex behaviors may not occur at all. The answer to the question is that the experimenter reinforces partial behaviors that are in the appropriate direction. By reinforcing successive approximations, it is possible to shape the desired behavior.

Let us assume that a child does not have a particular sound or phoneme in his repertoire. Through a gradual process of reinforcing successive approximations and ignoring or extinguishing incorrect behaviors, the child is taught the sound. The production may be broken down into its components: closing the lips, vocalizing, building up air in the mouth, and so on. Each close approximation is reinforced when it appears.

GENERALIZATION

Behavioral responses tend to generalize or spread from the original stimulus to similar ones. This principle was illustrated in the GSR auditory testing when the child was conditioned to a 1000 Hz tone and later her responses generalized to the 500 Hz tone. In most cases generalization is highly desirable. For instance, after the child learns to produce the correct [s] phoneme in a few key words, much effort is expended to encourage him to use the correct [s] in new words on which he has not been instructed and in new situations.

DISCRIMINATION

In generalization the person responds to the similarities in stimuli, but there are times when a response to differences in stimuli is desired. This process is called discrimination or differentiation and is learned by selective reinforcement of some responses and extinction of others. In some programs of articulation therapy the child is initially taught to discriminate between the correct sound and the error. The procedures for achieving this discrimination of auditory stimuli are to reinforce the child's correct responses and not to reinforce the incorrect ones.

The processes of generalization and discrimination may be seen at work in the behavior of the infant. At 3 months he will smile when a face appears—even a mask at the end of a broomstick. By 8 months, however, the infant has discriminated the significant faces in his environment, and when a stranger appears, he may show fear.

MODELING

Bandura (1969) has investigated an aspect of learning which he has called *modeling*. In Chapter 3 we pointed out that the child learns about his world in the early years as a result of the modeling of the parents, particularly the mother. Bandura refers to the process as a form of *imitation* of appropriate models. Others have called it identification, copying, vicarious learning, social facilitation, and role playing. Each of these terms gives nuances to the meaning and reveals different theoretical orientations. Bandura has given the concept of modeling a research foundation and has demonstrated its relevance to behavior modification, that is, the application of learning principles to the improvement of human functioning. He says that modeling "demonstrates that virtually all learning phenomena resulting from direct experiences can occur on a vicarious basis through observation of other people's behavior and its consequences for them."

Bandura has also noted that in naturalistic settings the behavior of the model which the child reproduces may not have an immediate reinforcement. In fact, some behaviors remain latent and are performed many months later. Immediate reinforcement does not seem necessary for its learning, although it may be given when the behavior is performed.

Modeling is one of the basic processes in socialization of the child. To enable the child to function within a society he must learn the behaviors appropriate to his society. Language is one of the key social behaviors that must be learned.

THE BEHAVIORAL LEARNING MODEL OF PSYCHOPATHOLOGY

The behavioral learning model of psychopathology states that abnormal or maladaptive behavior results from inadequate learning or learning from inadequate models during development. From this point view there is no underlying cause within the individual. Rather, at a time when proper learning should have taken place there was no model for adaptive behaviors, adaptive behaviors were inadequately reinforced, or maladaptive behaviors were taught instead. In any event the behavior of the person is inadequate for proper social interaction. The principle applies whatever the area, whether it be speech or sexual behavior. Therefore, during intervention the problem behavior itself is dealt with, rather than some hypothetical disease entity. The behavior therapy is carried out, using principles derived from research, to extinguish maladaptive behaviors and to reinforce new skills.

PROGRAMS OF BEHAVIOR MODIFICATION

Programs of behavior modification stem directly from the basic assumptions and principles which have been presented above. Such programs represent a systematic application of the principles of learning. The material to be learned is carefully arranged so as to guide the learner through tasks that follow a logically and psychologically sound sequence of activities and experiences. These should lead the learner step by step to the desired behavior. The programs are structured to provide sufficient learning so that the behavior does not extinguish easily. Habituation is essential. They also provide for the maximum amount of generalization of the desired behavior. The most highly structured programs have been repeatedly tested and revised to increase their efficiency. A large number of such programs have been developed in all areas of communicative disorders. Some of them will be discussed in Chapter 7.

LEARNING THEORY AND STUTTERING

The application of learning principles to communicative disorders, especially stuttering, has had a comparatively long history, considering the age of the discipline itself. Our examples will be drawn from the literature on stuttering. Dunlap (1928) wrote about negative practice in stuttering.

We do not know what causes suttering, even though there has been more research in this area of speech breakdown than in any other. Nevertheless, a vast store of information has accumulated which has helped in preventing stuttering and in intervention with stutterers. A well-founded theory of causation exists in each area, documented with clinical and experimental evidence. Sheehan (1970) has reviewed this literature for the interested reader.

On an observable level stuttering is seen as a frequent disruption in the relative continuity or fluency of speech. It is characterized by repetitions and prolongations of sounds and syllables and hesitancies in the utterance of sounds, syllables, and words (Wingate, 1962). In some cases there are interjections of unnecessary sounds, as well as associated eye, lip, or head movements.

On a more covert level the stutterer usually anticipates when he is going to stutter and attempts to avoid it by increasing the tension in the speech mechanism and disrupting his breathing pattern. The speech situation is accompanied by an increase in anxiety.

There are inconsistencies in the speech. There are more words on which the stutterer is fluent than on which he stutters. He is fluent when talking to himself, to children, to animals, to those in an inferior status position. He is fluent when he can speak in a sing-song rhythmic fashion or with other distraction devices. Stuttering tends to increase during telephone speaking or when the stutterer talks to a nonreceptive audience.

Stuttering usually begins between the ages of 3 and 5, but may begin earlier. It is more prevalent in males than in females. Its onset is insidious, making it difficult for parents to pinpoint its beginnings. It is found in all cultures throughout the world, though its frequency differs. It seems to run in families, although the validity of such a statement is presently in dispute. Many children who are diagnosed as stutterers recover spontaneously.

A great deal of activity has centered on an attempt to identify stuttering as a learned behavior, to explain its acquisition and maintenance, and to utilize behavioral principles in its modification. Johnson and his students (1959) conducted a 30-year program of research into the nature of stuttering and much of their effort was directed toward the application of learning theory. Johnson emphasized two findings: the adaptation effect and the consistency effect.

If a stutterer gives successive readings of the same passage, he shows a gradual decrease in the frequency of stuttered words. This is called the *adaptation effect*. If after a lapse of time he is asked to read the passage again, the frequency of his stuttering returns close to its original level. Johnson felt that adaptation might be equated with experimental extinction (reduction of conditioning as a result of nonreinforcement). It follows then that the recovery of the frequency of stuttering after a time interval could be viewed as spontaneous recovery.

Johnson also pointed to the *consistency* effect, a finding that stutterers tend to stutter on the same words or in response to the same cues or stimuli. Both the adaptation and the consistency effects suggest that stuttering is a learned response. More recent experiments have challenged the validity of equating adaptation with extinction. The question still remains unanswered.

If a stutterer can predict the words on which he is going to stutter, then the idea of his trying to do something about it makes sense even if his efforts make matters worse. Both Bloodstein (1958) and Johnson (1967) evolved concepts of stuttering along the lines of an anticipatory struggle reaction. Bloodstein wrote that stuttering is a

> habit of making elaborate preparations for speech on the assumption that it is a difficult and treacherous process. In his very anxiety to articulate words or syllables adequately, the stutterer makes certain he will fail to do so, like the frightened and inexperienced swimmer whose struggles to stay afloat serve to drag him down. In a word, stuttering is the speech difficulty of a person who tries to speak not wisely but too well" (p. 5).

Johnson (1967) said that "stuttering is an anticipatory apprehensiveness, hypertonic, avoidance reaction." If a stutterer can predict stuttering, he can anticipate it, become anxious about it, and tense his speech muscles in the attempt to avoid stuttering. Thus stuttering is a behavior that the stutterer has learned in order to avoid stuttering.

Wischner (1952) was concerned with the maintenance of stuttering. He wondered why stuttering was so hard to eradicate if it was a learned phenomenon. He suggested that the perpetuation of stuttering was in part due to the self-reinforcing nature of the behavior itself. During the stuttering block the stutterer is in a state of heightened anxiety. On completion of the stuttered word he feels an immediate reduction in anxiety. Mowrer's (1948) hypothesis is that anxiety reduction is a reinforcement for whatever precedes it. The stutterer, therefore, may be reinforcing his stuttering every time he completes a stuttered word.

Sheehan (1958), in his first theory of stuttering, presented two propositions to encompass both the anticipatory struggle and the anxiety reduction concepts. He hypothesized first that the stutterer is engaged in an approach-avoidance conflict—a conflict between speaking and not speaking, between being silent and not being silent. The hypothesis is based on Miller's learning theory formulation (1944). Sheehan's second proposition is the fear reduction hypothesis. "The occurrence of stuttering reduces the fear which elicited it, so that during the block there is sufficient reduction in fear-motivated avoidance to resolve the conflict, permitting release of the blocked word" (p. 125). Fear reduction, therefore, reinforces stuttering.

Shames and Sherrick (1963) were among the first to make a direct application of Skinner's operant conditioning model to stuttering. They explained the development and the maintenance of stuttering in Skinnerian terms. Goldiamond (1965) noted that if we consider stuttering an operant learned behavior, then it must be under stimulus control. On that basis he illustrated some possible conditions for learning stuttering, especially in homes where stuttering "runs in the family." Stimulus control rather than genetics may be involved in the observation that stuttering runs in families.

Ingham and Andrews (1973) reviewed thirteen years of research on behavioral therapy including operant procedures for the treatment of stuttering. Their conclusions are somewhat discouraging. They say, "Few have convincingly demonstrated that a procedure or a set of procedures can reliably establish durable normal speech in patients." Especially lacking are studies which demonstrate generalization of therapeutic gains outside the laboratory.

The therapeutic techniques that have been employed varied and showed considerable ingenuity on the part of clinicians in applying behavioral principles. Nevertheless, after studying the reported results, the authors state, "At this time there seems little justification for concluding that behavior therapy has made a major contribution toward providing clinicians with effective and reliable therapeutic procedures."

PIAGET'S COGNITIVE THEORY

Piaget, the Swiss psychologist, has provided the clearest and most complete theory of the intellectual development of children. His research and theorizing on the way in which the individual acquires knowledge spans a period from the 1920s to the present time. In recent years there has been a renewed interest in Piaget's formulations, especially among educators and psychologists. Much of what Piaget has written has direct application to curriculum development for normal children, assessment of intellectual development, and planning of educational programs for exceptional children. The impact of Piaget's findings is only now being felt in the field of communicative disorders. Present indications are that his material will be integrated into the body of knowledge required of speech pathologists and audiologists. His material is essential for the understanding, assessment, and therapy of children with language and cognitive problems including the emotionally disturbed, mentally retarded, socially disadvantaged, learning disabled, and the deaf.

Piaget's theory deals with the cognitive aspects of development. Cognition includes all the means whereby the individual represents anything to himself or uses these representations as a means of guiding his behavior (Leeper, 1951). Cognition includes the psychological processes that give meaning to our sensory impressions, organize them through some coding method, hold them until needed, and select them for use at an appropriate time. Perception, concept formation, problem solving, memory, and thought are among the various cognitive processes. If we look at Piaget's cognitive theory from a slightly different point of view, we might say that it helps us to understand and chart the stages through which the child passes on his way to a discovery of and adaptation to reality (Church, 1961).

As the foundation for his theory, Piaget assumes that the infant is born with a genetic hereditary endowment which will facilitate his making contact with the reality of the world. The neonate has inherent structures which somehow preadapt him to a primitive reality and predispose the direction and quality of his cognitive development.

THE SCHEME

STRUCTURE OF THE SCHEME

In discussing the physical determinants of speech, we noted that there are anatomical structures, such as the lungs and the larynx, which are organized to perform certain functions of breathing and voice production. By analogy Piaget postulates that there are cognitive structures that perform mental functions. These cognitive structures are called schemes.

The scheme is a basic intellectual structure of the individual. It is by means of these structures that the individual interacts with his environment in an organized and adaptive fashion. As such the scheme may be thought of as a structure within the individual that mediates or intervenes between environmental stimuli and the adaptive responses of the individual.

Schemes help the individual by providing him with a conceptual framework for apprehending and interacting with the world in an orderly and organized way. For example, schemes help reduce the complexity of the world by enabling the individual to see relationships and thereby organize his perceptions into classes, categories, and concepts. They also provide for generalization in his responses to the environment.

Basically, the scheme represents an organization of three groups of processes: (1) receptive, (2) central, and (3) expressive. The receptive processes of the scheme involve the organized input of the data from sources within and outside the individual. We recognize the psychological processes of attention and perception as belonging to this category. The central processes of the scheme serve to assimilate, associate, and integrate the input data. The psychological processes of "intellectual work" (Kagen, 1966) belong here, including memory, recall, learning, concept formation, and other psychological functions of thought. The expressive aspects of scheme involve the choice and guides for behavior and action. This includes most motor behavior, visceral reactions, and speech behavior.

Schemes undergo many transformations during the life of the individual as a result of biological maturational influences, physical experience, social interaction, and an inborn motivation toward adaptation. Some of the important schemes include those of time, space, identity, classification, number, combinations, negation, probability, and quantity (Furth, 1969).

FUNCTION OF THE SCHEME: ADAPTATION AND ORGANIZATION

There are two functions of the scheme: adaptation and organization. Although the structure of the scheme changes during each developmental stage of life, its basic functions of adaptation and organization remain the same.

Adaptation consists of two processes: assimilation and accommodation. *Assimilation* is the psychological process of taking things into the structure of the scheme from the environment. On a biological level the lungs take in air from the environment, oxygen is extracted and carried by the blood to organs of the body, and the oxygen is assimilated into these structures. On a psychological level assimilation refers to the incorporation of the results of experiences into the schematic structures. Assimilation takes place especially where there are novel elements in the environment, when there is a partial transfer of elements from a similar past experience, or when emotionally meaningful elements are discovered.

The psychological processes of discrimination and generalization are involved in assimilation. The type of material assimilated varies with the level of development of the scheme. During the first few years of life predominantly sensory experiences and motor actions can be assimilated; in adolescence verbal concepts and ideas are assimilated into existing schemes.

Accommodation refers to the process of the modification of an existing scheme to take into account more knowledge or the creation of a new scheme to deal with a newly discovered environmental demand. On a biological level accommodation can be seen when a need for an increased assimilation of oxygen into the respiratory system of an athlete in training brings about an enlargement of lung capacity. The alteration in structure allows the athlete to respond to the new environmental demands. On a psychological level accommodation can be seen in the modification of a reflex behavior into a voluntary action, as when reflexive vocalizations in infancy become modified into babbling behavior and echoic imitation of adults, and in the addition of new behavioral repertoires or modification of old as a result of environmental situations.

Organization refers to the process of integrating psychological structures into a functional whole. This tendency toward integration of structures and functions can be seen on both biological and psychological levels. On a biological level the separate structures for breathing, vocal fold movement, hearing, and movement of the lips, tongue, jaw, and palate become synthesized after successive stages of organization into the system we recognize as the speech mechanism. Psychologically, the organization of the processes of speech, language, and cognition is necessary for communicative behavior.

Through the adaptive functions of assimilation and accommodation the schemes of the individual move toward a state of *equilibrium* with the environment. Equilibrium is achieved when the schemes effectively deal with environmental situations commensurate with their developmental level. This, of course, is almost impossible to achieve since each time a scheme reaches equilibrium, it is in a state to discover inconsistencies and deficits in its structures which must be dealt with. New assimilations and accommodations become necessary. Movement toward equilibrium thus may be likened to a motivational state. Relative equilibrium is said to occur following the completion of each developmental stage.

Maladaptation takes place when the individual has severe deficits in his schematic structures or functions and thereby is prevented from achieving a state of equilibrium. In childhood problems such as autism, learning disabilities, and social and emotional deprivation the individual is in a constant state of maladaptation or disequilibrium. Disequilibrium may also be seen in the adult problems of aphasia and schizophrenia.

STAGES OF DEVELOPMENT

The cognitive development of the child follows orderly and predictable stages which are clearly reflected in the quality of the child's intellectual behavior. The stages follow a genetic-developmental pattern. Each stage represents the achievement of a new organization of intellectual structures and lays the foundations for the stage to follow. It is not possible for the child to skip stages or to change their order. The stage concept means that there are not only quantitative increases, but also qualitative changes in complexity, organization, and integration with development.

Piaget recognizes four main periods of cognitive development: sensorimotor, from birth through 2 years; preoperational, from 2 to 7 years; concrete operational, from 7 to 11 years; and formal operational, from 11 years on. These periods are not considered to be developmental norms in terms of ages. The ages are approximate, but the sequence of development is invariable.

SENSORIMOTOR PERIOD: BIRTH TO 2 YEARS

The sensorimotor period, referred to by Piaget as the "cradle of intelligence," is the first period in the child's cognitive development and lasts from birth to approximately 18 to 24 months. Development during this period is remarkable when we consider the magnitude and variety of behavioral changes that take place in so short a time. The infant enters the world interacting by means of primitive reflex mechanisms. By the time he completes the sensorimotor period, he is employing newly developing symbolic schemes for mediating his interactions with the environment. As the name implies, the child's mental development takes place through the development and coordination of schemes based on sensory input and motor movements. Throughout the six stages of this period the child builds schemes of action which serve as the foundation for later intellectual life.

Stage 1: Birth Through 1 Month. At birth the infant interacts with his environment solely on the basis of innate reflexive behaviors. The infant comes into the world with a variety of reflexes, some of which form primitive schemes for survival. For example, the scheme for food intake consists of the rooting reflex, a rotating head movement for seeking the breast. When the cheek touches the breast, snapping reflex movements of the lips take place until they surround the nipple, whereupon sucking reflexive movements bring in the milk.

These reflexes rapidly become modified through the processes of assimilation and accommodation and become organized into a food-seeking strategy. Within a few weeks the infant anticipates feeding when he is held and approches the nipple directly and commences sucking. The reflexive schemes become transformed. They are more intentional and efficient and soon organize into larger coordinated schemes.

Among the reflexive schemes of interest to speech pathologists are the noncrying and crying vocalizations which appear in the earliest hours of life and undergo repeated processes of differentiation and integration.

Stage 2: 1 to 4 Months. During stage 2 the infant engages in the *primary circular reaction*. This is the first of three circular reactions of the sensorimotor period. In the process of assimilating a new behavior into his schematic repertoire, the infant produces circular reactions which are highly stereotyped repetitions, somewhat like a chain of imitations.

The primary circular reaction is centered around the infant's own body. The sources of the behavior are accidental variations of reflex responses, which seem to delight the child and demand repetition. The newly discovered behaviors are reinstated again and again. As an example, the infant accidently strikes his feet against the bars of his crib, and the crib begins to rattle. He does not know exactly what has created the noise, but he likes it. He bangs his feet again and again with apparent pleasure. The behavior becomes organized into a coordinated sensorimotor scheme

In the latter part of this period the infant begins to imitate and reimitate in a circular fashion sounds that he has accidentally produced.

Stage 3: 4 to 10 Months. *Secondary circular reactions* develop in stage 3. Like the primary circular reactions these are highly repetitious behaviors, but unlike the primary circular reactions, which center around the infant's own body, these involve things in the child's environment. Again by chance action the child produces some interesting effect that pleases him, but this time he sees a connection between his unintentional actions and the effect. He is therefore able to reproduce them. The repeated behaviors become assimilated into sensorimotor schemes of action. Learning through secondary circular reactions is limited in that it is based on accidental discoveries and hence lacks an intentional goal-directedness such as searching for a means to do something.

Vocalizations are included in the secondary circular reactions. The child will imitate sounds in his environment, provided they are part of his repertoire.

Stage 4: 10 to 12 Months. At this stage the child begins to show signs of intentional, goal-directed behaviors which Piaget feels are among the first signs of true intelligence.

If the child sees a toy that he wants, he will intentionally pull on the string attached to the toy to bring it closer to himself. In this action he reveals some interesting developments: (1) he can engage in purposeful, goal-directed behavior and (2) he has learned the means for achieving his goal. This implies the beginning of the development of a scheme of causality since his actions produce a result.

During this stage the child will freely initiate sounds from a model, even if they are not part of his current repertoire.

Stage 5: 12 to 18 Months. In the *tertiary circular reactions* which occur during stage 5 the child once again manifests highly repetitious behaviors, but there are important differences. The child does not merely repeat accidental behaviors, but makes strong efforts to seek out and accommodate himself to things in his environment. He manipulates things and then tries to reproduce his actions and make them part of his behavioral repertoire.

He integrates novel elements into existing schemes by combining them with previous behaviors. The experimental nature of the tertiary circular reaction gives variety to the repertoire and thus it differs from the stereopathy found in the earlier circular reactions.

At this stage the child also reveals that he is developing the scheme of the permanence of objects; he is beginning to understand that things have existence independent of his own immediate sensory awareness.

Stage 6: 18 Months to 2 Years. This is considered an important transitional stage between the sensorimotor and preoperational period which follows. The major development is the child's initial use of mental symbols or representational thought. Objects may be out of sight, but the child can refer to them because he can use words as anchors for his thoughts. He is no longer bound totally by the here and now sensory and motor images for his internal representations.

Related to his ability to keep things in mind even if they are absent is the child's use of deferred imitation. The child can hold in mind things that he has seen, practice them mentally, and imitate them at a later time.

Overview of Development During the Sensorimotor Period. A review of some of the major aspects of the child's cognition during the first two years of life includes the following.

1. The development of schemes moves in stages from innate reflexive through sensorimotor to the beginnings of coordinated schemes mediated through symbolic representations.
2. The child's speech develops from innate reflexive vocalizations through imitative circular reactions of sounds to words.
3. The child gradually develops the scheme of object permanence. He learns that things exist even if not immediately visible and that they retain the same identity even though they appear different when viewed from varying positions or distances.
4. The child makes headway in the development of spacial schemes to the point of symbolic representations of space, but his schemes of time are limited to revealing knowledge of future by anticipation and the past by memory.
5. The child's actions progress from reflexive through accidental to intentional. They become goal-directed; his means are sensorimotor schemes. The relationships between his intentions, means, and goals reveal the development of the scheme of causality.
6. The child develops from being bound and limited to the exploration of concrete here and now objects in his visual field to the first stage in the manipulation of things out of sight through words.
7. Until the conclusion of the period, when he becomes aware of the independence of objects from the self, the child's orientation toward things and people is almost entirely subjective. The child first sees things as extensions of himself and later sees himself as the center of the world.
8. The child does not differentiate inner experiences from outer reality. His very limited ability to classify and categorize causes him difficulty in differentiating imaginary versus real, animate versus inanimate, and pictures versus things. This fusion of all things at the same level of reality is called *realism* by Piaget.

PREOPERATIONAL PERIOD: 2 TO 7 YEARS

During most of the first two years of cognitive development the child employs sensorimotor schemes for his adaptation to the environment. Bruner (1966) calls the mediation of the sensorimotor schemes *enactive representation*, since they are based on a process of motor manipulation of actual objects. Toward the end of the sensorimotor period the child begins to alter his schemes by utilizing a new type of symbolic representation. The sources of these schemes are found during the sensorimotor period in the child's imitation and delayed imitation of behaviors he has seen. The fact that the child can reproduce motor actions which he has previously seen without the original model being present is an indication that he has at his command a prototype of symbolic representation which he can manipulate mentally.

A transitional stage appears near the close of the sensorimotor period and the beginning of the preoperational period. It is signaled when the child's delayed imitation of things is internalized into signifiers (symbols). These signifiers are composed of perceptual images of significates (objects and things that are symbolized). The child's storage and later use of these signifiers reflect a giant step forward in development. It is this ability which differentiates the child from other animals—the ability to represent reality symbolically. Bruner (1966) calls this type of representation of perceptually linked symbols *iconic representations.* A word is attached and becomes an integral part of the icon.

While the preoperational iconic representations are a major achievement over the sensorimotor enactive representations, the child's cognitive ability is still lacking in two major attributes. (1) There are limitations in the child's ability to perform higher mental operations because iconic representation is tied to perception which limits the amount of abstraction possible. (2) The child's word meanings are largely private and cannot be readily shared with others.

Phillips (1969) notes that the deficits in the preoperational child's cognitive abilities center around a group of related concepts: concreteness, irreversibility, inability to

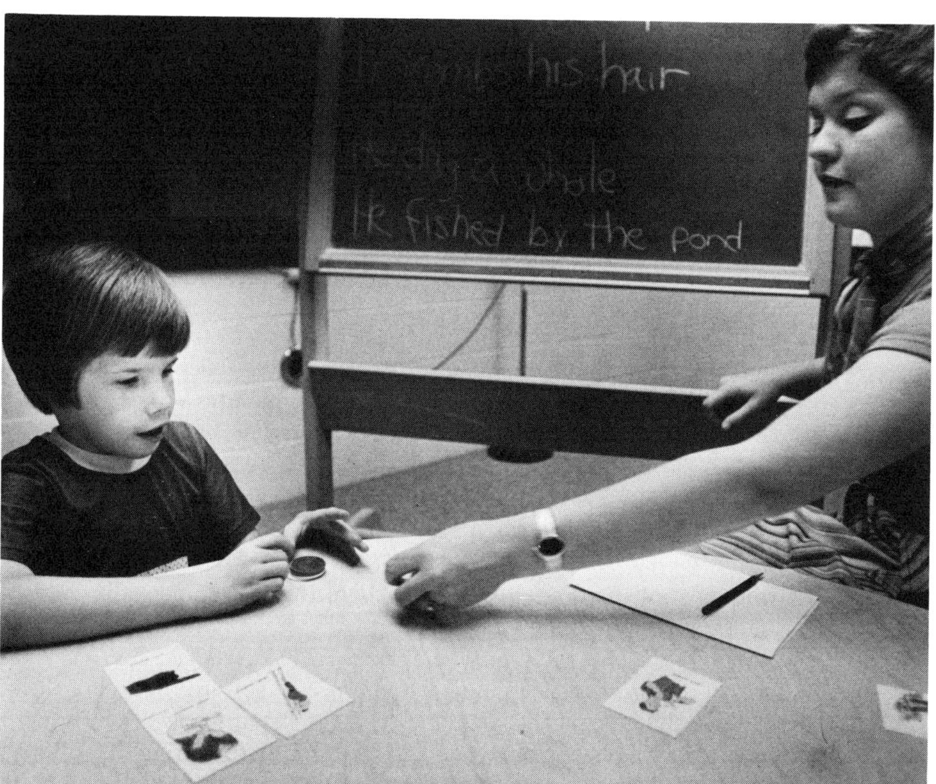

take into account more than one variable at a time, inadequate classification, and egocentrism. To illustrate the way in which the preoperational child is bound by his concrete perceptions, the child is shown two equal lengths of track that are parallel. The child agrees with the experimenter that they are the same length. When one track is rearranged, before the child's eyes, in a zigzag fashion, the child insists that the tracks are now of different lengths because they appear that way.

When presented with another problem in which two factors must be integrated for a proper solution, the child will attend to one variable only and come to the wrong conclusion. The child confirms that two balls of clay are equivalent in mass, but he changes his mind when one ball is flattened into a sausage shape before his eyes. He is not yet capable of the logical thinking necessary to conclude that greater length is compensated for by a reduction in thickness. Furthermore, he is still dominated by his visual perceptions. At this stage visual perceptions prevail over logical operations.

Reversibility is the ability to follow through a problem mentally and then return to the starting point. It is beyond the preoperational child's ability to reverse in his thinking. For example, we know that if $2 + 6 = 8$, we can reverse that operation to obtain the statement that $8 - 6 = 2$. The child cannot follow such a reversal, not because he lacks arithmetic knowledge, but because his mental limitations prevent reversal operations.

The preoperational child also lacks the ability to combine classes of things into a hierarchy. The child will identify a pigeon as a bird, thus indicating that he understands classification, but when he is asked the question, "If all pigeons in this world were to die, would there be any birds?" he would most likely answer "No." He does not really understand the concept of grouping subclasses into supraclasses nor the reversibility of taking away one of the subclasses and still having things left in the supraclass.

Piaget notes that the preoperational child's orientation is egocentric. This aspect of his functioning is so pervasive that it influences all facets of his thoughts, language, and interpersonal relationships. The child is so immersed in himself that he views everything in relation to himself. He fails to see that others may think differently than he does or that there may be other points of view. Egocentrism is not based on a motive of selfishness; rather it is founded on a lack of awareness that other points of view do exist. At the same time the child is not critical of his own thinking. In fact, he may not even be sufficiently aware that he has a self that is thinking or that he has a point of view.

From a Piagetian orientation "language is viewed essentially as a symptom of underlying intellectual activities" (Flavell, 1963). Accordingly, the child's language reflects the underlying state of his thought development. The egocentric nature of the preoperational child's orientation is seen in his use of egocentric speech. Egocentric speech lacks communicative intent and does not recognize that the listener has a point of view. The message is not coded in a language that the listener can understand. The end result of egocentric speech appears to be selfishness, but this is not its purpose. The child is incapable of using the mental operations necessary to put himself into the listener's frame of reference.

Another aspect of egocentrism is the private nature of the meanings of words which the child uses. The word meanings are based on perceptual representations and are highly personal. These private meanings cannot be shared with others. It will take many years for the socialization of the child's word meanings and language.

CONCRETE OPERATIONAL PERIOD: 7 TO 11 YEARS

The concrete operations which the child from 7 to 11 employs provide him with more effective means of adapting to the complexities of his environment. His grasp of reality improves as he develops improved schemes of time, space, number, and causality. The mediational aspects of these schemes are in terms of highly organized and integrated representational verbal thought. The child's adaptive behavior reflects his intellectual growth.

Flavell (1963) states, "the concrete operational child behaves in a wide variety of tasks as though a rich integrated assimilatory organization were functioning in equilibrium or balance with a finely tuned, discriminative accommodatory mechanism" (p. 165). The child develops the ability to place things in an order based on comparisons and relations among variables. He can at this stage deal with more than one variable at a time and is capable of reversibility. This is shown in his development of concepts of mass, weight, number, area, and length. He understands that changing the shape of a substance does not change its weight or volume, that the length of a line remains constant despite changes in spacial arrangements or shape, and that area covered remains constant despite rearrangement of parts. Other logical operations that the child acquires include combination of subclasses into supraclasses and the breaking down of supraclasses.

Despite all the operations mentioned as a part of the new knowledge of the concrete operational child, he still has intellectual limitations for he must employ concrete materials to work with. He must use materials tied to his own experiences. He cannot deal with abstract problems. Abstract approaches to adaptive problems require a new type of operation which emerges in the following stage.

The child's communicative ability becomes less egocentric and more social during the concrete operational stage. Because of his ability to reverse operations and deal with several factors at the same time and to go back and forth between these factors, the child can shift his concentration from himself to his listener and back again during conversation. In addition to his new approach to interpersonal relations in conversation, the child's word meanings become less personal, thus improving his communication. His words are now based on socially shared meaning which the child has learned in his interactions with others in his society.

FORMAL OPERATIONAL PERIOD: FROM 11 YEARS

At approximately age 11, the individual begins the final stage of his intellectual development, the use of formal operations which provide the tools to deal with adaptation in an abstract way and with a high degree of generalization.

The child's solution to problems is independent of and transcends such concrete factors as immediate perceptions, the here and now of practical situations, and specific content. Because of flexibility of thought, the individual can compensate through symbolic representation for any perceived transformations such as shape, length, or height. Thus, by using formal operations the individual is capable of going beyond the perceptual data.

Using abstract thought the individual is capable of problem solving through hypothesis, using inductive and deductive reasoning, and all of the operations necessary for scientific thought.

The high degree of flexibility of thought removes the last vestiges of egocentrism and makes full relativism possible. Relativism is the ability to see things from another's point of view, independent of one's own. This, coupled with the socialization of language and thought, leads to mature social communication.

THE REPRESENTATIONAL MEDIATION OF BEHAVIOR

Bruner (1966) takes the position that inner language or verbal mediation of behavior is but one of three major types of thought. At each stage of development one type predominates. During the sensorimotor period the infant employs enactive mediation. Sensory images and motor movements become internalized and represent his actions toward things in his immediate physical and temporal environment.

During the preoperational period the child employs iconic representation. Perceptual images are used to signify things, groups of things, or happenings that the child has meaningfully experienced. Toward the end of the preoperational period and the beginning of the concrete operational period the type of mediation which will characterize all subsequent development appears—*symbolic representation* in the form of language. Language or verbal mediation is the most explicit and organized mediational form. Bruner notes that the use of conceptual language as an instrument of thinking is required for the logical operations used in advanced modes of reasoning.

Vygotsky (1962) gives us a clearer picture of how thinking becomes verbal. He also agrees that there are many types of thought, only some of which are verbal. He hails the development of verbal thought as the most momentous achievement of man and one that differentiates him from all other animals. Verbal thought must undergo elaborate stages of development before it can emerge as an instrument of social communication. He describes a preintellectual period of speech development in which speech sounds are without meaning and a preverbal stage in thought development in which cognition is devoid of language symbols. He sees speech and thought as having independent origins and parallel stages of development with many intersections of the processes before they ultimately become synthesized into a union of verbal thought and rational speech.

The semantic aspect or word meaning of the linguistic code is the point where a unity of speech and thought takes place. Word meanings are so closely related to speech and to thought that it is not possible to determine whether it is a phenomenon of speech or of thought. He identifies the word meaning as a generalization or a concept. These concepts are not static; rather they change with development and experiences. Each developmental stage of the concept brings about a new relationship between speech and thought.

In a series of research studies on the development and decline of egocentric speech in the child, Vygotsky takes the idea of egocentric speech that had been reported by Piaget and comes to different conclusions as to its function. Vygotsky identifies egocentric speech as the precursor of what will gradually be transformed and finally internalized into inner speech or verbal mediation. Between the ages of 1 and 7 the child employs a type of speech characterized by Piaget as egocentric. It consists of three types: (1) repetitions, including echolalic repetition of what the child hears, what he says, and what he has heard or said in the past; (2) monologue, talking when alone; (3) collective monologue, two or more children talking in each other's presence but without attending to the other's speech.

The peculiar grammatic structure of egocentric speech is important, according to Vygotsky. Pronouns and demonstrative adjectives are used inaccurately without indicating the referents. Cause and effect relationships are incorrect or muddled. Many parts of a story or explanation are omitted. The utterances seem to be unrelated parts strung together without logical order.

The complexity of the grammatical structure of egocentric speech increases gradually from age 1 to 3 years. At that time the structure of the egocentric speech and the child's social communicative speech are the same. Then, from 3 to 7 years, egocentric speech shows a gradual transformation until it becomes almost unintelligible to others. It becomes elliptical, telegraphic, predicated with subject and referents omitted, and devoid of causal explanations. It is at this point that Vygotsky feels that egocentric speech, which he sees as a thinking aloud and not intended for others, becomes fully internalized into inner speech or verbal thought. Verbal symbolic mediation predominates at this time, and the child's social speech, intended for communication with others, becomes almost identical in structure to adult speech.

THE RELATIONSHIP OF COGNITION TO LANGUAGE

LOGICAL OPERATIONS AND GRAMMATICAL FORMS

Problems concerning the relationship between language development and cognitive development have serious implications for programs of assessment and therapy for speech pathologists and audiologists. Does the development of cognitive schemes employing certain mental operations precede the development of logicogrammatical expression, that is, language which employs these operations? Are these cognitive schemes necessary for the development of such grammatical forms? Does the development of speech and language precede the development of logical operations and in fact facilitate acquisition of these cognitive structures? Do language and cognition have somewhat independent and parallel development? Might language and cognition have differential influence at various stages of development?

Piaget places a limited emphasis on language in the formation of mental operations, even at the concrete operational stage. According to Rees (1972), "Piaget makes it plain that language is insufficient for the formulation of vital operational structures like classification and seriation. Once these intellectual structures begin to develop from their underlying mechanisms, language plays a necessary but not sufficient role in their refinement and completion."

To explore the question of whether language is necessary to solve the type of thinking tasks Piaget describes, Furth (1969) conducted a series of experiments with children. He found that the deaf children, despite their linguistic deprivation, had all the important cognitive structures intact. Those differences which he found between the deaf and their hearing controls were due not to any failure in thought processes, but rather to unclear test instruction and a lack of social experience. Furth concluded that "language is not sufficient or necessary for the formation of concrete operations."

Another question we posed is whether the development of grammatical forms has as a prerequisite the existence of the presumed underlying cognitive structures. Carroll (1964) has summarized the various conceptual meanings which are presumed to underly grammatical form classes or parts of speech (Table 5-1). For example, the conceptual meaning of the class of nominals (nouns, pronouns, and noun phrases) involves underlying schemes of such cognitive structures as permanence of objects, identify, space, and relations. Thus, one might conclude that correct grammatical usage is based on adequately developed cognitive structures.

If passive understanding precedes active speech, can we assume that correct answers to questions in certain grammatical forms (indicating comprehension of language use) indicate the development of cognitive abilities which underly those grammatical forms? In other words, might the child have adequate cognitive ability but

Table 5–1. Major Form Classes and Their Conceptual Meanings

Class	Linguistic Manifestation	Approximate Conceptual Meaning—The Class of Experiences That Includes:
Nominals	Nouns, pronouns, noun phrases	Objects, persons, ideas, and relations whose location or distribution in space, actually or metaphorically, can be specified
Adjectivals	Adjectives, adjective phrases	Qualities or attributes perceived as applying to nominals, either on an all-or-none basis (presence-absence) or in terms of degree
Verbals	Verbs, verb phrases	Events, relationships, or states whose location or distribution in a time dimension can be specified
Adverbials	Adverbs, adverb phrases	Qualities or attributes perceived as applying to adjectivals and verbals, either on an all-or-none basis or in terms of degree
Prepositionals	Prepositions, prepositional phrases	Relations of spatial, temporal, or logical position relative to nominals
Conjunctives	Conjunctions	Logical relations occurring whenever any two or more members of any class (or construction) are considered together

Source: J. B. Carroll. ***Language and thought.*** © 1964 p. 92. Reprinted by permission of Prentice-Hall Inc., Englewood Cliffs, New Jersey.

reply incorrectly because of inadequate language comprehension or, on the other hand, might the child have inadequate cognitive ability and still reply correctly.

Wiig and Semel (1973), in a study of learning disabled children, interpret incorrect answers to questions in certain grammatical forms as an indication of and a result of poorly developed cognitive ability. The questions (or language concepts) and their related cognitive concept used by Wiig and Semel are:

1. Concept of comparative relationships
   Example: Are watermelons bigger than apples?
2. Concept of passive construction
   Example: Mary was pushed by Jane. Who was pushed?
3. Concept of relationship between sequential events
   Example: Does spring come before winter?
4. Concept of spacial relationships
   Example: The elephant sat on the mouse. Who was at the bottom?
5. Concept of family relationships
   Example: Give another name for your mother's father

Wiig and Semel found that learning disabled children showed more difficulties in comprehending than normal children. In family relationships answers of the learning disabled indicated logical operations at the sensorimotor or preoperational levels. The investigators attributed the language disabilities to inadequate cognitive abilities.

Langer (1969) notes that the child's comprehension is more advanced than his actual use of material, especially in the case of speech. But he sees that as a special case.

> The child's comprehension of speech is quasi-idosyncratic. On the one hand he seems to understand the meaning of relational terms, descriptive terms . . . when used by adults; he performs adequately when given verbal commands in which such words are used. Moreover, he can be trained to produce and to use more advanced terminology. On the other hand, his understanding does not affect his cognitive conceptions . . . even when he is trained to use the advanced terminology. (p. 136)

Langer (1969) interprets Piaget as saying that during the latter part of the preoperational period there are parallel changes in mental operations and language. The development of mental operations does not occur as a result of speech. The conceptual meanings which the child has for his language are reconstructed from environmental sources to be in accord with his developmental level. He utilizes or transforms meanings to conform with his existing schemes. Thus Piaget's belief is that cognitive development is an autonomous achievement based on its structure and function, whereas systems such as language and perception are "subordinate to intelligence" and can be influenced by factors such as maturation, experience, and social communication. Piaget does not see language as playing a central role in the development of the child's cognition. The child may utilize the correct grammatical forms before he has comprehended the logical operations on which the language is based.

Stendler (1969) in the films *Classification* and *Conservation*, in which children are tested with Piaget tasks, notes that the children give the right answer for the wrong reasons. They have acquired the language without having developed the cognitive foundations on which the answers are based. "Piaget's studies proved that grammar develops before logic and that the child learns relatively late the mental operations corresponding to the verbal forms he has been using for a long time" (Vygotsky 1962.)

CONCEPT FORMATION AND LANGUAGE

Concepts are part of the central or mediational aspects of schemes. As such the processes of concept formation constitute some of the intellectual work of cognition, a part which Furth calls "active knowing." Concepts reduce the complexity of sense data by categorizing the diversity of objects and events with which the individual must deal (Bruner, Goodnow, and Austin, 1956).

Werner and Kaplan (1963) observed that in the development of the child's concepts there is an increasing movement away from the concrete, perceptual motor experience out of which the concepts are originally created toward a grouping of classes of an abstract nature. This development is reflected in the child's definitions of words. At one stage a child's definitions are concrete and context-bound, for example *orange* might be defined as "you eat it." After considerable development definitions reflect the more abstract grouping of classes of concepts; the child is then able to say, "An orange is a citrus fruit."

Vygotsky (1962) points out that early in a child's concept development, when he is developing a vocabulary, his concepts are pseudoconcepts. Outwardly they appear to be similar to adult concepts, but they are radically different. Since adults cannot impart concepts to a child, concepts are autonomous achievements of the child himself. The adult supplies instead ready-made word meanings around which the child builds a pseudoconcept. The ready-made meanings are of a denotative type, naming an objective reference. These words aid in the communication between the child and the adult, but abstract qualities and connotative meanings of the words are absent. As Vygotsky says, "The child's and adult's words coincide in their referents but not in their meanings."

Brown (1973) refers to speech used by the child which is based on pseudoconcepts as *randomly adaptive*. Adults must project meaning into the speech from a knowledge of the child's background and from the context of the situation. They double check their responses through expansions of the child's utterances.

According to Bruner (1960) concept development is an inventive and creative process concerned with the coding aspects of classifying and categorizing the input data into a coding system. Bruner says that "the coding system is the person's manner of grouping and relating information about his world and it is constantly subject to change and reorganization."

Miller (1956), in his fascinating article *The Magical Number Seven Plus or Minus Two*, explains how the severe limitation of the human brain for storing information is overcome by recoding of information employing a verbal code. He says, "Our language is tremendously useful for repackaging material into a few chunks rich in information. The abstract concepts, with their classification and reclassification of data, given language labels are the very lifeblood of the thought processes."

OTHER POINTS OF VIEW

Church (1961) takes an extreme point of view on the importance that language development has on the individual.

> We must emphasize that language is not just one function among many. One does not speak in the same sense that he walks, or eats, or makes love. Language is an all-pervasive characteristic of the individual, such that he becomes a verbal organism whose walking, eating, love-making, and the rest are altered in keeping with his symbolic experience" (p. 94).

Thus Church feels that once language is learned, the individual's behavior is gradually transformed in all of its characteristics because the underlying mediating behavior has become symbolically directed. He emphasizes that language is both a means of education and, in contrast to Piaget's thinking, a vehicle for cognitive development once it has been learned. Adults . . . "impart typical verbal operations which he (the child) takes over and uses for himself: making comparisons, passing judgment, pretending the contrary of what is so, narration, generalizing, exaggerating, wishing, classification, hypothesizing, and so forth" (p. 108).

Both Vygotsky (1962) and Luria (1961) have written about the directive function of the child's inner language on behavior and the control of expressive behaviors. This type of verbal mediation brings behavior under control of cognitive processes. This point of view is similar to that of the psychoanalytic writer, Rapaport (1951). He differentiates the sensorimotor nonverbal thought as being a primary process. The child's behavior is ruled by his impulses. As the child's cognitive and language abilities increase, his behavior is brought under a secondary process, which is verbally mediated. The child's behavior is more in tune with environmental demands. His use of his cognitive abilities to control behavior is called *reality testing*.

COGNITIVE DEFICITS

Cognitive dysfunctions may be revealed in low scores on intelligence tests, tests of abstraction, categorization, and concept formation. Piaget-type tasks are also revealing of cognitive development or retardation. Behaviorally, distortions in concepts of time, space, and identity result from cognitive malfunctioning.

MENTAL RETARDATION

Cognitive deficits are one characteristic of mentally retarded persons. The group is a heterogeneous one in terms of the origins of the problems and adaptive levels. Schiefelbusch (1972) feels that the cognitive deficits should be regarded as a failure of the child or adult in developing learning sets or learning how to learn. These cognitive deficits make subsequent learning difficult. Schiefelbusch is also in agreement with Vygotsky that the failure in the language area is a contributing factor to the cognitive retardation.

Siegel (1964) cautions us not to utilize intelligence test scores as an explanation for language deficits. It is not correct to say that speech problems result from low intelligence, since intelligence is a descriptive term rather than an explanatory concept.

Spreen (1965, 1966) reviewed the research literature on cognition in mental retardation and found that the great diversity in the population requires a somewhat generalized picture of their cognition. He reports that studies on the cognitive abilities of this group have led writers to conclude that the children are deficient in what he calls the abstract attitude. They manifest concreteness of behavior such as would be found on the sensorimotor and preoperational levels. Nonverbal forms of mediation predominate. Rigidity of behavior is indicated by an inability to consider more than one factor at a time and an inability to shift from one thing to another. Deficiencies in verbal mediation were found in a number of studies. Mentally retarded children are inferior to normals on tasks requiring verbal mediation, even when the children are matched on the basis of mental age with younger normals. Their abilities in the verbal sphere tend to be retarded more than in other cognitive areas.

Woodward (1959) tested 147 children aged 7 to 16 years who were severely or profoundly retarded, using Piaget-type tasks. She found the levels of responses mirrored those which Piaget found with normal infants and further that the operations used by the retardates were consistent with their developmental levels.

CHILDHOOD PSYCHOSES

A diagnosis of psychosis, schizophrenia, or autism in children indicates serious cognitive involvement. It appears that the cognitive breakdowns are at the very core of childhood psychoses. The children do not seem to have mastered the stages of development as outlined by Piaget. Bettelheim (1967) writes, "To discuss fully the many parallels between our findings on infantile autism, and those of Piaget on the intellectual development of children would again make voluminous reading" (p. 443). He points out the breakdowns in assimilation and accommodation and illustrates with case studies the faulty development of schemes of permanence of objects, time, space, and causality. Goldfarb, Mintz, and Stroock (1969) discuss the lack of development of essential adaptive functions and the primitivity in the content of the child's causal thinking. Goldfarb's case of the 7-year-old boy Peter is a good illustration of the latter.

Peter, a 7-year-old schizophrenic child who had just washed himself in preparation for lunch, commented to his child care worker, "Is it night time?" He had looked out the window and noted that the sky was darkening, signaling an impending storm. Despite reassurances from the worker that it was not night, Peter persisted in his belief and became increasingly fearful as the sky continued to darken. The worker explained that it was still daytime and that the cloudy sky indicated rain. Peter cried fearfully, "But it's dark out so it must be night." Correcting his error, the worker once again commented that it was daytime and then in an attempt to reorient him to the day, she outlined the activities of lunch and school which would soon follow.

Peter's reasoning, "But it's dark out, so it must be night," is an example of transductive reasoning which is characteristic of the preoperational stage, age 2 to 4 years. It is a reasoning by analogy. A is like B in one respect; therefore A must be like B in other respects. It is dark out; since it is dark at night, it must be night. In this type of preconceptual thinking the child reasons from the particular to the particular.

Halpern (1966) studied a 15-year-old psychotic boy who had been found to be of normal intelligence on a number of standardized intelligence tests. Yet when he was given the Piaget tasks, he was found to be functioning well below his chronological age and revealed a primitivity in thinking in certain areas. His responses to the concept of life were precausal in nature and the content of his cognition indicated animistic thinking. Although the intelligence test scores seemed to indicate adequate intellectual development, his responses to Piaget tests placed him at a level below the stage of formal operations in some areas.

Kates and Kates (1964) reviewed a number of research studies on the concept formation and categorization abilities of psychotic children. All the studies showed serious cognitive deficits in their use of narrow and in adequate categories and idiosyncratic categorization with bizarre content. The authors concluded that these cognitive deficits represent a lower adaptive functioning of the children.

Disturbances of thought are reflected in speech. The child may possess a large and complex vocabulary, yet not be able to combine the words into usable sentences. He may show echolalia, bizarre and irrelevant word choice, pronominal reversals, madeup words, logorrhea (oral diarrhea), confusion, inhibitions, and blocking. Speech may cease in the middle of a thought, only to be resumed with an apparently unrelated subject. All of these reveal severe distortions and disorganization of the thought processes. They result from breakdowns in cognitive awareness of reality and especially breakdowns in the function of synthesis. At the same time these thought disturbances reflect idiosyncrasies in the use of the linguistic code which impairs communication.

INSTITUTIONALIZED INFANTS

In the 1940s attention was draw to a group of children who had suffered emotional and cognitive breakdowns as a result of varying periods of institutionalization during early infancy (Spitz, 1946). The children had been placed in hospitals or orphanage nurseries immediately following birth or after a period of weeks or months with their natural mothers. The deleterious effects of separation from the mother or from the impersonal care they received in an antiseptic, nonstimulating environment ranged from death after a wasting-away disease to retardation in cognition and language. A film entitled *Maternal Deprivation in Young Children* (1952) shows a number of such children up to the age of 5. They appear to be functioning at the sensorimotor level of development. They were physically stunted in growth and showed little evidence of intellectual and language development.

The findings of numerous studies tend to emphasize the importance for proper cognitive and language development of both emotional relationships and intellectual stimulation during the critical early years. Deprivation of these experiences may result in intellectual retardation with specific defects in perception, memory, concept formation, schemes of time and space, and language (Goldfarb, 1955).

LEARNING DISABILITIES

Wiig and Semel's (1973) study of children with learning disabilities showed that they had cognitive defects especially in the ability to use and understand the logical operations which underly certain grammatical forms. Other investigators, such as De Hirsch (1957), Johnson and Myklebust (1967), and Lerner (1976), have reported dysfunctions in the skills of concept formation and its components of abstraction and generalization.

Moorhead and Ingram (1973) report several studies of language retarded children who were given Piaget-type tasks. In the studies by Inhelder (1966) and Ajuriaguerra (1966) the children had normal operative or base intelligence, but they showed disturbances in the area of representational mediation, as shown in language, delayed imitation, imagery, and symbolic play. These studies suggest that children with learning disabilities do not develop in a bizarre fashion, but rather development proceeds with a normal sequence, with delayed onset and at a slower rate. These conclusions are in sharp contrast with those of Moran (1975) to which we referred in Chapter 3. She reported that the children she studied were using different morphologic rules from those of their normal counterparts.

PSYCHOANALYTIC THEORY

Freud's theory of psychoanalysis as a theory of personality and a theory for therapy for emotional disturbances is still being utilized today. Its development has been continuous and there have been adjustments and revisions of the theory as a result of research. When these alterations are incorporated, the theory is considered to be neo-Freudian. Freud and the neo-Freudians have provided us with the most meaningful approach to the study of emotional development of the individual, and the theory has been particularly helpful in explaining breakdowns in development such as neuroses and psychoses. We shall be applying this theory to speech and hearing.

THE PSYCHODYNAMIC MEDICAL MODEL OF PATHOLOGY

Psychoanalytic theory was developed out of the clinical experiences of Freud in Vienna in the 1890s. Because the theory evolved out of Freud's medical practice with severely emotionally disturbed individuals, it places a strong emphasis on explaining the pathological forms of personality as they would be found in psychiatric practice. The theory explains psychopathology by utilizing a form of the medical model. As we have seen earlier, the medical model utilizes concepts derived from the diagnosis and treatment of diseases of the body. The physician assumes that the signs of illness that he observes are the result of an underlying disease process which must be differentiated carefully from similar diseases by means of a differential diagnosis. The patient's complaints are merely symptoms of the underlying process and the treatment must be directed toward the elimination of the disease rather than the surface symptoms of the disease. If the treatment is successful, the symptoms will disappear without direct therapy on the symptoms.

In applying the medical model to emotional disturbances, Freud reasoned by analogy. The patient presents complaints which are disturbing to him and which he believes are the emotional disturbance itself, but careful, diagnostic study by the psychiatrist will reveal an underlying conflict of which the patient is not aware. The patient's complaints are the symptoms of the underlying emotional disturbance. Treatment, especially in the early stages, concentrates on unearthing and giving the patient insight into the unconscious conflicts. Symptoms will disappear when the conflict has been resolved. We have labeled this view of psychopathology the psychodynamic medical model of pathology.

In recent years there has been considerable disenchantment with this conceptualization of emotional disturbances. The idea of *mental* illness which it evokes is an anathema to some psychiatrists and psychologists.

BASIC ASSUMPTIONS

The set of assumptions on which psychoanalytic theory is based center on the concept of multiple determination of behavior (Rapaport, 1960). The psychoanalytic view is that the behavior of the individual at any given time may be explained on the basis of a number of determinants. All behaviors, despite differences in magnitude, no matter how trivial or serious, simple or complex, have an underlying cause or determinant. No behavior, from suicide to a slip of the tongue, is spontaneous, without stimulus or cause.

LEVELS OF CONSCIOUSNESS

It is possible for behavior to stem from any level—from deeply unconscious to superficially conscious. Thus, the individual may have varying degrees of awareness of the reasons for his behavior, whether it is normal or abnormal. The most crucial determinants are thought to be unconscious. Neurotic behavior is determined by conflicts of which the individual is not aware. If we consider stuttering to be a neurosis, which is the prevalent view of psychoanalysts, the stutterer himself is not aware of the underlying reasons for his stuttering. The conflict basis of his behavior is unconscious.

THE CRITICAL PERIOD ASSUMPTION

The underlying neurotic conflicts as well as all determinants of psychic life are assumed to have their origins during the earliest stages of life, especially during the first five years of childhood. The person is most vulnerable to conflict during this critical period for personality formation. Experiences during the critical period of life are still operative and influence all subsequent behavior on into adulthood. The critical experiences around which conflicts develop are the interpersonal relationships which accompany feeding, cleanliness training, sexual training, and the control of aggression.

PSYCHOSEXUAL DEVELOPMENT

Freud outlined the critical periods of development of the personality. His sequence describes the way the individual personality unfolds through stages to reach its goal of adult maturity. The complex theory has been modified and now takes into account biological, psychological, and cultural factors.

In addition to critical periods in psychosexual development Freud postulated that there are critical zones of the body that are invested with libido (sexual-type energy) and around which the major events of development are centered. The following is a brief overview of the stages of development. From birth until about the first birthday the infant is in the *oral stage*. It is named because the libidinal pleasure is experienced when the region of the mouth is stimulated. Initially there is pleasure in sucking, and later in biting and in other oral activities. Mother-child interpersonal relations during feeding and other activities are of great significance. Adequate mothering with a fusion of gratification of needs and sufficient tolerable frustration leads to normal development and the establishment of a life-long trust in other people. The quality and quantity of mothering at this and subsequent stages is influenced by the following factors: (1) biological factors such as the physical health of the child and mother; (2) the mutual interaction of the child's temperamental endowment and the mother's personality; (3) the child rearing practices dictated by the culture as well as the stability of the culture itself. The degree of the mother's identification with the culture and her socializing effects on the child will influence how well he or she adapts to the society at that and subsequent stages.

Breakdowns in development at this stage are thought to be caused by excessive oral gratification, excessive frustration, or an alternation between the two. Development may cease partially or totally, and this arrest in development is called *fixation*.

During the second year of life there is a shift of interest, and the child enters the *anal stage*. He or she derives libidinal pleasure from holding on and letting go of feces. This is the period when the mother begins toilet training of the child and the child asserts the need for autonomy. These factors add up to a possible interpersonal struggle between mother and child. One child development film has referred to this period as "terrible two's." Proper handling of this period leads to the establishment of a sense of autonomy in the child that stems in part from the mastery over his or her own bowels. Failure leads to the development of feelings of shame and doubt about the self with symptoms of obsessiveness and compulsivity about cleanliness and punctuality. These may be generalized to all facets of the thought processes. Severe breakdowns may result in *regression*—a return to the behaviors that were more appropriate in an earlier developmental stage when the child experienced more success.

From age 3 to approximately 5 years the child's interest centers around the genital zone, which becomes endowed with sexual energy. This is the *phallic stage*. Freud postulated that during this stage of budding sexuality the child experiences the Oedipus complex. This is a fantasied love relationship with the parent of the opposite sex and a competitive ambivalent desire to be rid of the parent of the same sex. After some vagaries, including a threat of castration and abandonment the Oedipus complex passes and the child identifies with the parent of the same sex. Identification involves a transformation of the self to become like the loved or feared person and includes a simulation of attitudes, values, and behaviors. Hence, with the resolution of the Oedipus complex the child internalizes the social values and carries social control within. This frees the child to develop initiative, imagination, and creativity. Failure at this stage leads to feelings of guilt and inadeqacies in sexual identity. The pregenital period—the oral, anal, and phallic stages which we have discussed—seems to be the most critical for personality formation both in its normal and abnormal aspects.

There are two additional stages, latency and genital stages. During the school years until puberty no new zone emerges and the child is in a period of *latency*. All sexual energies become available in sublimated form to be used in learning and other social activities. Achievement in the school areas instills a sense of accomplishment. On the other hand, speech, language and other learning disabilities at this stage may engender feelings of inferiority which could color all subsequent stages of life.

The *genital stage*, which has several substages, begins during adolescence. Adult genital sexuality emerges at this time. Adequate interpersonal experiences based on a foundation of success at earlier stages leads to a sense of identity in an adult role in society.

Application of a psychoanalytic theory of psychosexual development to speech and language pathologies has been made by a number of speech pathologists and other writers. Wyatt (1969) has shown the relationship between language disturbances and stuttering to breakdowns during the pregenital stages of development. Travis (1957) and Glauber (1958) discussed stuttering and pregenital neuroses. Rousey (1969) and Rousey and Moriarty (1965) have demonstrated that specific voice and articulation problems may be traced to conflicts arising during each stage of development. Shervanian (1967) has explained certain aspects of pathological speech and language found in childhood psychoses as fixations and regressions in psychosexual development.

DRIVES, ENERGY, AND ADAPTATION

The psychoanalytic theory postulates that there are forces within the individual which are called *drives*. These drives or needs constitute the motivation for action toward a goal. Behavior is pictured as being determined by drives. The drives are of a sexual and aggressive nature or derivatives of these. Conflicts can occur between the components of the individual's personality or when the drives meet thwarting demands from the society.

Drives are assumed to have psychic *energy* at their disposal to spark the action toward an object or goal. The drive energy is directed toward or invested in a loved or hated object. The fulfilment of a goal results in a discharge of energy, whereupon the individual feels a tension (energy) reduction which is pleasurable. If the drive energy cannot be directed toward or invested in an object because of conflict or unavailability of the object, the person experiences the heightened tension as painful anxiety. He is then in a state of disequilibrium.

Attempts of the individual to achieve equilibrium within the self and between the self and the environment are aspects of a process of adaptation. Behavior is determined by the efforts toward adaptation. The social and cultural demands of physical reality which are made on the individual thus become determinants of behavior.

THE PSYCHIC STRUCTURE

The personality is said to be organized into hypothetical structures called the id, the ego, and the superego.

The Id. The id is totally unconscious. It is the source of the basic instinctual drives of the person. There are two basic drives—the sexual or libido and the aggressive or death instinct. The drives are characterized as having source of energy or excitation, and an aim or direction toward an object (person or thing). When the aim of the drive is achieved, there is a reduction in the drive tension and this is experienced as pleasurable. If the tension is maintained, the experience is one of pain. The id operates in terms of the *pleasure principle*, that is, the demand for immediate gratification of needs.

Since the id is unconscious, it utilizes images and symbols that are nonverbal. Most of the symbols are private, although some are socially derived. The operation of the id is a *primary process*, that is, it is independent of logical rules for the manipulation of concepts of time, space, identity, and causality. Opposite feelings and meanings, such as love and hate, can exist side by side toward the same person.

Since many of the psychological determinants of behavior are found in the id, it follows that many feelings and actions have irrational sources that are not known to the individual.

THE SUPEREGO. The superego represents the internalized values, restrictions, moral demands, and ideals of the society. These are partially conscious and partially unconscious. The superego includes what is commonly called the conscience. The values of the society are learned from the parents and other agents of socialization in the community, such as teachers and religious leaders, very early in life. This learning keeps sexual and aggressive drives in line with the dictates of society.

When the individual manifests behavior which runs counter to these internalized values, he experiences feelings of guilt or shame.

THE EGO. The ego is a structure which serves as a mediator between the drives of the id, the controls of the superego, and the demands of reality. It operates in a *secondary process* fashion, employing all the logical processes at its disposal. In its function as mediator between the id and the external environment, the ego cannot utilize the immediate need gratification of the pleasure principle. Instead it operates in terms of the *reality principle*, that is, delayed gratification through postponement, substitution, or other compromises.

The three major functions of the ego are: (1) cognitive appraisal of reality, (2) synthesis of behavior, and (3) selection of responses. We will consider these and their speech and language components.

COGNITIVE APPRAISAL OF REALITY

The developmental stage of the individual's ego structures will determine how well he appraises reality, since, according to Piaget (Ginsberg and Opper, 1969), "reality is determined by the structures with which it is apprehended." For example, the reality of money varies with each stage of development. Money for the 2-year-old in the anal stage is something to play with or even tear up in a destructive way. To a 6-year-old in the latency stage it represents a means to purchase candy to share with peers. To a 19-year-old it is something to use as a down payment on a car, an object that is both useful and enhancing of his social image.

One's appraisal of the environment requires perceptive discrimination and judgment, faculties that take a long time to develop. It is necessary for the ego to select from the myriad of stimuli in the environment those things which have significance to the self, to abstract the relevant material from the irrelevant, and to counteract the distractions within and outside the self because of aggression. Thus cognitive appraisal of physical reality includes judgments about those things in the world which are potentially beneficial, sources of gratification, or self-enhancing. Conversely, the ego must be aware of those things in the physical environment which are potentially dangerous. The perception of the act of driving at breakneck speed down a highway as gratifying or self-enhancing may be the result of an ego defect; this repression of the facts of mortality may very well create a situation in which no further learning about reality can take place.

The ability to discriminate between constructive and destructive events and actions involves judgments about cause and effect relationships. It also has components of time and space. Thus the ego's appraisal of physical reality must include concepts of time, space, and causality. In this regard there is an overlapping with Piagetian theory. However, psychoanalytic writers explore these concepts not only in terms of their influence on adaptation, but also in terms of their conscious and unconscious components and their relationship to drives or motives.

Cognitive appraisal also includes awareness and judgments about social reality. This involves knowledge of the social institutions of role, status, family, education, religion, and law, as well as the social mores. Knowledge of these institutions and the variety of interactions that are possible with them is extremely important for proper adaptation. As we shall see later, each of these social institutions has its own language and communicative norms. Adequate functioning within a society requires awareness about which actions are socially appropriate and which would cause social ostracism and punishment.

Cognitive appraisal of the reality of the self is yet another aspect of the ego's judgment function, a requisite for adaptation. *To thine own self be true* is quite meaningless if it is not accompanied by self-awareness. Self-knowledge must precede integrity. This means knowledge of one's own self as a sentient being, acting autonomously from others and from the environment. It includes awareness of the body's physical needs for food, elimination, heat and cold avoidance. It especially means cognizance of the emotional needs for sexuality and aggression. The concept of the body and its separateness from others is a prerequisite for the development of communication.

SOME FACTORS OF LANGUAGE AND CONCEPT FORMATION WHICH INFLUENCE APPRAISAL OF REALITY

Language and communication play important roles in the adaptive function of cognitive appraisal of reality. The relationship of language and cognition previously discussed applies also to the development of cognition in the task of conceptualizing reality. In addition there are these factors.

Validation of Concepts of Reality. How does the child or adult know that the concepts he utilizes for appraising reality are valid? Since these concepts serve as the basis for selecting his behavioral responses, the concepts must be in tune with social and physical reality for adequate adaptation. Language and communication probably lead to the validation of the individual's concepts and their subsequent behavior. The verbal prohibitions, guidance, and encouragement serve to shape the individual's concepts of reality with a specificity that would otherwise be impossible. Reality concepts are relative to the culture in which they are formed. Checking concepts of reality in terms of the behavioral consequences leads to a consentual agreement about concepts and brings them in line with those shared by others in the society. In this way the individual does not have too many private or idiosyncratic concepts. Unfortunately, if this socialization process is carried too far, it stifles creative thinking. Private concepts may be seminal for creativity in science, art, and literature.

Facilitation of the Mastery of Complex Parts of Reality. Bettelheim (1967) points out that "the more complex parts of reality are best mastered through language" and that "ego growth depends on correct concept formation based on language." The formation of language or verbal concepts allows the individual to become aware of reality far beyond anything he could achieve through the use of sensory and perceptual information. While the sensory input of data has importance initially for the child to allow him to make contact with the environment, symbolic and finally verbal symbolic concepts allow the child to go beyond the raw sensory data.

The statement of Bettelheim that the more complex parts of reality are mastered through language has profound implications for communicative disorders. Helen Keller, without sight and hearing, achieved a keen appreciation of social and physical reality once she had developed a symbolic language through her tactile sense. In her autobiography (Keller, 1936) she clearly reveals that the discovery of symbolization was one of the most dramatic moments of her life.

Stabilization and Orientation of Perceptions. Language helps the child in his adaptation to reality by stabilizing his perceptions and by verbal orientation to surroundings. Rapaport (1951) notes that labeling of perceptions, especially for the child between the ages of 2 and 4, tends to mobilize attention, stabilize the perceptions and aids in the categorization and classification of things. The *naming game* has implications for bringing the child into a keener awareness of the physical and social environment and of his own body. Furthermore, this process of labeling lays the foundation for true concept formation.

Luria (1961) studied 5- to 7-year-old children in problem-solving situations. He found that they employed a type of talking to the self in which they identified things and relationships in the environment that would help them out of their difficulty. He called this use of egocentric speech a verbal orientation to surroundings.

The Influence of Repression. Repression is a defense mechanism which can influence the perception of reality and the recall of memories in such a way as to keep the individual from cognitive awareness of aspects of external and internal reality. Repression can lead to ignorance of significant knowledge of the self and the environment and result in maladaption in the behavior of an otherwise intelligent individual. It can work to prevent the validation of concepts and behavior in interpersonal relationships. Knowledge, presented by others through language in social, educational, or psychotherapeutic communication, may help to overcome the blocks in perception and memory which repression can establish within the self (Rapaport, 1951).

However, knowledge alone is insufficient. A person might be able to catalogue all kinds of information about himself and reality and still adapt inadequately. What is needed is knowledge applied in an insightful and emotionally meaningful fashion to the totality of the personality.

Identification of Symbolic Forms. Dollard and Miller (1950) describe a variety of symbolic forms which are in varying degrees connected with language and memory. They feel that these symbolic forms exist at a number of levels of consciousness, from deeply unconscious to fully conscious. The determining factor in level of consciousness according to them is the degree to which the symbols have been made into language symbols. Full consciousness is only possible with language.

Since the adaptive behavior of the individual is influenced by these forms, whether conscious or unconscious, the person may be symbolizing things that influence his actions without being aware of the source of these influences. The source of a great deal of maladaptive or neurotic behavior is not known to the individual himself. Dollard and Miller contend that a major part of psychotherapy has to do with providing the patient with proper labels and sentences "which will match the events going on within and without him." With new vocabulary and sentences for formerly unconscious material, the individual will be able to employ higher mental precesses such as reasoning for solving the conflicts which produce his maladaptive behavior. Thus, language and labels will make the individual more cognitively aware of the reality of the self and the environment.

Dollard and Miller recognize the following symbolic forms as determinants of behavior. (1) Rational verbal thought is the subject and product of higher cognitive processes. The person is fully aware and can use formal operations for problem solving. (2) Isolated verbal fragments are bits and pieces of things and ideas remembered by the individual, but they are not coherently organized and remain incomplete and unconnected. Labels are necessary to organize these fragments and make them available to the individual. (3) Screen memories are also fragments of thought, but they are unlabeled memories based on sensorimotor enactive images that were experienced before language was learned. These primitive thoughts need labeling, since they may be the source of much neurotic conflict. (4) Emotional and operant responses are triggered by memories of specific environmental events that have not been labeled. The person is aware of his responses to specific events, but not the reason for his emotions or actions. The responses have become disconnected from their origins. These need labeling. (5) Lost symptoms are responses which are symbolic of underlying conflict but the person is not aware of what has triggered the memory or symptom. These too need labeling. (6) Dreams or nonlanguage memories have their sources in past or present experiences. The person is not aware of their underlying meaning for they are not labeled. They have idiosyncratic meanings and are condensed and syncretic.

SYNTHESIS OF BEHAVIOR

The synthetic function of the ego is primarily an adaptive function. Through its processes of organization, integration and differentiation of cognitive structures, affective needs, and social values, it brings about an equilibrium of the structures within the individual and with his environment.

Rapaport (1951) indicates that language plays an important role in the synthetic processes since so much of the work of synthesis utilizes verbal conceptual symbols. Language is an efficient means by which new information and experiences, which are the raw materials for concepts, are acquired and also the medium which lends itself to codification into highly abstract verbal concepts.

The synthetic processes of the ego are, of course, not subject to direct inspection. We become aware of the end result when the child or adult achieves a new level of adaptive equilibrium. Spitz (1957) calls the resultant signs of adaptive equilibrium *indicators*. They include such things as the smiling response at 3 months of age, showing that the infant is "aware" that there are things outside of the self; the meaningful use of *no* against the mother at 15 months of age, indicating that the child is beginning to develop the rudiments of concept formation.

Breakdowns of the synthetic processes are easily seen in the regression and dedifferentiation which accompany the "falling to pieces" of the personality.

SELECTION OF RESPONSES

Another function of the ego is the selection of responses. The individual, in addition to being cognitively aware of reality, must select responses in each situation from his behavioral repertoire. We noted earlier that behavior is determined by a large number of factors. We will be concerned with those that are influenced by the ego.

Some responses have become so automatized that they require no conscious thought, but most responses are chosen with varying degrees of awareness. Higher mental functions may be involved in the selection of carefully reasoned behaviors with consideration being given to all components of reality. Or the selection of a response may be impulsive and based on the wish for immediate need gratification. Redl and Wineman (1951) identify two types of responses: reality based and defensively based.

All responses, including reality based ones, utilize some degree of defensive processes. However, reality based defenses have socially learned goals. For example, in the process of socialization which continues throughout life the individual learns to inhibit and modify needs which may not be immediately acceptable. The individual must learn to substitute for things that are socially prohibited. He must learn patterns of behavior, physical and emotional, as well as the timing of these behaviors, so as to fit into the society (Kluckhohn and Murray, 1950).

The process of utilizing socially acceptable behaviors with proper timing is called sublimation. Sublimation is a process of giving up direct expression of basic drives in exchange for cultural achievements which are valued. Most of our educational systems are geared to teaching the child sublimation of needs in favor of social learning.

Table 5–2 lists ego defenses. In general they are employed by the individual when he perceives a threatening situation. These responses are based on an attempt to avoid anxiety. Defensive responses are learned early in life and tend to become habitual in response to any threat of anxiety or feelings of guilt. Defensive responses may be symptomatic of underlying neurotic conflicts.

As the child learns language, it aids in the development of social control of be-

Table 5–2. Mechanisms of ego defense.

1. *Identification:* Transformation of the self by unconsciously adopting the behavior, attitudes, feelings, and other attributes of a loved or hated person.
2. *Incorporation:* The taking of something in orally and making it a part of the self.
3. *Repression:* A psychically motivated forgetting in order to exclude from consciousness thoughts that are too painful to face.
4. *Undoing:* Behavior usually ritualistic that is intended to prevent, avoid, or atone for impulses or thoughts which are not acceptable.
5. *Intellectualization:* The isolation of the emotional significance of an experience by dealing only with the cognitive or intellectual aspects of it.
6. *Regression:* A return to a more primitive form of behavior when activities or development have thwarted or threatened the individual.
7. *Fixation:* Behavior that stems from an earlier stage and results from a cessation in development.
8. *Displacement:* Gratification of an emotional need by shifting it toward someone or something which is more available and less anxiety-provoking.
9. *Reaction Formation:* Disguising of an unacceptable motive by adopting behavior that is the opposite of what is wished.
10. *Projection:* The attributing of unacceptable impulses to others in order to avoid accepting them as part of the self.
11. *Sublimation:* The discharge of an unacceptable drive by adopting indirect, socially approved behavior.

havior. The language itself is a socially learned response and a medium for learning more about reality and facilitating the selection of responses. There is an increasing richness in responses mediated through language.

NEUROSIS

Neurotic conflict results when the ego employs habitual patterns of repression against unacceptable sexual or aggressive id drives to prevent their discharge. Feelings of anxiety, shame, and guilt may be experienced when the repression is not entirely successful, as is often the case. The individual is not aware of the reasons for these feelings since the underlying conflict is unconscious.

The background for neurotic conflict is laid down in the earliest period of development—during the oral, anal, and phallic periods. Partial fixations and regressions in development at these stages are centered around conflicts in the feeding situation, toilet training, sexual training, and control of aggressive behavior.

Neurotic behavior is expressed in one or more of the following ways (Dollard and Miller, 1950).

1. The person expresses feelings of unhappiness and misery and seems to get little satisfaction out of life. He feels frustrated and thwarted in his actions.

2. When the behavior of the individual is examined, some actions, especially in interpersonal situations, appear to be not in his best interests. Yet he does not know why he persists in these actions for he is an otherwise intelligent individual.

3. The individual may have general feelings of anxiety, guilt, or shame. Once again he is not aware of why he has these feelings for they are without any objective source.

4. The individual may employ a pattern of defensive mechanisms whenever he feels the threat of anxiety. These defensive responses become organized into a habitual cluster and become identified as the overt personality characteristics of the individual.
5. The individual may show defensive behaviors which are likely to be identified as symptoms of disturbance. These vary with the type of conflict and the age of the individual. They include: eating and sleeping problems, phobias, bed wetting, stealing, tics, excessive shyness, bullying, psychosomatic illnesses, and speech and hearing problems.

SYMPTOMS OF NEUROSIS

Symptoms of neurosis are an indirect result of unconscious conflict and are frequently symbols of the underlying conflict. They may be read as a type of language. For example, mutism may be found in children who are physically competent to speak. When children of this type and their mothers were examined by Wilcox (1956) psychoanalytically, he discovered that the symptom was unconsciously chosen by the child and unconsciously encouraged by the mother in order to avoid destructive communication between them. The interpersonal relationship between mother and child was so impaired that hostile use of speech could have completely severed the relationship. By not speaking the mother and child could continue the relationship, and the child would receive the maternal care he needed.

This study illustrates another component of symptoms. Every symptom of conflict is a mechanism of adaptation to the environment. Mutism represents a neurotic adaptation, but it may be the only possible adaptation at a time within the mother-child relationship.

There are three other aspects of symptoms which are especially germaine to communicative disorders. They answer the question as to why the neurotic may continue to manifest symptoms despite his conscious wish to be rid of them because of the negative social reactions they elicit. First, symptoms develop in response to anxiety and at the same time serve to reduce it partially. Tension reduction reinforces the symptomatic behavior.

Second, despite all the negative reactions to symptoms there are some positive reactions, referred to as secondary gain, which partially outweigh the negative. For example, symptoms call attention to the differences of the individual so that he stands out from others. They may also be a source of extra attention. The child with stuttering symptoms may be treated deferentially.

Third, symptoms may be maintained because they have become habitual or automatized. It is possible for symptoms to be perpetuated long after the neurotic conflict that brought them into being has been resolved. This concept of the functional autonomy of motives and autonomatization may explain why stuttering once learned as a symptom becomes difficult to eradicate (Allport, 1937; Rapaport, 1951).

NEUROSIS AND SPEECH

A large number of studies have been summarized by Markel (1969) that show that the personality of the individual influences all aspects of his expression in speech and language. We might think of the variability we hear in speech and language as personality reflections of individual differences.

If we ask to what extent speech and language pathologies are symptoms of neurosis, the research provides almost no answers. Methodological problems and the inadequacy of standardized personality tests give confusing and ambiguous answers (Bloch and Goodstein, 1971). While the research seems to give little help, the vast clinical data indicate that there are some predictable connections between speech pathologies and neurosis. Neurotic breakdowns of speech are found primarily in the paralinguistic structures. The voice may reflect neurosis through aphonia (loss of voice); phonatory quality problems, especially of hoarseness; and pitch problems, particularly during adolescent mutations. Other problems include stuttering, mutism, and possibly articulation disorders.

Most neuroses affect the content of speech rather than its linguistic structure. They influence the attitudes, ideas, and feelings that are being verbally expressed. By comparison with other symptoms of neurosis, the speech mechanism is rarely involved in neurotic conflict. For any number of reasons the linguistic and auditory structures are resistant to noticeable breakdowns. We do not say they are never involved, for the clinical literature contains examples of such breakdowns. Nor do we mean that the function of the speech mechanism is not influenced by emotional states. Under conditions of anger, fear, and anxiety there are demonstrable changes in the cycle of breathing, pitch, quality, loudness, rate, resonance, and articulation. These emotional states affect the speech, but they are of a temporary nature and do not reflect the individual's habitual mode of speech.

There are, however, some severe neurotic emotional conflicts which involve the speech and hearing mechanism directly.

Neurotic Voice Disorders. Conversion neuroses belong to a class of psychosomatic illnesses. The physiological malfunction may be traced back to an unconscious emotional conflict. The individual cannot satisfactorily deal with a problem so he unconsciously chooses an illness as a method of coping. Thus, conversion symptoms of voice "provide a solution, unconsciously determined, to situations with which the patient cannot deal effectively in any other way" (Aronson, 1969).

Aronson gives protocols from the case of a 26-year-old policeman who developed aphonia as a conversion illness. He had had several previous occurrences from which he had recovered spontaneously. This time he found himself in a bind which he had not been able to verbalize. He disliked his work and wished to quit, but was reluctant to disappoint his parents who took pride in his work. Specific aspects of his work ran counter to his personality. Basically he was a "quiet, unaggressive person," who wanted to be liked by people. He experienced extreme discomfort when he had to reprimand pedestrians or ticket motorists. If they persisted in arguing with him, he would lose his temper, and when he did, he "shook and became livid with rage." The psychiatrist viewed the aphonia as a socially acceptable excuse for quitting his job.

Wolski and Wiley (1965) present a case report of a 14-year-old boy who was being treated for aphonia and other conditions by both a speech pathologist and a psychiatrist. The psychiatrist's report on the psychodynamics of the case stated that the boy's neurosis centered around ambivalent feelings of love and aggression toward his mother. He had been very close to his mother until he was 12, when these feelings gradually changed. He was able to express his negative and hostile feelings about her to the psychiatrist. "He expressed contempt for his mother together with some suspicion that in some way she had disposed of his father so that 'she could have me for herself' " (p. 72).

With the advent of puberty and the reemergence of the Oedipus complex, he feared that he might express his incestuous feelings toward his mother. His behavior changed to hostility in a reaction formation against prohibited sexual feelings. This was effective until his voice began to change and he became increasingly anxious. His aphonia at this point "represented a further attempt to deny forbidden sexual impulses which were to him symbolized by a deep bass voice" (p. 73).

Therapy, which successfully removed the voice symptom, was directed toward resolving the sexual and aggressive conflict and increasing masculine identification.

STUTTERING. Fenichel (1945) defines stuttering as a pregenital conversion neurosis. The term pregenital implies that the emotional conflicts are formed during the oral, anal, and oedipal periods of development. Glauber (1958) suggests that the neurotic conflict is revealed as a desire to speak and a fear of speaking. The stutterer fears that he will express primary process archaic meanings through his speech. These could include aggressive impulses, maschochistic impulses, voyeuristic expressions, simple desires to be loved, to be potent, to be castrated—all of which stem from the pregenital periods. Their expression is unacceptable to both ego and superego.

SUMMARY

A well-rounded approach to the psychological determinants of communicative disorders requires a background in the normal developmental aspects of speech, language, cognition, and personality. In addition we need to know the principles by which these components are learned. Since a global theory which will account for all of these factors does not exist, we have chosen to present three well-known theories: a learning, a cognitive, and a personality theory. Each of these helps us to gain a perspective on the psychological components of communicative disorders and suggests an approach to therapy.

Two models emerge from these theories—the behavioral-learning model and the psychodynamic medical model. Both of these working models are used in contemporary speech and hearing programs.

REFERENCES

Ajuriaguerra, J. D. Speech disorders in childhood. In C. Carterette (Ed.), *Brain function: Speech, language, and communication* (Vol. 3), Los Angeles: University of California Press, 1966.

Allport, G. *Personality*. New York: Holt, Rinehart & Winston, 1937.

Aronson, A. E. Speech pathology and symptom therapy in interdisciplinary treatment of psychogenic aphonia. *Journal of Speech and Hearing Disorders*, *34*, 321–341 (1969).

Bandura, A. *Principles of behavior modification*. New York: Holt, Rinehart & Winston, 1969.

Bettelheim, B. *The empty fortress*. New York: Free Press, 1967.

Bloch, F. and Goodstein, L. D. Functional speech disorders and personality. A decade of research. *Journal of Speech and Hearing Disorders, 36*, 295–314 (1971).

Bloodstein, O. Stuttering as an anticipatory struggle reaction. In J. Eisenson (Ed.), *Stuttering: A symposium*, New York: Harper & Row, 1958.

Brodbeck, A., and Irwin, O. C. The speech behavior of infants without families. *Child Development, 17*, 145–156 (1946).

Brown, R. *A first language. The early stages*. Cambridge, Mass.: Harvard University Press, 1973.

Bruner, J. S. *The Process of Education*. Cambridge, Mass.: Harvard University Press, 1960.

Bruner, J. S., et al. *Studies in cognitive growth*. New York: Wiley, 1966.

Bruner, J. S., Goodnow, J. J., and Austin, J. A. *A study of thinking*. New York: Wiley, 1956.

Carroll, J. B. *Language and thought*. Englewood Cliffs, N.J.: Prentice-Hall, 1964.

Church, J. *Language and the discovery of reality*. New York: Random House, 1961.

De Hirsch, K. Tests designed to discover potential reading difficulties at six year old level. *American Journal of Orthopsychiatry, 27*, 566–576 (1957).

Dollard, J., and Miller, N. E. *Personality and psychotherapy*. New York: McGraw Hill, 1950.

Dunlap, K. A revision of the fundamental law of habit formation. *Science, 37*, 360–362 (1928).

Fenichel, O. *The psychoanalytic theory of neurosis*. New York: Norton, 1945.

Flavell, J. H. *The developmental psychology of Jean Piaget*. New York: Van Nostrand Reinhold, 1963.

Furth, H. G. *Piaget and knowledge*. Englewood Cliffs, N.J.: Prentice-Hall, 1969.

Ginsberg, H., and Opper, S. *Piaget's theory of intellectual development*. Englewood Cliffs, N.J.: Prentice-Hall, 1969.

Glauber, I. P. The psychoanalysis of stuttering. In J. Eisenson (Ed.), *Stuttering: A symposium*, New York: Harper & Row, 1958.

Goldfarb, W. Emotional and intellectual consequences of psychological deprivation in infancy: A reevaluation. In P. H. Hoch and J. Zubin (Eds.), *Psychopathology of childhood*, New York: Grune & Stratton, 1955.

Goldfarb, W., Mintz, I., and Stroock, K. W. *A time to heal*. New York: International Universities, 1969.

Goldiamond, I. Stuttering and fluency as manipulable operant response classes. In L. Krasner and L. P. Ullman (Eds.), *Research in behavior modification*, New York: Holt Rinehart & Winston, 1965.

Halpern, E. Conceptual development in a schizophrenic boy. *Journal of the American Academy of Child Psychiatry, 5*, 66–74 (1966).

Ingham, R. J., and Andrews, G. Behavior therapy and stuttering. *Journal of Speech and Hearing Disorders, 38*, 405–441 (1973).

Inhelder, B. Cognitive development and its contributions to the diagnosis of some phenomena of mental deficiency. *Merrill-Palmer Quarterly, 19*, 299–319 (1966).

Johnson, D. J., and Myklebust, H. R. *Learning disabilities: Educational principles and practices*. New York: Grune & Stratton, 1967.

Johnson, W., et al. *The onset of stuttering*. Minneapolis, Minn.: University of Minnesota Press, 1959.

Johnson, W., et al. *Speech handicapped school children*. New York: Harper & Row, 1967.

Kagan, J. A developmental approach to conceptual growth. In H. J. Kansmeier and C. W. Harris (Eds.), *Analysis of concept learning*, New York: Academic, 1966.

Kates, W., and Kates, S. Conceptual behavior in psychotic and normal adolescents. *Journal of Abnormal and Social Psychology, 69*, 659–663 (1964).

Keller, H. *The story of my life*. Garden City: Doubleday, 1936.

Kluckhohn, C., and Murray, H. A. *Personality in nature, society, and culture*. New York: Knopf, 1950.

Langer, J. *Theories of development*. New York: Holt, Rinehart & Winston, 1969.

Leeper, R. Cognitive processes. In S. S. Stevens (Ed.), *Handbook of experimental psychology*, New York: Wiley, 1951.

Lerner, J. *Children with learning disabilities*. Boston: Houghton Mifflin, 1976.

Lovaas, O. I. A program for the establishment of speech in psychotic children. In J. K. Wing (Ed.), *Childhood Autism*, Oxford: Pergamon, 1966.

Luria, A. R. *The role of speech in the regulation of normal and abnormal behavior*. New York: Liveright, 1961.

Markel, N. N. *Psycholinguistics*. Homewood, Ill.: Dorsey, 1969.

Miller, G. A. The magical number seven plus or minus two. *Psychological Review*, *63*, 81–97 (1956).

Miller, N. E. Experimental studies of conflict. In J. McV. Hunt (Ed.), *Personality and the behavior disorders*, New York: Ronald, 1944.

Moorhead, D., and Ingram, D. The development of base syntax in normal and linguistically deviant children. *Journal of Speech and Hearing Research*, *16*, 330–345 (1973).

Moran, M. *Verb inflections of normal and learning disabled children*. Doctoral dissertation, University of Kansas, 1975.

Mowrer, O. H. Two factor learning theory reconsidered, with special reference to secondary reinforcement and the concept of habit. *Psychological Review*, *63*, (1948).

O'Neill, J., and Oyer, H. J. *Applied audiometry*. New York: Dodd, Mead, 1966.

Phillips, J. L. *The origins of intellect: Piaget's theory*. San Francisco: Freeman, 1969.

Rapaport, D. *Organization and pathology of thought*. New York: Columbia University Press, 1951.

Rapaport, D. The structure of psychoanalytic theory. *Psychological Issues*, *2*, Monograph No. 2 (1960).

Redl, F., and Wineman, H. *Children who hate* New York: Free Press, 1951.

Rees, N. Bases of decision in language training. *Journal of Speech and Hearing Disorders*, *37*, 283–304 (1972).

Rheingold, H. L., Gewertz, J. L., and Ross, H. W. Social conditioning of vocalizations in the infant. *Journal of Comparative and Physiological Psychology*, *52*, 68–73 (1959).

Rousey, C. *A theory of speech*. Paper presented as the convention of the American Association of Psychiatric Clinics for Children, Boston, 1969.

Rousey, C., and Moriarty, A. E. *Diagnostic* implications of speech sounds. Springfield, Ill.: Charles C. Thomas, 1965.

Schiefelbusch, R. Language disabilities in cognitively involved children. In J. Irwin and M. Marge (Eds.), *Principles of language disorders in children*. New York: Appleton, 1972.

Shames, G., and Sherrick, C. A discussion of nonfluency and stuttering as operant behavior. *Journal of Speech and Hearing Disorders*, *28*, 3–13 (1963).

Sheehan, J. Conflict theory of stuttering. In J. Eisenson (Ed.), *Stuttering: A symposium*, New York: Harper & Row, 1958.

Sheehan, J. G. *Stuttering: Research and therapy*. New York: Harper & Row, 1970.

Shervanian, C. C. Speech, thought and communication disorders in childhood psychoses: theoretical implications. *Journal of Speech and Hearing Disorders*, *32*, 303–313 (1967).

Siegel, G. M. Prevailing concepts in speech research with mentally retarded children. *Asha*, *6*, 192–194 (1964).

Spitz, R. A. Anaclitic depression. In *The Psychoanalytic Study of the Child*, New York: International Universities, 1946.

Spitz, R. A. *No and Yes*. New York: International Universities, 1957.

Spreen, O. Language functions in mental retardation: A review of language development, types of retardation and intelligence level. *American Journal of Mental Deficiencies*, *69*, 482–489 (1965).

Spreen, O. Language functions in mental retardation, a review. II. Language in higher level performance. *American Journal of Mental Deficiency*, *70*, 351–362 (1966).

Stendler, C. B. in Davidson Films, *Piaget's Developmental Theory: Classification*. San Francisco, Cal., 1969.

Stendler, C. B. In Davidson Films, *Piaget's Developmental Theory: Conservation*. San Francisco, Cal., 1969.

Travis, L. E. (Ed.). *Handbook of speech pathology*. New York: Appleton, 1957.

Vygotsky, L. D. *Thought and language*. New York: Wiley, 1962.

Werner, H., and Kaplan, B. *Symbol formation*. New York: Wiley, 1963.

Wiig, E. H., and Semel, E. M. Comprehension of linguistic concepts requiring logical operations by learning-disabled children. *Journal of Speech and Hearing Research*, *16*, 627–636 (1973).

Wilcox, D. E. Observations of speech disturbances in childhood schizophrenia. *Diseases of the Nervous System*, *17*, 20–23 (1956).

Wingate, M. E. Evaluation and stuttering. III. Identification of stuttering and the use of a label. *Journal of Speech and Hearing Disorders*, 27, 244–257 (1962).

Wischner, G. Anxiety-reduction as reinforcement in maladaptive behavior. Evidence in stutterers' representations of the moment of difficulty. *Journal of Abnormal and Social Psychology*, *47*, 566–571 (1952).

Woodward, M. The behavior of idiots interpreted by Piaget's theory of sensorimotor development. *British Journal of Educational Psychology*, *29*, 60–71 (1959).

Wolski, W., and Wiley, J. Functional aphonia in a fourteen-year-old boy: A case report. *Journal of Speech and Hearing Disorders*, *30*, 71–75 (1965).

Wyatt, G. L. Language learning and communication disorders in children. New York: Free Press, 1969.

THE SOCIAL DETERMINANTS
Chapter 6

Language is a social phenomenon. It has its origins in the social history of the species and must be learned by each individual. All aspects are socially derived, including sounds, words, grammar, and meanings. These elements of language must be used in highly consistent and predictable ways, in order to have communication in a culture. Too great a variation would restrict the use of language for its supreme purpose–social communication.

Mature social communication in humans may be thought of as the prime example of the organism's tendency to organize and synthesize its structures and processes into coherent functional systems. Through this integrative tendency speech, cognition, and the interpersonal-emotional developmental processes combine to form the communicative process. Each of these processes must undergo its own independent development. However, fusion with one another is necessary if social communication is to take place.

Before an individual can sustain a high level of social communication, he must achieve maturation of the speech mechanism, cognitive development to the level of formal operations, competence in understanding and performance of the linguistic code, maturity of interpersonal relations based on development and differentiation of the self and an awareness of self and others. Communication represents the ultimate in adaptation of the organism to the environment and at the same time, during its development, communication contributes significantly to the process of adaptation.

THE STRUCTURE OF COMMUNICATION

Human communication, an interpersonal act, takes place when a message has been created and transmitted by one person and received and understood by another.

Markel (1969) illustrates the minimal model for communication in Figure 6–1. It consists of an encoder, a person who initiates the communication. Utilizing the cognitive and emotional processes of his nervous system, he formulates a message. Impulses travel from the central nervous system through his efferent nervous system to activate muscles and glands. The action of the muscles and glands is the source of the message. The destination of the message is a sensory receptor of the decoder. The channel of communication thus involves the source (sounds, gestures, and so forth) and the appropriate receptors. Nerve impulses from the receptors are transmitted by the afferent nervous system to the central nervous system where, through the psychological processes of cognition and emotion, the message is interpreted. The entire act is repeated by a reversal of the roles.

Speech is the major channel for transmitting a message. In the preceding chapters we have given detailed descriptions of the speech mechanism as the source of speech and the ear as its sensory receptor. We have also considered the cognitive and emotional influences on the structure of speech and its content.

Other sources of communication which are nonverbal include body movement, with *kinetics* as the channel. Birdwhistle (1970) has shown that this area is rich with communicative meaning. The body surface through the channel of *touch* has communicative significance especially in early life (Frank, 1971). Body placement with the channel of *proxemics* has been explored by Hall (1959) and found to be meaningful to birds as well as to businessmen.

In addition, Egolf and Chester (1973) refer to *organismics*, the effect that our

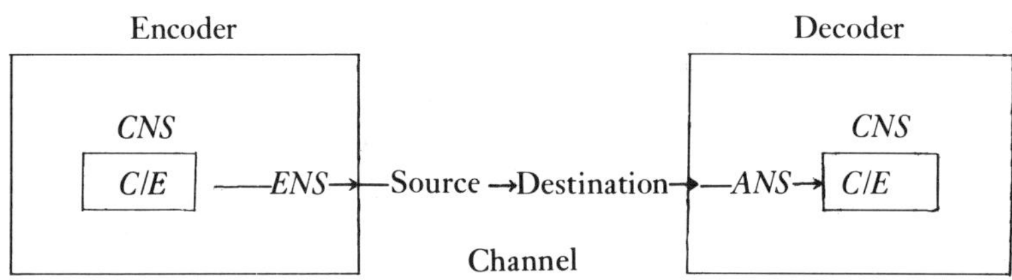

CNS: Central nervous system—the brain and spinal cord
C: Cognition—the process of knowing or perceiving
E: Emotion—the process of feeling or affect
ENS: Efferent nervous system—nerve fibers carrying neural impulses from the CNS to muscles and glands
ANS: Afferent nervous system—nerve fibers carrying neural impulses from sensory receptors to the CNS
Source: Muscular movement, glandular secretion, or biochemical change which originates a message
Destination: Sensory receptor which can respond to a message
Channel: Medium which carries messages from encoders to decoders

Figure 6–1. Minimal model of communication. (N. Markel. *Psycholinguistics*. Homewood, Ill.: Dorsey, 1969.) Reprinted by permission.

"relatively physical attitudes" have on communication, and *vocalics*, the influence of vocal quality on communication. Mehrabian (1968) says that vocal quality accounts for 38 percent of the affective attribute of the message.

THE FUNCTIONS OF COMMUNICATION

Communication must be recognized as a means to an end, not an end in itself. It is a process for encouraging joint action for fulfilling needs. Hence it is a social phenomenon. "It comes into its first use at a time when joint action is the only means whereby the young organism can survive" (Bruner, 1965). Communication has the following functions.

TOOL FOR ADAPTATION THROUGH SOCIAL INSTITUTIONS

Communication is the major means for facilitating the socialization of the child and development of his personality. Socialization is the result of a long and varied communication with members of the society, or agents of socialization, such as parents, peers, and educators.

Socialization is a process of teaching the behaviors and ways of thinking which will allow the child to grow up and function in a society in accordance with the values of that society. The learning in socialization is a function of social interaction. As the child interacts with members of the family, peers, and others, he learns the sounds, intonations, words, syntax, and denotative and connotative meanings of words in order to communicate in the society.

Just as there is a physical structure that determines speech, there are also social structures that determine the speech, language, and thought employed by the child. These structures include the family, the peers, school, church, social class status, and role. All of these social institutions work toward socialization of the child.

Many variations of speech and language have origins in the social environment. Sociologists discuss social structures as behavioral patterns that are used by groups or classes of people. These structures influence the development of group differences in speech, language, thought, and communication. The differences are reflected in the individual. As Sapir (1927) indicated, society speaks through the individual. Furthermore, the interrelationships are such that human beings do not exist out of society. The person in isolation is still in society in the sense that he carries with him patterns of thought that were formed in a society.

ROLE. Role differences are clearly reflected in speech. The role we play comes with its linguistic and paralinguistic usages. These are learned by the individual. We tend to think of sex differences in speech as being physically determined, yet many of the differences result from social learning and identification. In a recent case of surgical sex change in a male transvestite, the speech pathologist had to teach the individual the proper role-determined pitch, intonation, stress, and quality of voice.

People who have authoritative roles also have to learn differentiating characteristics of speech. Moses (1954) said: "The male teacher, lawyer, judge, the preacher often use a low voice to express authority, utilizing the deepest part of their potential range" (p. 43).

Cameron (1944) felt that the learning of role plays an important part in the development of social communication. Not only is it essential for the individual to assume an appropriate role for himself but he must also learn to become aware of and identify with the roles of others. A person must empathize with and experience the other person's attitudes and reactions. These actions allow the individual to predict the responses of others to his messages and facilitate appropriate social communication. It is through this type of knowledge of the role of others that allows a speaker to send a message "in the most appropriate form for conveying intended meanings to a particular person for particular effects." (Muma, 1975). Cameron hypothesized that it was a lack of role taking skills that resulted in the inability of the adult schizophrenic to communicate and resulted in his social isolation.

Dialects: Multidimensional Variations in Language. *Dialect* refers to a mode of speech or language. It is homogeneous in itself, is spoken by a considerable number of people, and differs appreciably from analogous forms of the language from which it is derived. Dialects may differ in the structures of prosody, phonemic aspects, morphology, syntax, and idiom. The term is not used in a disparaging sense, but represents a variation in speech which has evolved because of geographic and social separation, mixtures of languages, or political, economic, educational, and religious influences (Gray and Wise, 1946).

In the United States there are three major dialects and a number of lesser dialects. The Eastern dialect is spoken primarily in the New England area. An example is the speech of the late President Kennedy. Southern American is used primarily in the states that made up the Confederacy. George Wallace's speech is an example. General American is spoken in the rest of the nation. The lesser dialects include Pennsylvania German, Milwaukee German, Appalachian, Black, Cajun.

Social Class and Mode of Socialization. The groundwork for communication is laid in the social interaction between the mother and child during the early critical period in the child's development. One might think of these important maternal socializing efforts as a preparation for educability or, as some writers put it, a "learning how to learn." This idea may be expanded into learning how to learn in order to learn how to live in a given social structure—that of the mother's social class and social status.

Class differences are socially determined and are independent of racial and ethnic differences. They are determined by membership in social institutions, not genetic endowment.

Extensive research has been carried out on the modes of socialization used by the mother through speech, thought, and interpersonal communication. Bernstein (1961) and Olin, Hess, and Shipman (1967) have studied how mothers from different socioeconomic levels utilize different codes to communicate with their children. For example, Bernstein labels the working-class code as the restricted code and the middle-class code as the elaborated one. The restricted code used by the working-class mothers is employed in the context of specific situations. It is concrete in terms of situation and level of explanation, but at the same time it lacks specificity and exactness in explanations. The motivational basis for the control exercised by the mother is unspoken, and the authority for the control is vested in the mother by virtue of her position. Bernstein (1961) describes the linguistic structure of the restricted code as:

1. Short, grammatically simple, often unfinished sentences with a poor syntactical form.
2. Simple and repetitive use of conjunctions (so, and because).
3. Little use of subordinate clauses to break down the initial categories of the dominant subject.
4. Inability to hold a formal subject through a speech sequence, thus facilitating a dislocated informational content.
5. Rigid and limited use of adjectives and adverbs.
6. Infrequent use of impersonal pronouns as subjects of conditional clauses or sentences.
7. Frequent use of statements in which the reason and the conclusions are confounded to produce a categorical utterance.
8. A large number of statements and phrases that signal a requirement for the previous speech sequence to be reinforced. Examples are: *wouldn't it*, *you see*, *just fancy*. This process is termed sympathetic circularity.
9. Individual selection from a group of idiomatic sequences will occur frequently.
10. The individual qualification is implicit in the sentence organization: it is a language of implicit meaning. (p. 297–298)

The elaborated code employed by middle-class mothers in socializing their children differs significantly from the restricted code. It too is concrete in terms of specific situations, but the control is differentiated by taking into account the context, the subject matter, and the individual. The motivational base for control is explained and the implications are discussed. Stress is placed on internalizing controls through mediation of well-reasoned concepts.

Hess and Shipman (1968) have shown that there are significant differences not only in cognitive style employed by the mothers in socialization, but also in the linguistic structure. The teaching behavior of the lower-class mothers is "deprived of meaning." Behavior is controlled through the status role of the mother rather than through understanding of the future implications of present behavior.

Some writers have pointed out that there are serious deficits in this mode of communication, which result in inadequate concept formation and schemes in the child. They assert that it does not provide an adequate base for future development of problem solving or reasoning, so necessary for school learning.

TOOL FOR EDUCATION AND TIME-BINDING

Communication allows the individual to go beyond his own limited personal experiences and to derive knowledge from the past and present to enlarge his concepts. All the accumulated knowledge of the past, its wisdom, methods, science, art, and values as well as prejudices, are passed on to each generation, which in turn adds to the store of knowledge for the succeeding generation (Korzybski, 1933). It is by means of this time-binding capacity that man differs from other animals. In literate societies such as our own both spoken and written means are used to communicate past information, whereas in nonliterate societies knowledge and tradition are passed on orally.

TOOL FOR SOCIALIZATION OF THOUGHT

Social language is the major medium for adult communication. The language code in all of its components is a product of social learning. The semantic meanings of words and the language signs that are associated with representational processes reflect a stability of learning experiences within a given culture, so that the meanings of the most common words will be highly similar among people in the same culture and cultural subgroups (Osgood, Suci, and Tannenbaum, 1957). Word meanings therefore are indexes of social affiliation (Abercrombie, 1969).

Yet the early development of the child's thought, as we have discovered, holds many idiosyncratic meanings, which undoubtedly are based on individual experi-

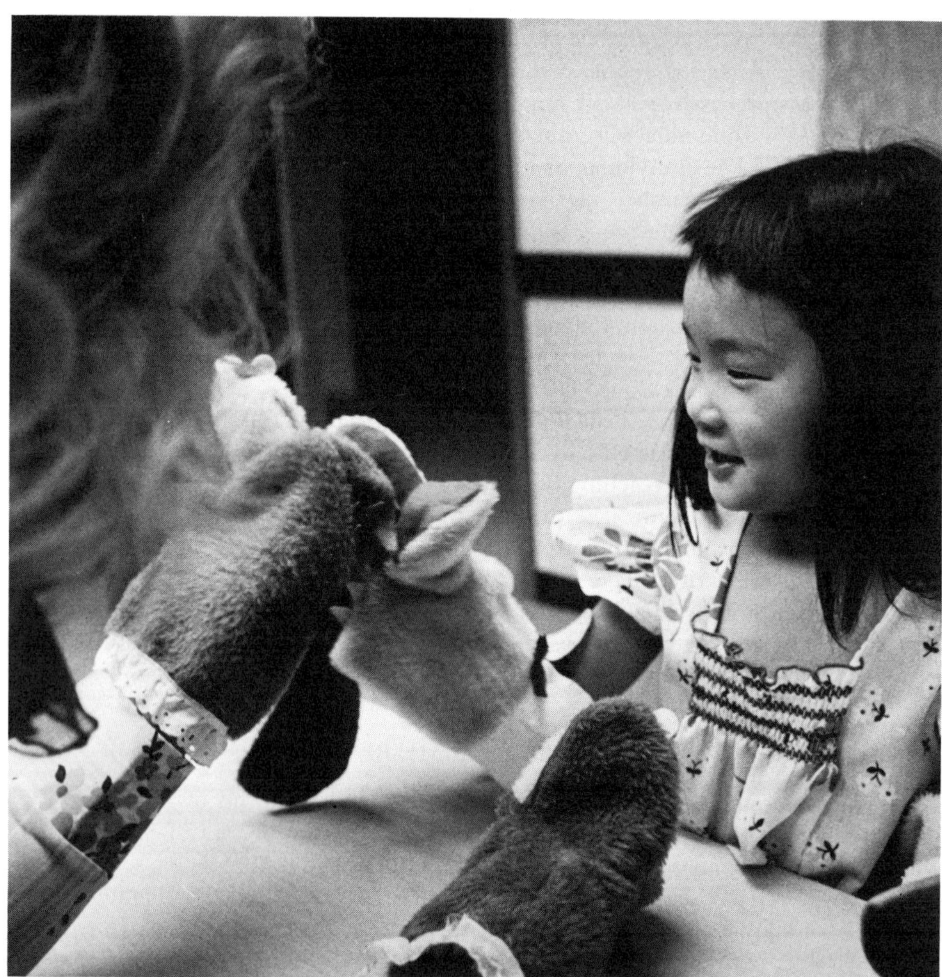

ences. Piaget stresses the egocentric and idiosyncratic nature of the child's thought during the sensorimotor and preoperational periods of cognitive development. In referring to the child's concepts Piaget and Werner both discuss its syncretic nature. Flavell (1963) has defined syncretism as:

> a type of thinking or perception which assimilates reality into global, undifferentiated schemas; the individual contents of the assimilated reality interpenetrate and fuse with one another, anything being joined to or combined with anything else simply by virtue of common membership in the loosely bounded schemata potpourri. (p. 273)

Syncretic thinking and perception of reality are based on private experiences. This makes conceptual social communication extremely difficult. We employ language and communication as tools for socializing percepts and concepts. In this way a high degree of standardization of meaning can exist between people in the same culture.

Whorf (1956) feels that language shapes man's concepts and percepts of reality. The language and its structure guide the individual's cognitive processes. He says:

> "We dissect nature along lines laid down by our native languages. The categories and types that we isolate from the world of phenomena we do not find there because they stare every observer in the face; on the contrary the world is presented in a kaleidoscopic flux of impressions which has to be organized by our minds—and this means largely by the linguistic systems in our minds. We cut nature up, organize it into concepts, and ascribe significances as we do, largely because we are parties to an agreement to organize it in this way—an agreement that holds through our speech community and is codified in the patterns of language. The agreement is of course an implicit and unstated one. *But its term are absolutely obligatory;* we cannot talk at all except by subscribing to the organization and classification of data which the agreement decrees. (p. 106–107)

Thus, through the processes of language communication concepts and percepts become social by being formed into a "shared subjective reality of a linguistic community" (Bruner, 1965). Osgood, Suci, and Tannenbaum (1957) have shown through the use of the semantic differential that members of a social community agree on word meanings.

SOME FACTORS IN THE DEVELOPMENT OF COMMUNICATION

Communication develops out of an interpersonal relationship of the mother and child. Her efforts are twofold. (1) The mother has her role to play in nurturing the highly dependent infant to insure his survival. The human infant belongs to the class of mammals which are relatively helpless at birth and require a long period of maternal protection and nurturing for survival. (2) The mother is the key agent of socialization in the early period of the child's life to prepare the child for existence in a society. She must teach him the behavioral patterns and norms appropriate for the social structure he has to enter.

Communication is both a behavioral pattern and a tool by which behavioral patterns are most readily learned. The child's learning of communication is a long-term process that entails concurrent physical development of the speech structures, acquisition of the linguistic code, cognitive development, emotional development, and the establishment of interpersonal relationships. We have previously dealt with each of these factors. Here we will explore some of their interrelationships in communication development.

THE NONVERBAL PERIOD

The nucleus out of which communication grows can be found in the process of need fulfillment in the interactions of the mother-child matrix. At birth the child is totally dependent on the mother for gratification of all of his needs. Spitz (1957) emphasizes the importance of the long-term biological and psychological dependency as a necessary precondition for establishing interpersonal relationships and communicative behavior. These social forms develop out of a state of helplessness. The infant cries when he is hungry or disturbed. His cries are a symptom of his distress. The mother reads his cries as a sign of heightened needs and relieves him of his discomfort.

Gradually the infant learns to cry not merely as a reflex response to discomfort, but as an intentional signal toward the mother. He has acquired a vague notion that cries bring relief from outside himself. There is no specificity to the child's crying; the mother can recognize only that the child is in need.

Bettelheim (1967) has stressed the active role that the infant plays in expressing his wants and in taking relief when it is offered to him. He also pictures the mother as deriving gratification from performing the role of providing relief. Communication between mother and child becomes a mutual effort, gratifying to both partners and engendering trust. This relationship serves as a model on which subsequent communicative relationships are built. It should be noted that defects in the original model adversely affect future communicative relationships.

Main (in Mussen, 1975) studied 12-month-old babies through intensive observations of the mother-child interactions. Major interest was focused on attachment and feelings of security of infants with their mothers.

At age 21 months, the infants were studied again, this time in a social interaction with an adult playmate. Main found that infants who were securely attached to their mothers at 12 months reacted positively to the adult playmates, whereas infants who were insecurely attached avoided or related poorly to the adult. When communicative skills in the children were studied, it was found that the securely attached children's group "had larger vocabularies, spoke more words, used more morphemes per utterance, and a larger number of different words."

It appears from this study that the quality of the early mother-child relationship is prognostic of the ability of the child to relate socially and utilize verbal skills in that relationship.

Nonverbal communication uses the media of bodily movements, tactile and thermal senses of skin contact, and the vocal sounds of the mother which accompany her actions. Egolf and Chester (1973) think that these nonverbal media are more effective in conveying affect and feeling than the cognitive language forms. Voice, movement, and touch convey emotion better than words, and the nonverbal messages are received through empathy and intuition (Rapaport, 1951).

As the infant moves on to more symbolic forms of communication through gesture, imitation, identification, and then speech, these forms require the development of a concept of self and self-identity and a recognition of the separateness of others. Mahler (1968) has referred to this development as the separation-individuation process and it is closely related to the emotional development of the child.

SOMATOPSYCHOLOGY

Individuals with speech and hearing problems, especially those with observable physical disabilities such as cerebral palsy, frequently are placed in an inferior status position in our society. This status position carries with it certain psychological reactions which may handicap the individual far beyond the disability itself. A study of this area of social psychology is called somatopsychology. It deals with "those variations in physique that affect the psychological situation of a person by influencing the effectiveness of his body as a tool for actions or by serving as a stimulus to himself and others" (Barker, Wright, and Gonick, 1953, p. 1).

Goffman (1963), in enlarging on this concept, has referred to the social reaction to perceived differences in individuals as a *stigma*. He defines the stigma as "a negative attitude toward someone not quite like ourselves." Stigmas may originate in physical handicaps, behavioral differences, or racial and class differences. When these are perceived as stigmas, the belief is that the person is "not quite human."

SOMATOPSYCHOLOGICAL MODEL OF PATHOLOGY

Speech and hearing problems may have a serious effect on communication by impairing intelligibility, reception, or comprehension of the message. Malfunctioning of the speech and hearing mechanism is an objective basis for difficulty in communication. However, emotional overlays, such as devaluation of the speaker by the listener and acceptance of the devaluation by the speaker, contribute to additional impairments of communication. Consideration of the subjective or emotional basis of breakdowns in communication is the foundation of the somatopsychological model of pathology. The effect of a speech or hearing problem on communication is compounded by social and psychological factors, which increase the difficulty in communication, and so on in a vicious circle. The medical, behavior-learning, and psychodynamic medical models of pathology deal with the original speech or hearing deficit. The somatopsychological model deals with the additional complications that arise once the deficit has appeared.

SOMATOPSYCHOLOGY OF SPEECH AND HEARING

Wright (1960) gives details of the social and psychological impact of physical disability. We shall relate her findings to speech and hearing deficits. Depreciation often takes the form of jokes. Jokes about the speech of the stutterer, the cerebral palsied, the child with cleft palate, the lisper, and the foreigner are rampant. Children who lisp are sometimes taunted by their peers. Expressions and actions of a devaluating nature adversely influence social and occupational status and may have an adverse effect on a person's choice of sexual partner. McDaniel (1965) writes about the wide variety of vocational problems of the individual with a cleft palate, a hearing loss, or a stuttering problem. He decries the tendency to stereotype the deaf and hard-of-hearing into a specific occupation. Johnson (1960) described the substantial nature of the vocational handicap for stutterers.

The literature indicates that many people find stuttering behavior aversive, and they reflect this attitude by talking less, interrupting, and moving and looking away when talking to a stutterer. They harbor feelings of pity, sympathy, surprise, and embarrassment toward the one who stutters. Giolas and Williams (1958) indicate that even very young children are aware of and disapprove of stuttering.

Current trends to mainstream handicapped children may have some positive effects in changing attitudes. The grade school boys in the Woods' (1974) study did not differentiate their classmates who stuttered and those who did not in ranking social position. The children were aware of the deficit and did evaluate stutterers as poorer speakers than those who did not stutter.

There is a large body of literature that points to negative evaluations of stutterers. Unlike the boys in the Woods study many people look down upon and devalue the person who stutters. Tape recordings of psychotherapeutic sessions with Jim, a young stutterer, reveal how devaluation and patronizing attitudes of others may be perceived and internalized.

> Everybody else thinks I'm, "Oh well, he's crazy," or there's "something's wrong with him, he can't talk right, he can't do anything right. So we simply let him go. Oh, well, I guess we'll be nice to him, but he's no good, he's just sorta worthless." That's the way I feel people think about me; they think I'm crazy or something; I don't know, I guess I am (Seeman, 1957, p. 8).

We see many parallels between the research data on stuttering and Wright's somatopsychological findings. Stutterers experience feelings of shame, self-pity, and guilt. They feel anger towards themselves based on their acceptance and internalization of the negative evaluations of the normal majority. Many accept the inferior status position where they have learned to "feel and act like a less fortunate being." They revere normal standards of speech, making it difficult for them to accept aspects of themselves. Their anger is directed at the listener and this further aggravates the speech situation and the interpersonal relations. Jim, the stutterer, comes to the painful conclusion that he is expressing aggression through his stuttering:

> Well, ah, I've been th-thinking about my ag-gression. It's—I'm beginning to s-s-s- well, I'm not beginning to see more, I'm beginning to feel more that I might be showing a lot of aggression in my st-stuttering toward other people because I know now, ah, the other person suffers even more than I do sometime. And it's, I don't know, I guess I am doing it to make the other person suffer. I mean this is something I could never—I could never admit before. I mean, I mean, it would—if I just said it, it would just be a lie, but I'm beginning to see now maybe it isn't a lie, maybe I do have a lot of aggression in myself. That's the way I'm showing it toward people. I know I used to feel quite bad about my speech. But, ah, it's, it's something s-so new that I'm probably showing aggression in my speech. I need to say it over and over again. It's, I'm just trying to work it through. I-It surprises me so much. (Seeman, 1957, p. 10).

The somatopsychological effect of alaryngeal speech is shown in the Gilmore (1974) study. Using two excellent alaryngeal speakers as subjects, Gilmore studied how a large group of business and community leaders compared them to normal speakers in terms of social and vocational acceptability. The speakers were consistently evaluated as less acceptable than the normal speakers. They were thought less capable of handling jobs; those jobs that they were thought capable of managing were of significantly reduced prestige and involved considerably less public contact. When judges were informed on the nature of the disorder, this information further increased the rejection of the speakers from public contact, but it did increase their acceptability in other areas. Gilmore concludes: "Intelligibility and fluency of esophageal speech is important, but not enough for vocational rehabilitation."

When Malone (1969) reported on the psychological and social attitudes of relatives of 20 persons who had become aphasic, he said that severe disruptions of family life were found. Especially prevalent were guilt feelings toward the aphasic, manifested by "a feeling that 1) they were responsible for the patient's problem; 2) that the aphasia was a punishment for wrong-doing; and 3) that they were not doing all they should be doing for their relatives." Social changes included disclosures that friends stopped coming for visits and an attempt by one wife to hide her husband from the family and friends. These attitudes of rejection and shame are frequent.

Wright (1960) has provided some positive rehabilitation procedures for dealing with somatopsychological problems. Especially important are changes in self-concepts which will lead to acceptance and better adjustment.

THE SOCIAL-CULTURAL MODEL OF PATHOLOGY

The social-cultural model of pathology states that pathologies are determined by conditions in the social or cultural environment—social class, role, caste, family, or any other institutions such as education or religion. These conditions may be related to attitudes, interests, values, and intrinsic and extrinsic support for the functioning of the institutions.

As the research has accumulated, different points of view have emerged concerning report of failure in academic achievement of many children from the lower socioeconomic levels. One point of view stresses the findings of serious deficits among these children. They lag behind middle-class children in most aspects of cognitive and language development. Bereiter and Engelmann (1966) point to the inadequacies of experience coupled with deficits inherent in the cognitive and language socializing models. Raph (1967) has commented on the language of lower-class children as "meager, restricted in variety of vocabulary, repetitious, with incorrect grammar, pronunciation and articulation, and with poor syntactic form."

Another point of view interprets the speech of children of lower socioeconomic levels as a nonstandard form of language which nevertheless is well developed and complete. It is merely different from that of middle-class children. So-called deficits found in the language are attributed to the tester's employment of standards for comparison based on middle-class criteria. Adler (1971) stresses that we are not a homogeneous population, but a pluralistic society, and we must recognize the cultural differences in speech and language.

Baratz (1968) has presented the point of view that children of lower socioeconomic levels have fully developed speech and language, but it is a nonstandard variant. She says that the child does not speak standard English because it is not spoken in his environment. According to Baratz (1970), deficits in cognition and language do develop because of factors within the educational institutions and their curriculum. The linguistic structure and pronunciation of the middle-class teachers' speech differ from that of the child. In addition, the syntactic structures and content of the reading materials differ significantly from the child's own language and experiential background. The child experiences an alienation from the educational system which does not utilize his own language and which places a negative value on his communication system. These add up to a rejection of the child's identity.

Failure in cognitive development, especially in language and reading, may stem from the discontinuity in cultural training which takes place when the child reaches school. He is placed at a disadvantage by being asked to change from one linguistic system to another and from one cognitive style to another. Those who fail become alienated from the system after having experienced feelings of inferiority. Erikson (1963) has pointed out that the school-age child has an ego need for industry. There are strong drives for learning of every kind including all the school subjects. Failure, for whatever reason, results in feelings of inferiority which influence the child's subsequent development.

SUMMARY

We have explained the social determinants from several approaches. We examined the structure of communication which is a social achievement in terms of its functions and development. We considered the impact of a number of social structures such as social class and role on language and communication, as an aspect of the socialization process. Pathologies of speech, thought, and communication were examined in terms of the somatopsychological model of pathology and the social-cultural model of pathology. In our discussion of the speech and language of lower-class children we presented two points of view, one which sees the application of the social-cultural model and the other which stresses the differences which are reflections of normal variations between social groups.

REFERENCES

Abercrombie, D. Voice quality. In N. Markel (Ed.), *Psycholinguists*, Homewood, Ill.: Dorsey, 1969.

Adler, S. Pluralism, relevance, and language intervention for culturally different children. *Asha*, *13*, 719–723 (1971).

Baratz, J. D. Language in the economically disadvantaged child. A perspective. *Asha*, *10*, 143–145 (1968).

Baratz, J. C. Teaching reading in an urban negro school system. In F. Williams (Ed.), *Language and poverty—Perspectives on a theme*, Chicago: Markham, 1970.

Barker, R. G., Wright, B. A., and Gonick, M. R. *Adjustment to physical handicap and illnesses: A survey of the social psychology of physique and disability*. New York: Social Science Research Council, 1953.

Bereiter, C., and Engelmann, S. *Teaching disadvantaged children in the preschool.* Englewood Cliffs, N.J.: Prentice-Hall, 1966.

Bernstein, B. Social class and linguistic development: A theory of social learning. In *Education, economy and society.* A. H. Halsey, J. Floud, and A. Anderson, Eds. New York: Free Press, 1961.

Bettelheim, B. *The empty fortress.* New York: Free Press, 1967.

Birdwhistle, R. L. *Kinesics and context.* Philadelphia: University of Pennsylvania Press, 1970.

Bruner, J. S. *On knowing.* New York: Atheneum, 1965.

Cameron, N. Experimental analysis of schizophrenic thinking. In *Language and Thought in Schizophrenia,* J. S. Kasanin, Ed. Berkeley: University of California Press, 1944.

Egolf, D. B., and Chester, S. L. Nonverbal communication and the disorders of speech and language. *Asha, 15,* 511–518 (1973).

Erikson, E. H. *Childhood and society.* New York: Norton, 1963.

Flavell, J. H. *The developmental psychology of Jean Piaget.* New York: Van Nostrand Reinhold, 1963.

Frank, L. K. Tactile communication. In *The rhetoric of nonverbal communication,* J. Bosma, Ed. Glenview, Ill.: Scott Foresman, 1971.

Gilmore, S. I. Social and vocational acceptability of esophageal speakers compared to normal speakers. *Journal of Speech and Hearing Research, 17,* 599–607 (1974).

Giolas, T. G., and Williams, D. Children's reactions to nonfluencies in adult speech. *Journal of Speech and Hearing Research, 1,* 86–93 (1958).

Goffman, E. *Stigma.* Englewood Cliffs, N.J.: Prentice-Hall, 1963.

Gray, G. W., and Wise, C. M. *The bases of speech.* New York: Harper & Row, 1946.

Hall, E. T. *The silent language.* Garden City, N.Y.: Doubleday, 1959.

Hess, R. D. and Shipman, V. C. Maternal influences upon early learning: the cognitive environments of urban preschool children. In *Early education,* R. D. Hess and R. M. Bear, Eds. Chicago: Aldine Press, 1968.

Johnson, W. *Speech handicapped school children.* New York: Harper & Row, 1960.

Korzybski, A. *Science and sanity.* Lancaster, Pa.: International Non-Aristotelian Library, 1933.

Mahler, M. S. *On human symbiosis and vicissitudes of individuation. Infant psychosis,* Vol. I. New York: International Universities, 1968.

Malone, P. L. Expressed attitudes of families of aphasics. *Journal of Speech and Hearing Disorders, 34,* 146–150 (1969).

Markel, N. N. *Psycholinguistics.* Homewood, Ill.: Dorsey, 1969.

McDaniel, J. W. Current status of vocational rehabilitation for disorders of hearing and speech. *Journal of Speech and Hearing Disorders, 30,* 17–31 (1965).

Mehrabian, A. Communication without words. *Psychology Today, 2,* 52–55 (1968).

Moses, P. J. *The voice of neurosis.* New York: Grune & Stratton, 1954.

Muma, J. R. The communication game: dump and play. *Journal of Speech and Hearing Disorders, 40,* 296–309 (1975).

Mussen, P. Communication and the development of prosocial behavior. *Asha, 17,* 324–330 (1975).

Olin, S. G., Hess, R. D., and Shipman, V. C. Role of mothers' language styles in mediating their preschool children's cognitive development. *The School Review, 75,* 414–424 (1967).

Osgood, C. E., Suci, G. J., and Tannenbaum, P. H. *The measurement of meaning.* Urbana: University of Illinois Press, 1957.

Rapaport, D. *Organization and pathology of thought.* New York: Columbia University Press, 1951.

Raph, J. B. Language and speech deficits in culturally disadvantaged children. *Journal of Speech and Hearing Disorders, 32,* 203–214 (1967).

Sapir, E. Speech as a personality trait. *American Journal of Sociology, 32,* 892–905 (1927).

Seaman, J. The case of Jim. An annotated script of a record on counseling. Nashville, Tenn.: American Guidance Services, 1957.

Spitz, R. A. *No and yes*. New York: International Universities, 1957.

Whorf, B. L. A linguistic consideration of thinking in primitive communities. In *Language, thought, and reality: selected writings of Benjamin L. Whorf*. John B. Carroll, Ed. New York: Wiley, 1956.

Woods, C. L. Social position and speaking competence of stuttering and normally fluent boys. *Journal of Speech and Hearing Research*, *17*, 740–747 (1974).

Wright, B. A. *Physical disability*. New York: Harper & Row, 1960.

APPROACHES TO INTERVENTION Chapter 7

Three groups of people contribute directly to effective teaching of communication skills—clinicians, teachers, and parents. As we indicated in Chapter 1, the group specifically trained to deal with these problems are the speech and language clinicians. They can assess all the parameters of communication, make some comprehensive judgments about the nature and degree of severity of the problem, and plan therapy programs when they are indicated.

Without the aid of the other two groups, however, the work of the clinician may be unproductive or even impossible. Teachers work with children for two to six hours a day, depending on whether the children are in preschool or regular full-time school programs. During that time teachers are communicating with children on many topics at different levels of complexity. We view the teacher's role as twofold: (1) to complement the clinician's work with those who have communication deficits and (2) to utilize the language arts curriculum to improve communication skills of all the children. Clinicians should work with teachers on both of these aspects. Teachers who know which children have communication problems and the nature of their deficits, can aid those children tremendously. In addition, teachers can carry out speech and language development programs that are valuable for all children.

Before either the clinician or the teacher sees the child, the parents control his environment and his learning. They can encourage the listening, the speaking, the thinking processes of their child almost from the day of birth. They too must know how communication develops, how they can identify signs of slow development, and what they can do to enhance their child's talking.

There are many one-parent families in which it may not be possible for the mother to spend much time with her child. If she is working, she may take him to the babysitter, to the day-care center, or to a preschool where he will spend many hours each day. Those to whom she entrusts the well-being of her child should be carefully selected, so that they can provide the experiences necessary for the child's total development. That includes communication.

This chapter will be concerned with the roles of many groups in the development and maintenance of normal communication. The specific responsibilities of clinicians will be discussed in relation to employment settings, evaluation, intervention, and in-service training. Teachers' roles in instruction, carry-over, and development of curriculum guides for listening and speaking will be discussed. Parents' contributions from the beginning of life in their modeling of language through their alertness in noting whether their children are developing adequately are then presented. The individuals' needs—those of children, adolescents, and the aging—are considered. Finally, techniques for developing expressive language and some selected programs for aspects of oral language are reviewed. The chapter ends with material on listening programs.

THE ROLES OF THE CLINICIAN

The speech and language clinician has many roles, each determined to some extent by the setting in which he is employed. Regardless of settings, however, the clinician's primary responsibilities center around evaluation and intervention. A third role, related to both, is to provide in-service training to clinic staff members, parents, and others in the environment of the client who can help with the communication problem.

EMPLOYMENT SETTINGS

Clinicians are employed in many different settings. The largest number work in schools, hospitals, community centers, rehabilitation centers, universities, and private practice. A few work in departments of health and education at the state level and some in residential nursing homes. The clientele, teams of professionals with whom the clinician interacts, and the services required of the clinician vary in the different settings.

Community Speech and Hearing Centers. The clients in community centers come from a variety of sources. Some centers have contracts with other social agencies to provide speech and hearing evaluations and therapy. Depending upon the size of the center and its location, it may service adults who work in industry, children referred by the county health director, or children enrolled in the schools.

In addition to those who receive speech and hearing services as a result of contractual arrangements, the center accepts clients from many additional sources. Physicians in the community refer their patients for help. Parents who are concerned about their child's development request evaluations. Adults who are experiencing serious communication problems refer themselves to the center.

Many centers are partially supported by community charitable organizations such as the United Fund. In addition, fee schedules designed to take into account the income and expenses of the family are utilized. Medicare, Medicaid, and some health insurance plans which provide funds for speech and hearing services are tapped for appropriate patients.

Hospitals and Rehabilitation Centers. Clinicians in these settings usually work closely with medical and rehabilitation personnel. Not only do they provide evaluation and intervention, but they also help to plan total remedial programs for patients. They must understand the technical vocabulary, diagnostic techniques, and treatment programs of their colleagues and help to inform them about developments in the field of speech pathology so that comprehensive, feasible, and goal-oriented programs can be provided.

Most hospitals have teams that deal with special problems. As we indicated in Chapter 1, the teams consist of those persons who can provide input to the problems of the patient. The cleft palate team may include a pediatrician, plastic surgeon, orthodonist, prosthodontist, psychologist, social worker, audiologist, and speech clinician. Some teams have a geneticist available for consultation.

The team's goal of total rehabilitation of the patient is more likely to be achieved if all members understand the specific goals of each specialist involved. One team member may have to modify a recommendation because it is interfering with the achievement of other goals. For example, an 8-year-old cerebral palsied boy who lived in a small town needed a physical therapy program and a remedial reading program, but he could be enrolled in only one program at a time. The team decided to recommend remedial reading for the summer because of the importance of reading in his ongoing educational program. Since he made good progress, the team decided to continue him in that program for the entire year. The reading activities were utilized to strengthen carry-over of the speech and language units the clinician was teaching. Then, the following summer, he was enrolled in intensive physical therapy to improve his walking.

Clinicians must be capable of devising alternatives when a particular course of action is not feasible. Parents' feelings and beliefs influence decisions about their children's rehabilitation. For example, in response to a speech clinician's recommendation of an evaluation of their daughter's cleft palate by a plastic surgeon, one set of parents indicated that they would not permit her to have surgery because of their religious beliefs. As a result of this information, the clinician recommended that the parents arrange for the prosthodontist, a member of the cleft palate team, to evaluate their child for a prosthetic appliance to separate the nasal from the oral cavity and to help control the expulsion of the air stream through the nose by means of a bulb extension. The appliance provided an alternative to surgical repair.

The type of client in hospitals and rehabilitation centers varies. In veterans' hospitals, for instance, all patients with strokes, muscular deficiencies, laryngeal cancers, and similar medical problems are referred for evaluation and therapy. In children's hospitals perhaps only children with major speech or language deficits will be referred because therapy is available from other sources when they leave the hospital. In general hospitals clinicians may be assigned specifically to departments and to special clinic teams.

University Clinics. The university clinic may have full-time qualified clinicians on their staffs who carry out evaluations and therapy as a part of their university appointment. It is more likely, however, that such clinicians supervise the work of the students who are enrolled in clinical practicum. Many individuals request help in this type of clinic because of the expertise of the clinical staff.

As part of their practicum students are supervised on a regular schedule and discuss their work with their supervisors. Clients are informed of their student status and realize that their evaluation and therapy are being observed by a qualified clinician.

Private Practice. Some clinicians are in private practice, either on a full- or part-time basis. Those on a full-time basis maintain an office where patients come for help by appointment. Their clients come from a wide variety of sources, but most are referred by physicians. Some parents prefer private therapy for their child, so that he is not taken from class for his special speech needs.

Schools. More than half of all clinicians are employed by schools, particularly the public schools. Most state schools for the mentally retarded and some preschool programs, such as Head Start and day-care centers, have clinicians.

The procedure for referral of students with communication deficits differs among school districts. Some districts assign clinicians to evaluate the communication of prekindergarten children in the spring prior to school entry. Children who are identified as needing assistance may then be enrolled in a summer-speech program.

In some school districts all first-grade children and all transfers from other districts are tested in the fall. A screening procedure is utilized to obtain a sample of the child's communication skill. Children who fail at the criterion level set by the clinician or by specific tests are scheduled for a thorough in-depth study of the problems.

Other districts do not use any screening procedures, but rely on teacher referrals. Many utilize a combination of all the procedures—preschool evaluations, routine first grade and new student checks, and teacher referrals. The more opportunities the clinician has to evaluate pupils, the greater the chances for enrolling in therapy all those who need help.

School clinicians have an additional responsibility that is not shared with clinicians in other settings. They must also plan for students whose communication problem is secondary to a primary difficulty—whether it be mental retardation, learning disabilities, emotional disturbance, or orthopedic problems. Their role with these children, particularly if they are in special classes, is that of a resource person in evaluating and then planning appropriate programs with the teachers. With the current emphasis on keeping exceptional children in the regular classroom, clinicians need to be involved in the planning of the language arts curriculum, so that they can help teachers to meet the goals of the speaking and listening half of language arts.

EVALUATION

We introduced the role of the clinician as an evaluator in Chapter 1 and to some extent in the above section. The evaluation determines whether or not an individual has a communication deficit.

Screening. Evaluations may utilize screening procedures or in-depth study of the problem. Screening divides into two or three groups the individuals in a large population such as a school, day-care center, residential home, or hospital with special types of patients. The first group consists of those who do not have any deficiencies. The second group includes those who in the judgment of the clinician need further study. The third group consists of those who are scheduled for subsequent testing, for example, individuals with minor or temporary problems which may correct themselves without treatment or individuals who need periodic checking after therapy.

Screening can be carried out on an individual basis or in small groups. The clinician may have five or six children grouped at a table. While one is tested, the others listen and wait their turn. In that way directions do not have to be given quite so frequently. Screening of adults is almost always on an individual basis. Literate adults are asked to read a specially prepared paragraph; nonliterate adults are engaged in conversation.

In-Depth Evaluation. In-depth evaluation is a process whereby the clinician studies the speech and language behavior of an individual over a period of time. The clinician observes, tests, and makes judgments about the person's communication skills. The evaluation has several purposes.

1. To describe the communication problem in detail
2. To determine whether or not further evaluations by other professional persons are indicated
3. To provide a tentative prognosis about the effectiveness of therapy
4. To plan a therapy program
5. To provide educational and therapeutic guidelines for prevention of further disruptions in the communication of the individual and for prevention of potential dysfunctions

The initial step in evaluation requires that the clinician listen to and observe systematically the client's production and reception of speech and language. Is the message delivered fluently? Are the vocal characteristics of quality, pitch, and intensity adequate? Is he hearing? Tentative answers to these questions come from two sources: spontaneous speech samples the clinician hears and records unobtrusively, and free speech he engages in with the client prior to more formal testing.

Spontaneous Speech Samples. Planning for a spontaneous sample may provide the guidelines for the specific tests necessary. Wherever possible the samples are videotaped or tape-recorded for later review. Even if the clinician is taking careful notes, he will miss some of the deviations.

Except for adults who refer themselves, someone usually brings the client to a clinic for evaluation. The clinician has many choices of ways to get his potential client to talk freely in the reception room. He can ask a parent to encourage a child to talk; he can place toys, books, and magazines appropriate to the age and interest of the client in the room; or he can have an aide present to initiate conversations. In the school the clinician can observe the child in the classroom, on the playground, and in other situations in which the child is likely to talk naturally.

In initiating spontaneous speech, the clinician utilizes topics that will generate interest and enthusiasm. The question "Did you watch television last evening?" is not as fruitful as "Tell me about your favorite television show." The most productive techniques seem to be open-ended and situational questions, work on a puzzle or a game together, and viewing and talking about a filmstrip or a few slides. Clinicians new to practice sometimes tend to talk too much, leaving less time and opportunity for their client to be a verbal participant.

During later reevaluations spontaneous speech is the best indicator of the amount of learning that has taken place. We evaluate the changes in speech behavior during and at the end of therapy in terms of the amount of appropriate carry-over the individual has achieved in situations outside the clinic room.

Testing. A test is a systematic procedure that permits comparison of the performance of a specific behavior of two or more individuals or of the same individual over time. It elicits a representative sample of responses to a standardized set of stimuli. Most tests emphasize the content of behavior and not the cognitive processes which mediate behavior.

Testing of speech and language requires that the clinician know the available tests, how and when to use them, and what information they provide. A list of current tests, with some information about each, appears in the appendix. The list is not all-inclusive, but represents instruments to test a spectrum of the abilities we need to tap.

Training in both intra- and interreliability of judgments has been facilitated through the development of high-fidelity tape recorders that are portable and cost less than $500. Also, many schools and clinics now have their own videotape and videocassette recorders and playbacks, which can be utilized for sampling the reliability of evaluative judgments. Both audio- and videotapes have been used for practice and rechecks, but they can also be used for instruction in administering tests and for determining test reliability.

Many university clinics and instructional media centers keep a file of videotapes and videocassettes which demonstrate an expert speech clinician administering and scoring tests. These tapes can be dubbed with permission so that "refresher" programs can be planned for clinicians at regular intervals.

Articulation Assessment. An articulation assessment is a phonetic analysis by means of which the clinician determines whether each sound in the language is produced correctly. He may use sounds in nonsense syllables, words, sentences, or conversation. Children under age 4 are usually tested on their ability to echo or imitate the clinician's model; children over 4 are generally asked to name either objects or pictures; older clients are asked to read words or sentences or to describe objects.

During the assessment the clinician may test the phonemes in isolation and in the initial, medial, and final positions in words or in nonsense syllables in order to determine whether or not there is any consistency in the error pattern.

Most tests using words from which judgments about the accuracy of a phoneme in the three positions are to be made employ an extremely small sample—one word for each position of the phoneme, plus a few samples for the blends. As a result the clinician does not know whether the child has the phoneme in his repertoire in words that are not a part of the test. Administering a deep test, such as the one developed by

McDonald, which evaluates the phoneme in multiple contexts, increases the reliability of articulation assessment.

A CASE STUDY: EVALUATION OF BARRY. The following report on a 7½-year-old boy with normal hearing illustrates the use of procedures just described. The information is taken from the files of one of the authors.

Articulation. When Barry talked with his clinician prior to testing, he was difficult to understand. If the response was short, it was easier to figure out what he was saying. However, in the longer sentences that dealt with an unknown topic, his clinician could not follow him.

In response to the articulation test using pictures to elicit responses, Barry produced correctly all the phonemes in initial, medial, and final positions in single words up to approximately the 5-year developmental level. Blends were not tested. He made the following errors.

Substitutions: [tʃ] for [ʃ] and [z] in all positions; [tʃ] for [s] in the initial and medial; [tʃ] for [θ] in the medial and final; [f] for [θ] in the initial

Distortions: [l] in all positions

Barry was not able to produce any of his error sounds correctly in isolation, following the model of the examiner.

During the spontaneous portion of the evaluation Barry's articulation was punctuated with many additional sound errors. In free speech he either distorted [r] or substituted [w] for it. He also used [w] for [l] sometimes. He replaced [ð] with [d] inconsistently.

The results of the picture test indicated that Barry used [s] correctly in the word *bus*, yet he could not produce [s] in isolation, following the model for the examiner. Could he use this phoneme correctly in any other contexts? During spontaneous speech the clinician had not heard the [s] phoneme. The [θ] was not used either in conversation or on the picture test. Although he had acquired [r] for the three words on the test (*rabbit*, *carrot*, *car*), he did not use it in free speech for the most part. Nor did he use [ð] consistently. On the test he distorted [l], but in talking he sometimes replaced it with a [w]. On the basis of observing and testing thus far, his clinician recommended that the deep tests for [s], [r], [θ], [ð], and [l] be administered.

When Barry returned for his next session, deep tests for the [r] and [s], the two phonemes that appear most frequently in our language, were administered. On the McDonald Deep Test he used the [r] correctly in 10 of the 60 contexts and the [s] in 7. Deep testing for the other phonemes was postponed until Barry had acquired and automated these two phonemes in his conversation.

While Barry was talking freely and in the test situations, his clinician had observed no deviations in his use of the speech mechanism. Therefore the clinician did not formally assess the structures or his diadokokinetic rates.

Speech Sound Discrimination. Since Barry had substituted [tʃ] for [s] and for other sibilants both in the testing and in free speech, his clinician decided to test his speech discrimination. Even though he was producing [r] correctly in several contexts and was farther along in the acquisition stage, it seemed appropriate to test his discrimination on this phoneme also. Because his clinician wanted a measure that would provide specific information about [r] and [s], he gave him subtests D, E, and F of the Farquhar Discrimination Test (1961). On all three of these for [r] his scores were 100 percent. For [s] the situation was different. He was always able to identify the [s] when it was placed among vowels and among voiced consonants; but his score of 50 percent on the subtest where he had to select [s] from among the unvoiced consonants could have occurred by chance. His clinician then modified the Farquhar items to include the [tʃ], [f], [θ], [ð], and [s] only, and Barry could not select out the [s] phoneme.

Language. From the first observations of Barry in the reception room it was obvious that his level of language usage was below his age. In spite of the unintelligibility his clinician hypothesized that he had deficits in size of vocabulary, complexity of sentence structure, and syntactic use. Following is a summary of his performances on the various language measures.

On the Peabody Picture Vocabulary Test, Form A, his raw score of 52 converted to a comprehension or a receptive language age for single words of 5.4 years. His responses were quick and certain during the first 48 items. Then he began to hesitate, indicated he did not know the answer, failed 6 out of 8 consecutive items, and the test was terminated. Either he had limited experience with these words or with the pictures for which they are the representatives. In either case this test indicated that Barry was functioning two years below other children of his age.

The Illinois Test of Psycholinguistic Abilities, Revised Edition (1968) was also given to Barry. Since his clinician had heard many grammatical errors in his spontaneous speech, he started with this subtest. It requires the child to listen carefully to the examiner as he points to a picture and makes a statement about it. The child fills in the appropriate response for the second part of the picture. For instance, the examiner says, "Here is a bed," as he points to the bed. He then points to the two beds and says, "Here are two ______," and the child is to respond "beds." The child gets credit for his response even if he uses a sound substitution for [s] which he may not be able to produce. Barry gave the correct responses to 11 of these syntactic forms and thus obtained a score of 5 years on the subtest.

The other 11 subtests were administered in order. No pattern of strengths and weaknesses emerged. There was little difference between his use of visual and auditory channels. The two subtests that represented his highest and lowest scores were the manual expression and verbal expression. He received a language age of 6 years 1 month on the former and 4 years 10 months on the latter. He was able to communicate more effectively with gestures than he could with words. His total language age was 5 years 6 months.

Home and School Environment. The spontaneous speech situations and the testing are only a part of this process of evaluation. They provide detailed information about the speech, language, and hearing, but they give no information about the assistance which might be obtained from the child, his peers, parents, and school personnel. The people in Barry's environment must be considered both in planning a program of intervention and in prognosticating about the success of intervention.

Barry's teachers and principal were very interested in helping him. The principal had obtained permission from the parents to bring him to the clinic, since the school had no speech clinician at the time. He could not persuade either parent to accompany him and Barry, however. His kindergarten teacher had recommended that Barry be promoted to first grade so that he could have six hours of schooling rather than three, plus a hot lunch. In her school report she had said that he was not really ready for first-grade activities. He had made some gains in her program, in attending to his personal needs, in handling crayons and pencils, in learning to count to 5. However, he was never able to print his name or identify most of the primary colors. At the end of kindergarten he was at the bottom of his class of 25.

His first-grade teacher spent extra time with him while he waited for the bus after school to provide more reading practice. She reported, however, that in spite of his being a year older than the other first graders, he was not functioning on their level in anything—not even in motor activities on the playground.

Barry's peers did not accept him in school. It could be that they did not understand him and therefore could not relate to him. However, that is unlikely because children with no English can usually make themselves understood with gestures and they are accepted. Barry, like his older brothers and sisters in school, was ill-clad, unkempt, and dirty. When he came to the clinic for his initial visit, he was wearing a shirt with no buttons on it, torn jeans, and sneakers without laces. We saw him first in December, with temperatures below freezing, but Barry had on only a thin coat. He wore essentially the same clothes each time he came for further sessions.

Since Barry's mother did not come to school for teacher conferences about any of her children, the principal and a teacher visited her at home several times a year. They were never asked to go inside. They described the house as a four-room shack, with no plumbing. Kerosene was used for lighting and heating. There was some electric supply, however, for the television set. None of the teachers had ever seen the father, though the children talked about him a great deal. In spite of the poverty the family was not on welfare. It seemed unrealistic to hope that we could entice the parents to help us.

And what about Barry? Did he want any change in his speech? As his clinician listened to his chatter in the reception room, he seemed outgoing and eager. He took the clinician's hand as they walked to the clinic, told him his name, age, teacher's name, what he wanted to be when he grew up, why he thought his principal had brought him to this "school."

When they were seated at the table he accepted the invitation to play with the five family figures. He grouped the mother and father figures together at one end of the table and the three children forms at the other. When his clinician asked him to supply conversations among these family members, he had dialogues between mother and father and among the children. When his clinician asked him to have the mother and father talk with the children, he always had the father talk. The father's conversations ran like this: "Let's go to the store," "Put your coat on," "Get me my car keys." When Barry was prompted to tell what the mother said, he shrugged his shoulders and turned away from the table. Only once did he supply a comment made by the mother. In his play he reconstructed many family activities: getting up in the morning, eating dinner, watching television programs, working on the truck in the yard. He used many gestures to help his clinician to understand these conversations.

We can interpret these samples in many ways. Talking at home was not sufficient to provide either an adequate model or adequate practice for Barry. He may have more difficulty talking with his mother than with his father and the other children. In any event his home environment had not squelched him.

Would Barry be willing to work to change his speech and language without encouragment from his parents? According to his teacher, he had learned a great deal of speech during his kindergarten program and was always willing to try as often as necessary to make himself understood. When his clinician asked him if he wanted to learn to talk so that many people could understand him, he said that he did. His efforts during the evaluation sessions indicated that he could and would complete tasks that pushed him a little further than his usual performance. However, he did not tolerate lengthy periods of failure at a task.

Prognosis. Though Barry was willing to try, prognosis for change was guarded. He needed daily therapy, but he did not get to school every day for a variety of reasons. He needed psychological support for his efforts to change his communication. We had only a clinician and a teacher who would be providing positive feedback to him on a regular but limited basis.

Plan for Therapy. Based on this evaluation his clinician recommended that therapy begin with the goal of further acquisition of [r] in words, sentences, and spontaneous speech. He could produce this sound; therefore, time should not be spent on either phonetic placement or on discrimination learning, but rather on providing him with practice to stabilize this phoneme. Since his first and his family names contained [r] and since he pronounced both correctly only part of the time, the clinician began with these words. Other vocabulary for practice came from his reader, with the hope that this additional practice might improve his reading. Other words were selected from his own repertoire to be as functional as possible.

Therapy to modify the other phonemes was to be delayed until [r] was being carried over into conversation at least 90 percent of the time or until Barry and his clinician had reasons to work on [s].

Acquisition and carry-over of [r] should be meshed with work on the grammar and new related vocabulary. For instance, [r] words could be learned within the context of a simple sentence, such as "Dad's car is green," "My name is Barry."

When it was time to begin therapy on [s], the clinician would need to reevaluate his abilities to discriminate [s] from among the other sibilants. If he still could not make the necessary discriminations, his program might have to incorporate [s] discrimination training.

Prevention. We should consider prevention from two vantage points: (1) further disruptions in Barry's communication as he grows older and (2) referrals of other children for evaluation at an earlier stage in development. Barry made limited gains in his therapy program. His clinician could work with him only three times a week for an hour each session the second semester. Barry had no summer program because there was no facility or person to bring him to a center for continued therapy. His grammatical structures and [r] were modified to an extent that he was easier to understand in the classroom and with his clinician. The clinician introduced discrimination training on [s] before the end of the school year, hypothesizing that Barry might practice during the summer with his 14-year-old brother whom he had found to be an ally. Therapy for Barry must be continued for several years.

If Barry had received a nursery program and had therapy at age 4, he might have made gains like those we have observed with Head Start children. Research reports, as well as clinical studies, show that these children can gain as much as two years in a five-month period in vocabulary and other psycholinguistic skills with a daily program with planned objectives.

Evaluation as a Continuous and Dynamic Process. We have attempted to demonstrate what kinds of information must be gathered and how the pieces are fitted together in a complete evaluation. More precise observations, additional speech mechanism data, more detailed testing of linguistic units, information about the early childhood development, premorbid performance and interests, medical reports about the nature and progress of the problem, additional knowledge about the psychological status of the person—for some clients all of these or selected aspects may also be necessary.

When evaluations are conducted in clinics devoted to special problems like cleft palate, cerebral palsy, or laryngectomy, team members are usually selected to cover the wide range of problems of the individuals who are evaluated. Decisions then are made by the team following the staff discussions of their findings.

In the case of Barry the members who brought information about his performance and provided the setting and support for his speech and language program constituted part of an informal educational team. The examiner, the school's speech clinician, the principal, and the first-grade teacher were functioning as a problem-solving group with Barry. An older brother joined the team later. Had his parents been willing, they too would have been a part of the team. As reevaluations are carried out, the team members will change; the process of evaluation is continuous and dynamic.

INTERVENTION

Clinicians plan therapy or intervention programs for those who have a communication disorder. The individual may be dysfluent or may have a voice deviation, a language deficit, an articulation problem, or a combination of these. Clinicians have priorities in selecting those with whom they work. Their employment setting and the time they have available will set a limit on the number whom they feel they can serve.

Most clinicians take into account the following criteria:

1. Relationship between the chronological age and the speech and language age
2. Severity of the problem
3. Prognosis for the life style of the individual
4. Suitability for an already existing speech, language, voice, or fluency group
5. Research considerations
6. Attempts to include some individuals from each unit (class, ward, floor, etc.)

General Principles Underlying Intervention. The first basic principle of intervention is that any program must recognize the uniqueness and individuality of the person. Each person has a personality that must be dealt with. The personality and situation of the individual must be considered in determining the approach to attain communication goals which are set for that individual.

A second principle is that practice makes permanent. Errors in speech production, misuse of the voice, dysfluency, and language deficits may be stabilized unless intervention is initiated. The lisp of the lovely 5-year-old may continue on into adulthood and be a barrier to social and professional opportunities.

A third principle is that a program must instruct the individual in basic rules of speech and language so that he may apply them in new situations. We cannot teach all the nouns that require [s] for plurality, but we can teach categories of nouns that take [s], [z], [əz], and zero inflections for plurality. We can modify the fluency of the speech the individual uses in therapy, but we must teach the rules for maintaining that fluency in all situations.

A fourth principle is that the program must encourage successful performance. Failure does not facilitate learning. The program should be structured to build on what the individual can already do and to introduce new skills gradually. All of us profit from encouragement, whether it is internal or external. Social rewards expressed as words of praise or a nod of the head may be all that is necessary. For others the pure joy of learning and achieving is sufficient encouragement to stay with a task. For others, particularly for retarded children, concrete and tangible token systems are needed.

A fifth principle is that language is our major medium for communication and for thinking. We recognize that some deaf persons use sign language and some of us use a limited set of gestures for communication. We do not require language for thinking at the early stages of child development, but we certainly need language to express our thoughts to others. Language becomes increasingly more important to learning and thinking as we get older.

The sixth principle is that children can learn. A program based on realistic goals, appropriate selection of materials, and an encouraging setting and reward system will bring about changes in their communication skills.

Progress in Therapy. In the process of achieving normal speech, the individual may go through various stages. For some the production may be slow and also labored. For instance, the child who has been substituting [θ] for [s] may still have difficulty keeping the front teeth together to prevent tongue protrusion as he makes the [s] sound. Other children may have no problem with the actual production, but may not know in what contexts to use the newly acquired response. The child who has just learned to add [z] to signify plurality at the end of certain words may overgeneralize and use the ending incorrectly.

Some individuals can use the new learning only in a specific setting or with a specific person. Sometimes the clinic room or the clinician is the reminder that they must communicate in a certain fashion or use certain syntactic structures that they have just learned. Therapy programs therefore encourage clients to practice in other settings, particularly in the classroom and in the home (Bankson and Byrne, 1972). When children say, "Oh, I only have to do that when I'm in speech therapy," we can be sure that they have not learned to automate the new response.

Carry-Over. Carry-over is the client's use of a newly taught response (a sound, a word, a syntactic unit, a new pitch level) appropriately and routinely in spontaneous conversation. Such use demonstrates that the new response has become an established pattern. The task of the clinician is complete when the individual demonstrates carry-over.

Some individuals reach this point in a few lessons, but others never quite achieve it. The clinician must be able to determine when the individual is using the skill as best he can. There are situations in which complete mastery may not be feasible and further work may even be detrimental. For example, children who have been in a therapy program for two years trying to learn to use subject-verb agreement in sentences may be so discouraged with their failures that it is better to discontinue that phase of language therapy. The clinician may work on some other aspects of their speech problems and later return to the syntactic problem.

An example of dismissal from therapy without complete mastery of the articulation function is the case of an 8-year-old boy who had learned to produce every sound correctly in short words, but could not maintain that level of correctness when he engaged in a conversation. His tongue movements were labored, and no amount of drill helped him to increase tongue mobility. Since the clinician felt that the boy was using his tongue as best he could, he terminated the therapy program and simply encouraged the boy to limit the length of his utterances.

Some clients exhibit carry-over but then slip back into their old habits once they are dismissed from their therapy programs. Perhaps they need to overlearn, in order to prevent the regression. Their speech should also be monitored by some one in their environment, such as a parent or teacher, so that they can be referred back for additional therapy as soon as they begin to regress to their old patterns.

There is still another group of children who have complete control of the responses but are unwilling to use them. In some situations the children will avoid talking completely. The emotionally disturbed child who gradually gives up oral communication of any kind is an extreme example. In one such case a clinician conducting an evaluation of a 7-year-old boy, obtained a 13-minute language sample that contained only a total of sixty words. Most of the utterances were phrases such as "I don't know" and "I told you" or single-word responses, such as "bathroom" and "tea." The psychiatrist, who had referred the child to the speech clinician, and the mother, who was in a program of family counseling, both reported that the boy had utilized much more language a year before the evaluation. He was gradually withdrawing from situations which required any interaction on his part, and this trend showed up in his very limited language in the sample.

A CASE STUDY: INTERVENTION FOR MAUREEN. When we evaluated Maureen the first time, she was 5 years old. Her speech was unintelligible because of the large number of phonemes that she either omitted or distorted or for which she used substitutions. Although she tended to use short sentences, we hypothesized that she might have utilized more complex sentence structures if she thought she could be understood. Her hearing and her speech sound discrimination were within normal limits. Her comprehension was excellent, and she was bright. She had misplaced and overlapping upper front teeth that made speech more difficult for her. Her parents were eager to do what they could for her.

We made two kinds of recommendations to the parents. The first was that they take Maureen to an orthondontist for evaluation of the teeth. It was important to get started on that project immediately to prevent any potential emotional problem that might ensue from the dental problem and Maureen's self-consciousness about smiling and to provide a more adequate dental alignment for speech production. Our second recommendation was that the parents bring Maureen back for therapy on a once a week basis. We would have preferred to work with her several days a week, but the family lived a hundred miles from the clinic and each visit required that Maureen's father take the day off since he was the only one who drove the family car.

The parents got started on both of these recommendations immediately. Within two months the orthodontist reported that the maxillary incisor was being moved to a normal position through the placement of an appropriate appliance.

We began a program to modify Maureen's speech immediately. We felt that the parents would have to carry out a large proportion of the therapy program at home because of their distance from the clinic. Therefore, we asked them both to observe Maureen as she worked with us in the clinic. It became obvious, however, that the father seemed the better of the two as a teacher and we therefore concentrated our attention on teaching him what we wanted him to do with Maureen. The mother said that she feared she would do the wrong things with her daughter. Because of her fear and because of her own problem of [s] production, we agreed that she should not work directly with Maureen, but should attempt to understand the nature of her total problem.

Our goal was to help the child to be as intelligible as possible. In therapy we began work on [s], because [s] is one of the phonemes used most frequently in the English language. Her program concentrated on production of [s] in words. Within seven sessions she was using it appropriately in the words that we taught her.

The parents were provided with a home program which they utilized until their next appointment three months later. When we saw Maureen then, her speech had improved considerably. The phoneme that was primarily defective was now the [r]. In addition she was confusing the [l] and the [j] in conversation, and her blends were still defective. However, during a one-hour session with her, we were able to teach her the [r] in a series of ten words such as *read*, *write*, and *run*.

We discussed with the parents the type of reading program that Maureen was getting in her first-grade class. They indicated that the teacher was using a phonics approach. Their impression was that Maureen was learning not only reading, but appropriate speech patterns extremely well as a result of this approach.

We wrote to the teacher to see if we could visit her classroom to determine how she was teaching reading and to give her some cues as to how she could help Maureen further in her communication program. During our visit Maureen, like others in her room, read for us. Maureen's speech pattern was very understandable, more so in the reading than in her sharing time presentation. We talked with the teacher later about the [r] and how she might encourage Maureen to produce it correctly in words in her reader. We decided that Maureen could underline words with [r] and her father would help her with the reading of those words each evening at home.

In order to determine whether Maureen should attend our summer session, we rechecked her in May, just one year following her visit to us. We recommended that she come into the summer program in order to get some additional intensive work on all of the sibilant sounds and additional help with the [r]. However, because of transportation problems, we saw Maureen only twice during the summer. Each time, however, her teacher was present and her teacher continued the speech activities each day with Maureen. Every three months we saw Maureen for additional checks and additional instruction. She learned rapidly and was an apt and very determined pupil. By the time she was 9 she routinely used all phonemes correctly and her spontaneous speech, regardless of topic, circumstance, or temporary tensions, was well within normal limits.

During those years the orthodontist worked on her dental problem and it was corrected by the time she was 8 years of age.

It would be difficult to project what might have happened to Maureen if she had not received speech therapy. She came to us at a time when she was highly motivated to learn, when her parents were willing to work with us, and when she had a teacher skilled in the teaching of phonics. The physical problem could have been much more serious if the treatment had been delayed. Maureen is representative of 1 to 2 percent of children who have serious communication deficits. Because she had learned the phonemes of English inappropriately, her communication was limited. As she or any other child her age gets older, the need for appropriate communication is more pronounced and penalties for inadequate communication begin to have more effect on a child. Maureen's progress resulted from the total involvement, commitment of time, and development of understanding of parents, teacher, principal, clinician, and child.

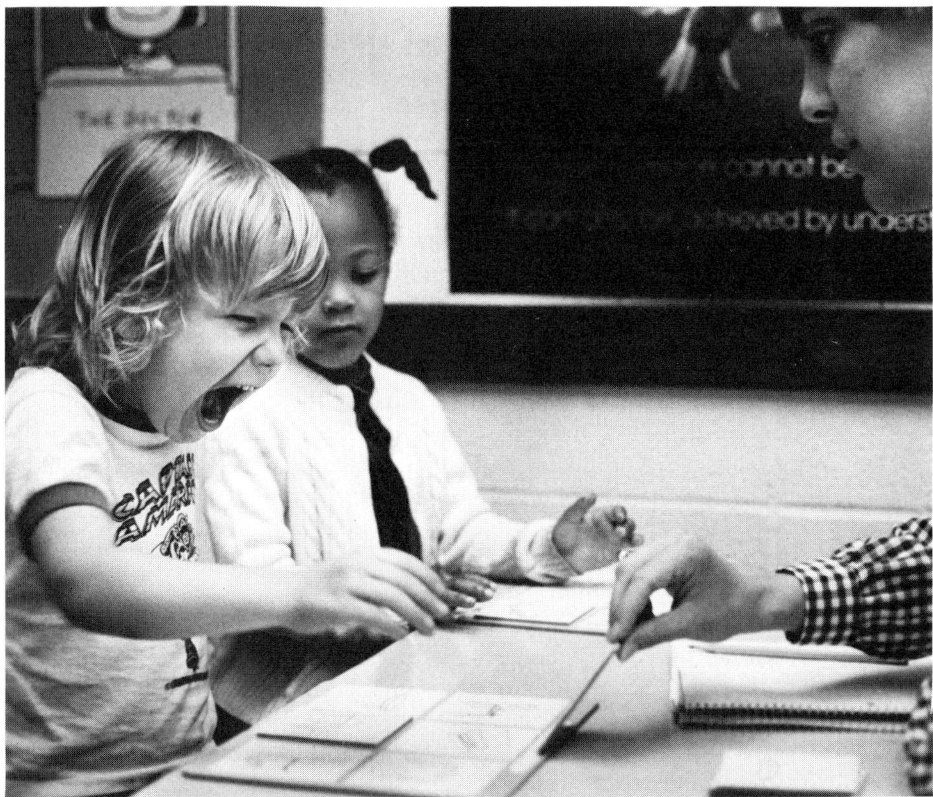

IN-SERVICE PROGRAMS

The clinician is responsible for in-service training of colleagues in the varying employment settings. The amount and the type depends on how much information various professional groups need in order to be able to make appropriate referrals and to work on selected goals of therapy for individuals.

Some clinicians routinely present a great deal of information about their work to groups of pediatricians, physical and occupational therapists, child-care workers, and others. Some provide needed information during the staffing of individuals.

School clinicians probably do the most in-service training. They are dealing with the largest number of pupils whose teachers can be excellent co-workers when they know what is expected of them. We shall deal with this aspect of the school clinician's role in greater detail in Chapter 8.

THE ROLES OF THE TEACHER

Loban (1969) made the following statement about the role of the teacher with regard to communication skills of children.

> Realizing that human worth cannot be measured by the language or dialect a man uses, teachers will be more likely to help children acquire a standard English without making them ashamed of their own language. Such acquisition, not improvement, is easier in situations where drill and directed efforts are oral, where they are linked to language expressing ideas, attitudes and values of genuine concern to the learners. To improve language ability a pupil must apply whatever is studied to situations in which he has something to say, a deep desire to say it, and someone to whom he genuinely wants to say it. (p. 109)

In this statement Loban is indicating that the teacher has a primary role in the modification of the communication skills of children whose language use is inadequate.

MODELING

Teachers are models whom children will imitate. Therefore, teachers must be aware of the volume, quality, and rate of their speech. They must also consider the content of their language. Vocabulary and complexity of sentence structure should be suited to the comprehension level of the students.

IDENTIFICATION OF DEFICITS

Since teachers observe children over a considerable period of time and in a variety of circumstances, from spontaneous interaction with peers to formal learning situations, they are in an ideal position to determine whether the children have any communication deficits. It is not necessary that they be able to identify specific deficits as defined by speech pathologists, but they should be able to recognize the presence of problems related to language, articulation, voice, dysfluency, and hearing difficulties. The more information teachers have about the nature of these problems and about the work of the speech clinician, the easier it will be for them to help the pupils.

GROUP INSTRUCTION

In carrying out language development programs at any level, teachers should plan activities that provide appropriate experiences in listening, thinking, and talking. The needs of both the group and each individual must be considered. The student who is having trouble comprehending needs to have his teacher begin with simple directions and move into more complex ones over time. The child who cannot follow sequences in a story will benefit if the teacher begins with simplified versions which he can monitor and then recall. Some children need to learn concepts such as *one* and *more than one*. The teacher must be concerned with those concepts that are expected of a child at the various grade levels. Most children need to understand the meaning of new words, and dictionary practice is a good technique to introduce to them as early as possible. Explanations of specific questions can be given in such a way that they help students to solve similar problems.

The "sharing time" can be structured so that only a few students talk each day. The teacher can use this informal situation to encourage all to listen to the speaker and to help the speaker to sequence his story about an experience.

When there are a few nonattending children as the teacher tries to tell a story, she can arrange the group so that the distractible ones are next to her or the most difficult to manage is sitting on her lap. Easy physical access to the teacher can encourage model behavior. The teacher must plan all activities in terms of the attention span of the group and in terms of ways to increase the attending time of the children.

CARRY-OVER OR GENERALIZATION ACTIVITIES

Children who are in therapy will improve faster if their teachers relate their class work to the clinician's program. For example, if the goal for a child is utilization of functional language, the teacher can concentrate on key phrases and sentences that are typically needed for use at school and at home and try to move the child along through the hierarchy of the functions of language as far as he can go. For children in first and second grade reading activities provide an excellent opportunity for additional practice. In addition, entire classes of children can engage in language development activities that will raise the level of communication for everyone and in particular aid the child with specific deficits.

Teachers can also provide a record of a child's progress toward the specific goals set by the clinician. For instance, if the clinician wants a child to be able to use correct plural forms of nouns, the teacher can select a group of nouns from the reader and check whether or not the student is reading them correctly. In addition, the teacher can provide an activity in which the child can demonstrate that he knows the difference between *one* and *more than one* when he uses the singular and plural forms of those nouns. The teacher's setting aside a few minutes each day to listen and record information about the goal toward which a child is working can be important in the intervention program.

Many activities that take place outside the classroom can be utilized to improve listening skills and speech development. For example, if the teacher and students eat lunch together, the students can be encouraged to talk about what and how they are eating, to comment about the food rather than hitting one another, pushing, and reaching indiscriminately for all kinds of food. The point is not to teach manners, but to teach simple skills, such as how to pour milk without spilling it, and to encourage verbal exchange in asking for and talking about things. When there are problem children in the group, the teachers can sit next to them, talk with them, put their arms around them, encourage them to enjoy the food which they need.

The bus ride to school can be another opportunity to carry out activities that enable children to achieve selected goals. Monitors can ask the students to observe and tell about what they see along the way—the trees in spring with their budding leaves, a man digging for something (worms for fishing), rain or snow storms. Children can discuss cause-effect relationships. For example, the bus driver approaches a green light, it changes to red, he stops the bus quickly; children jerk forward, some drop their books, and others stiffen. What is the cause-effect relationship among these incidents? The monitors can use the bus ride also to enhance concepts of color, sizes, shapes by having the students describe the buildings and fields that they pass. Children can be encouraged to read the signs of gas stations, stores, and advertisements. They can sing songs to improve their articulation and improve rhythm patterns.

CURRICULUM GUIDES

The curriculum guides that are a part of every school system are revised regularly. Teachers should contribute to the formulation of the school program so that it provides necessary experiences. For example, since listening and speaking are just as much a part of the language arts course of study as reading and writing, the curriculum should include activities designed to improve the listening and speaking abilities of children.

When teachers have an opportunity to write study guides, they can give examples listening and speaking activities. Some of these appear already in the curriculum guides. Others are a part of the language development programs that have been published. Many of these provide for responses in unison. In addition, however, there are opportunities for the child with the problem to be given a special chance to perform an activity.

Kindergarten and preschool group experiences usually involve some listening and speaking. Children gather for an assembly program to watch upper-grade children. They observe films about many topics. They take a trip to the fire station, to the local grocery store, or to a museum. They listen to records of their choice. There is always a story time for the children.

These listening and speaking activities can be utilized for maximum practice. Instead of just going to the fire station, the teacher can prepare the children for what they will see and hear through demonstrations with toys and through selected stories. After the trip the children can be encouraged to tell about what they liked and what they saw—how fires are extinguished, the other activities of firemen, and so on. This type experience can be used to extend vocabularies and logical thought processing.

Most of us learn best in a situation that is pleasant and provides encouragement and motivation. The old adage "Success begets success" is still a good principle for us to follow. When an individual's progress is praised, there is greater likelihood that he will keep on trying. When his attempts are ignored or deprecated, he is likely to respond in some negative fashion. In the film *Search*, prepared by the National Society for Crippled Children and Adults, a father is portrayed as so frustrated by his son's failure to get the blocks in the appropriate slots that he said to him, "No! No! No! You do it this way!" He took the blocks and proceeded to do the exercise that was planned to improve his son's muscular coordination. The occupational therapist who had been watching the situation called the father aside and asked him to play a simple tune on the piano. He started it, stopped, and tried again. She said to him, "No! No! No! You do it this way!" He answered, "Well, give me time and I'll get it." She then explained to the father how frustrating it was for his son who knew what he was supposed to do, but could not do it at this stage of his program. She was trying to help the father to see how recognition of an attempt and a positive reaction to it improve the chances of successful learning. All of us need to be reminded of this principle.

Most individuals need concrete evidence that they are learning a skill. In one language development program for 3- and 4-year-old children, the teacher drew smiling faces beside the names of the children who had performed appropriately during their language development lessons. Some "received" smiling faces for sitting in their chairs, others for attempting to answer questions, and others for telling about a picture. Each child knew for what he was being rewarded. Once the joy associated with learning for learning's sake had developed, this type of concrete evidence is no longer as necessary, but most people do enjoy some praise or indicator for a task well done.

Teachers who are understanding and kind to everyone in the classroom are likely to show compassion for the child or adult with special problems. Teachers establish the emotional climate in the class. If they ignore the individual who is different, deny him opportunities to take turns in recitations because he takes too long, or show displeasure when he cannot make himself understood, the other children will behave in a similar way.

Some teachers have said that they cannot spend time with a handicapped child because they have been hired to teach 30 or 40 students, not 1 or 2. There are ways to solve this problem. Older students or aides can work with the child under the teacher's direction. In university towns many undergraduates in education are assigned to teach individual children as part of their preparation for student teaching.

THE ROLE OF THE PARENTS

Parents and others in the home are the primary sources of language development and enrichment of young children. Parents provide the warmth and understanding that enhance the interpersonal relationships and set the stage for the learning of the structure and functions of language. It is in the home that young children first develop their cognitive sets; there they practice talking, to themselves, to their dogs, their play things, as well as exchanging ideas in words with the children and adults in the home.

Without opportunities for listening to language patterns and attending to the linguistic and paralinguistic structures of speech they have no pattern to follow. The exposure through hearing is essential to normal speech development.

Observations indicate that mothers talk to their babies from the time of birth. Ling and Ling (1974) studied the communication interactions of children 1 to 36 months with their mothers and reported that they tend to talk about immediate matters. The mothers tell the babies about what they are doing as they engage in activities. The study showed that 80 percent of their utterances are either comments or questions about objects and events in the immediate environment. The mothers use complex sentence forms, regardless of the age of the children. They physically manipulate toys and other objects as they show them to the children. They utilize many aspects of the paralinguistic—eye contact, facial expressions, body postures, marked stress and intonation patterns.

Analysis of videotapes of mothers who are just engaging their child in an activity or are teaching the toddler something shows an almost continuous flow of language. The child cannot possibly get more than a few items in the stream of language. As yet we do not know how the child processes or what keys are most critical for those under 2 years of age.

In most homes a great deal of talk goes on among the family members and friends. We hope the language model will be an accurate one, both semantically and grammatically, because the child's utterances will reflect what he hears. The fact that mothers talk more to a first child may be part of the reason that first children tend to have a larger vocabulary than others who come later.

As a result of attending and listening, the child builds a level of language comprehension. When he starts to talk, the parent corrects both grammatical and semantic errors. Parents tend to be more concerned with the semantic correctness. For instance, when the child says, "That a thing," the mother will reply, "No, that's a typewriter" or "No, that's a coat."

READING

Most young children learn about things and people not only through the mother's modeling, but also through books. Parents should read to their children regularly. Even if there are no books in the home, most communities have libraries where books can be obtained for family use. Children identify their favorites easily, and they should be encouraged to select those they wish to be read to them. One 3½-year-old child knows how many books his mother will read to him at bedtime by matching the thickness of the books with the space she demonstrates between her thumb and index finger. She will tell him "I'll read these many pages to you," as she separates the two fingers and shows him. Sometimes he will choose one thick book, and at other times he will pick two or three thin ones.

Parents know that their children have favorite books. They may get tired of rereading those stories night after night, but this activity and the opportunity it provides for developing and maintaining a close relationship is an important way for the child to increase his language comprehension and use. Children can retell the stories to their parents and younger siblings when they have sufficient words. Many children think they are "reading" when in reality they have associated the pictures with the words as they are read to them over and over again.

Just as there are times for eating, there must be time for reading. Each family should determine the amount and the schedule of reading to each child. If the children have similar interests, they may want to share the reading books and time. For the children 6 to 48 months of age reading time may increase from a minute or two to half an hour at a setting. Some parents try to provide two or three reading periods a day, followed by discussion time, and one at bedtime.

IDENTIFICATION OF A PROBLEM

Parents are usually the first to identify a child's lag in development. They may not be able to pinpoint the problem, but they can tell that something is wrong. When parents question whether or not a child is developing normal patterns, they usually can document their reasons. At that point they should seek appropriate evaluations and then follow through on the recommended programs. The next few examples are illustrative.

DYSFLUENCY. Parents may observe that breaks in the rhythm of talking are affecting the communication of a child. Some children are dysfluent during their early language learning, but seem to "outgrow" the repetitions. Parents can ignore this dysfluency completely, concentrating on the thought content of the child's message. In many instances this is just what is needed. Sometimes parents find that their children stop the repetitions of sounds and words when they are instructed to stop and start over again. Parents should seek the advice of a speech clinician if they are unable to help their child's "stuttering."

One set of parents, both college graduates, brought their 3½-year-old son, Bill, to a speech clinic for evaluation because, in their words, "he stuttered." The father was the principal of an elementary school and the mother was a homemaker. Bill's repetitions were very noticeable; some were effortless repetitions of the first sound in a phrase, but he struggled with others. The parents felt he was aware of his struggle to talk, and though they did not draw attention to his speech, they were concerned that his grandparents did.

The clinician talked about ways the parents could create an environment for easy talking—giving him time to talk, not attaching negative values to his disfluency—and suggested that the parents accept Bill's way of expressing himself and not ask him to change.

Six months later, when the clinician called the parents to find out if Bill should be reevaluated, the parents reported that the dysfluency had stopped and that their son was communicating with ease. The father indicated that he probably had felt anxiety about Bill's dysfluency because of two boys in his school. Both were severe stutterers, and he did not want his son to experience the struggles of these boys to make themselves understood when they were called upon in class nor the unwarranted sympathy expressed by teachers for their inadequate communication.

In two other cases the parents were nonplussed when the clinician called to make further appointments with them. Six months before the clinician had evaluated their preschool children because of their stuttering. In both instances the parents had forgotten that their children might have been labeled stutterers, for when the clinician called, the children were talking fluently.

Language is learned best in a home environment that encourages talking, with positive feedback and reciprocal exchanges with the parents and peers. In these three cases the parents had been asking their children to meet the standards of adult communication, and when the children blocked on words and repeated syllables, they were at a loss to know how to handle the situation. The parents became anxious, showed their concern, and the dysfluencies of the children became more noticeable and less acceptable.

College students and other randomly selected individuals report that they stuttered as children, but not at the time of the interviews. When asked to what they attributed the elimination of the stuttering, they said their parents made them stop and start over again when dysfluencies occurred and practiced and drilled them in the use of fluent speech. Some of their parents would say, "Don't do that." These parents were certainly not ignoring the problem; in fact, they were drawing the child's attention to it and asking him to modify his speech behavior. This is a direct approach, and it does work with some individuals.

There has been a decrease in the number of children who stutter. In some communities there are few if any who stutter when they enroll in school. Current child-rearing practices, which allow for an individual's development at his own rate and greater freedom in selecting activities and in decision-making of all kinds, are important in creating a home atmosphere that is conducive to fluency. Any environment that pressures the child beyond his tolerance level can contribute to speech dysfluency.

Hearing Impairment. Parents of hard-of-hearing and deaf children have a complex task of identifying the nature of the deficit. Many hard-of-hearing children begin to speech-read before they get any formal instruction. They look at the face of the person who is talking, they watch the person's mouth, his expression, and his actions in order to understand what is being said. Some are so adept at this activity that parents wonder whether or not the child has a hearing loss. If parents think their child has an auditory problem, they should ask their family physician, pediatrician, or well-baby clinic director to refer them to an ear specialist for an examination of the ears and for hearing tests. Early diagnosis and treatment may eliminate the problem. If not, an educational program must be initiated, preferably as early as possible.

The child may need amplification in order to comprehend and use language. The parents must be sure the sound of their voices and of the television set are loud enough, but not too loud, for their child's understanding. Parents must learn how to check the hearing aid for loudness, how to put in and test the batteries, and how to help their child put his ear mold in the external ear correctly. The preschool years are so vital for development of the child's language comprehension and use that daily teaching is required during that time. Every word and phrase may need to be taught if the loss is severe.

The television set can be modified to permit the hearing impaired child to use earphones as he watches and listens to his favorite programs. In this way the sound can be loud enough for him, without disturbing the rest of the family.

If a child is deaf, the parents need even more specific instructions for teaching their child. These can be supplied by directors and teachers of preschool programs for the deaf, state coordinators of speech and hearing services in the state departments of public instruction, and speech and hearing clinicians in the schools and in speech and hearing centers. Most states have a school for the deaf, whose superintendent can direct parents to the appropriate resources. The deaf child needs a language program immediately. The John Tracy Clinic has a correspondence course which many parents have taken. They use the lessons successfully with their deaf and severely hard-of-hearing children.

Because of the alertness of parents and the awareness of physicians of potential auditory deficits among their patients, many of these children are being identified before they are 6 months of age. When parents get started immediately with language teaching and work closely with a teacher of deaf children, the results can be dramatic. Some of the children are able to function with minimal school subject tutoring when they enroll in schools for nondeaf pupils.

MENTAL RETARDATION. There is at least some evidence that parents of retarded children can contribute to their infant's early development if they are taught what to do. There is no need to wait until the child is 3 years old. Studies of retarded children 3 to 5 years of age indicate that home programs with the parents as language teachers are effective (MacDonald, 1974). Mothers of three of these children observed and recorded what and how language was being taught in a clinic for two months, prè-pared appropriate materials, and carried out the lessons in their homes for the ensuing three months. Their children made tangible gains in length and complexity of their utterances in comparison with other similar children who had no language program. Children who began with single-word utterances, after five months, were putting two to four words together and had increased the frequency and range of grammatical rules in conversation.

THE NEEDS OF THE INDIVIDUAL WITH A DEFICIT

In the preceding material we have discussed the roles of clinicians, teachers, and parents. In this section we would like to focus on the individual with the problem at three different stages of life—as a child, an adolescent, and a senior citizen. We will consider the needs at each stage and suggest some ways in which we can contribute to adequate communication.

THE CHILD

Children who have been identified as either delayed or deficient in speech or language need many types of help. Whether they are in nursery or elementary grades, their teachers act as a major model for type of speech and language patterns as they give directions, tell stories, and provide all kinds of information orally. Young children tend to idolize their teachers anyway, and they will follow the lead of the teachers if they are encouraged to do so.

Children need to know what is expected of them in the classroom. They cannot guess what is required when they fail to carry out a direction or cannot be understood when they are telling a story or giving some information. They have the right to be told what is interfering with their failure to follow directions or to communicate orally.

Children also need opportunities in the classroom to listen, to talk, and to utilize experiences both in and outside the school. Many children with learning problems are carrying out primarily seat work. Some of them are in booths which isolate them from the other children during much of the day. Some teachers of these children report that there is almost no oral communication. The children learn to listen individually to the teacher, but they do not have an opportunity to talk with classmates or with the teacher and classmates in sharing verbally what they think and what they like. If they have language deficits, they are not in situations in which the teachers can identify specifically what is wrong or provide opportunities for improving the communication system.

Children need understanding and acceptance of their speech skills. There is nothing more demoralizing than being cut off in the middle of a presentation. They may be talking too long or are not being understood. In any event, termination of the oral situation should be handled deftly by the classroom teacher.

The child should be the center of attention. He is the one who is learning and makes the changes. If the program goals can be worked out as a joint endeavor of the teacher and child or the clinician and child, there is a greater likelihood of successful learning. Children like to be involved in the decision-making process. Parents use this principle when they ask the child which story he wants to hear at bedtime.

Children expect us to understand what they mean when they do talk. Though they use utterances that are not as definitive as we might wish, we are expected to get the point of what they are telling us. A clinician was talking to a very verbal 4-year-old child and her mother one afternoon. After the child told the clinician about a new toy she had brought with her, she climbed under the chair between her mother and the clinician. When the mother said, "Talk to the lady," the child answered, "I can't, Mommy, I'm under the chair." The clinician made another attempt to redirect the child's attention to her. As she gently pulled on the child's shoes, the clinician asked her if she could have them. Her mother said, "She is going to take your new shoes." The child turned on her back under the chair and giggled. She talked about the chair legs, about what she would do when she got home. Clinician and parent got the message. The child had "terminated" her direct talking to them.

THE ADOLESCENT

Although most of the speech difficulties associated with young children have disappeared by the time a student enters high school, a few serious problems will still be evident. Students with cleft palates or hearing deficits, those who stutter, and those whose language and articulation learning is faulty will be recognized during their first recitations in the classroom. Some of the students have known about their problems and refused help. Others have not been aware of the influence of their communication skills on eventual employment. The girl whose lisping may have been rewarded as a child because it was "cute" may now be penalized and labeled as immature. The boy whose hearing loss interferes with his ability to get signals on the football field may need considerable counseling before he accepts the needed hearing aid. The student whose surgical repair of a cleft lip has left visible scar tissue and prevented normal alignment of the lips may be very conscious at this age of the poor cosmetic effect. The black student who is using nonstandard morphology and syntax will have limited access to a vocational or college program if he does not get help.

In communities where there is no clinical speech program in the schools the communication deficits of the adolescent may not have been treated. As a result his speech pattern and his attitudes may be difficult to change. If there is no speech clinician in the school district, it is important that the teacher and other school personnel be familiar with the resources in the community and in the state for helping these young people.

Within the school setting the teacher can consult several professional colleagues. The school nurse can provide a great deal of medical history data about those students whose speech difficulties seems to be related to medical problems. The nurse can discuss a referral to medical specialists with the family. If the student has an open bite or another serious type of dental malocclusion which may be related to the speech problem, consultation with an orthodontist may be necessary. The student whose audiogram indicates a hearing loss needs to be rechecked for possible referral to an ear specialist. If the community is small and has no specialists, then the family physician should be encouraged to send his patient to the nearest community which has the required service. Arrangements can be made through county social agencies for financial assistance for those who cannot afford to pay for such services.

If the high school has a counselor, the teacher can utilize his skills in guidance for those students who are unable to cope with the communication deficit. The counselor can discuss attitudes with the student and can work with the school nurse in arranging for necessary evaluations and follow-up of the recommendations.

In high schools which are too small to employ counselors or have been unable to obtain such specialists, the principal should be familiar with the state resources and with some agencies which can provide the necessary information. The coordinator of the state's speech and hearing programs, who usually is a member of the staff of the division of special education in the state department of public instruction, can provide the names of qualified speech and hearing clinicians in specific areas of a state. Several colleges and universities maintain speech and hearing clinics to which students can be referred for both evaluation and therapy. The offices of vocational rehabilitation, with branches throughout a state, are concerned with those who can be given special training which will improve the individual's employment possibilities.

Most states have agencies designed to provide services for those students with a physical handicap, such as a crippled children's commission. Children born with handicaps, such as a cleft palate or orthopedic problem, can be referred to this agency and then sent to appropriate team clinics for evaluation and remediation.

Many young high school students with language and articulation difficulties could be aided if they desired help and knew of the resources available to them. Although high school students may be too busy with their individual programs during the school year, they can concentrate on their communication problems during the summer. Many universities sponsor summer speech programs which enroll these young people. Each state has some special resources for the high school student with speech or hearing problems that require specialized remedial programs. Encouragement and preliminary investigation may provide the impetus for major changes in the communicative facility of a student. Which of us can determine how much we may be contributing to the total learning and personality development of that student!

If there is a speech clinician in the district, he may be able to provide a therapy program for these students. If he cannot, because of his limited time, he can be a resource person to whom other school personnel can turn for sources of help.

THE SENIOR CITIZEN

The older person with a communication problem should receive an evaluation just as children do. Once the nature and severity of the communication problem is known, a program specific to the individual's needs can be planned.

The following suggestions will be useful regardless of whether the person is in a residential care center or in his own home. All of us should talk more slowly and in shorter sentences to the elderly with a communication problem. Also, if we expect to provide any practice for him, we must wait for his response. If he is hard-of-hearing, remember that talking louder will help some but not all such persons. We should look at the person as we talk to him. Also, we should check to make sure that if he is wearing a hearing aid, the batteries are working properly and the aid is turned on.

If a person is a cardiac patient and needs better breath control, we can help him to carry out exercises planned by the physical therapist and offer other suggestions. One person with limited breathing capacity found that she could walk up stairs and up hills if she let the person with whom she was walking do the talking. In that way, she conserved her energy and air until she reached a level surface.

Sometimes patients wear ill-fitting dentures or refuse to wear them because they hurt. The gums shrink with age and dentures that were made many years ago may no longer fit. Whenever possible the dentures should be fixed and the patients encouraged to use them. Teeth are important in speech production and their absence or the use of ill-fitting dentures will cause defective pronunciation. In addition, teeth add to personal attractiveness.

One of the most important needs of the aged is sufficient social stimulation, so that they do not slip into withdrawal. Communication is an important aspect of life, and it should be fostered. Stroke patients particularly need encouragement because many of them do not recover complete command of speech. Some patients who seem to have adequate recovery do not use language appropriately. A director of a nursing home reported that he had difficulty keeping aides on one floor because of the communication behavior of one of the patients. The patient would be talking in a sensible fashion and then suddenly begin to curse the aide. It did not matter which aide was on duty. In this instance the woman needed a therapy program to help her to differentiate between appropriate and inappropriate language use. Otherwise, she might have lost her chances to communicate. In addition the aides needed to understand that the cursing was not verbal abuse, but rather that those were the only words available to the woman at that time.

DEVELOPMENT OF EXPRESSIVE LANGUAGE

TECHNIQUES

There are procedures that are appropriate for teaching particular aspects of expressive language such as vocabulary, inflections, syntax, or sounds. Some of the techniques are more suitable for the slow developing child than others. The following list includes specific techniques that clinicians use in intervention and teachers utilize in classrooms.

1. Instruction through simultaneous demonstration and talking
2. Physical manipulation of a child to put him through a series of actions
3. Story telling
4. Group discussion
5. Drill
6. Expansion
7. Modeling
8. Prompting
9. Echoing
10. Questions in different forms to elicit yes or no answers, labeling, or open-ended responses
11. Commands which require an active or verbal response

Some of these procedures are either self-explanatory or have been described in the chapter on language acquisition.

An example of instruction through demonstration and talking would be the teaching of a safety lesson with stop and go signs. The instructor would explain in words what each means. Then he would have the children move or stop moving in response to the red and green signals as a demonstration of the meaning. This particular lesson would provide instruction not only in safety, but also in colors and commands.

Physical manipulation is particularly helpful with the slow learning child. If he is to be the policeman at the street corner, the teacher can take the child's arm and raise it to indicate that the children can now cross the street or extend it to keep the children from moving into traffic. She may even have him be the policeman in the classroom, utilizing those same actions to make sure he understands.

Story telling can be conducted in many different ways to serve different purposes. A technique designed to develop memory and sequencing of events involves using a series of large cards on which characters are carrying out a set of actions. A few sentences for the instructor to read appear on each card. When the listeners are asked to retell the story, the pictures can provide cues to help them recall the story and details of sequence. Stories can be told to develop children's ability to listen for content. The children may identify the characters, describe what each one did, and express ideas about why the story ended as it did. There are many reasons for telling stories and the instructor should be aware of all of them. The complexity of the story should, of course, be suited to the level of functioning of the children.

There are many situations in which the teacher acts as a group discussion leader. This activity is particularly useful with very bright children. It may be that the teacher wants them to decide how to handle a bus trip that the group is arranging. The children may determine that they want to go to a new section of the zoo or to a museum of natural history or an art museum. Group discussion can provide opportunities for everyone to talk and to use the most efficient language and correct structures.

Drill has been one of the mainstays of clinical activity. One program that we describe later is based on drill-group responses that are given immediately following the teacher's model. There is no doubt that drill can function as one of the means of practice. Saying a phrase or set of names for identification over and over again can help to stabilize the correct responses. However, we should recognize that it gets boring for the very bright child as well as for the developmentally slow individual.

The techniques of expansion, modeling, and prompting were described in the chapter on language acquisition. Most instruction provided by teachers falls into these categories.

Questions can be used to get a child to talk or to practice selected structures. The form of the question determines the type of response. Questions beginning with "what is" elicit one-word answers called *labels*. Questions beginning with the copula or an auxiliary, such as "Are you going home?" require a *yes* or *no* response. Both of these are important for the child who is in the early stages of language learning. Other forms of questioning allow for practice in longer responses. Questions beginning with *how* and *why* have open-ended responses and provide practice in lengthier explanations and descriptions which tend to be in the form of sentences.

Commands may be used to elicit a verbal response or to test or practice comprehension. The command most likely to be used for obtaining oral responses is, "Tell me about ______." When working on comprehension of commands, the teacher asks children to carry out actions, such as "drink your milk" or "come to the chalk board."

RESPONSES

The procedures we have just explained require various types of responses:

1. Imitation
2. Rehearsal to oneself
3. Self-correction
4. Practicing aloud
5. Sentence completion
6. Construction of spontaneous verbal responses
7. Retelling a story
8. Role playing

The first four responses are the primary tools of most children for learning. Imitation is one of the means a child has for learning a language initially. In addition, we can observe children rehearsing to themselves as they get ready to talk or explain something to an adult. We also note their self-correction while they are talking to both peers and adults. We can observe their practicing aloud whatever the verbal activity may be.

The other four response types are utilized in all settings—in the classroom, at home, or in the clinic. The child completes sentences when his mother asks him certain questions. Whenever he is talking to someone about what has happened during the day or wants to engage in a verbal interchange of any kind, he is constructing spontaneous verbalizations. Children retell stories they have heard to their parents, to their peers, and to younger children. Their role playing can be observed particularly in the games they choose to play. Creative dramatics of all kinds are particularly productive in the development of language for imagery. When the clinician wants the student to take over her role, the role exchange intrigues many of them. Any activity such as word bingo or games involving the exchange of pictures with which the person must do something represents some kind of role exchange also.

Although we have cited examples of ways in which children use these procedures, adults who are still mastering their communication patterns and those who are trying to relearn them will use the same ones. For example, the stroke patient may utilize a great deal of imitation if he is aphasic or may engage in practicing aloud if he is dysarthric.

COMPREHENSION VERSUS PRODUCTION APPROACHES TO LANGUAGE

There are two major points of view about the teaching of a language. Winitz and Reeds (1973) feel that normal children learn to comprehend language long before they are able to utilize more than simple word responses. Therefore, they feel whatever is being taught emphasis on comprehension must precede expression.

Other programs require imitative repertoires which the child produces without knowledge of what the words mean. Guess, Sailor and Baer (1974) have pointed out that children use words to which they attribute an incorrect meaning or no meaning at all and after acquiring the sound of the words through imitation eventually learn to attach the correct meaning to them.

Regardless of the approach, in the classroom situation comprehension of selected commands must be taught if the children do not understand them. The children's knowledge of their meanings enhances management within the classroom. They can be taught through demonstration with the total group. Commands such as "bring me, give me, show me, open the door, sit down, and close your book" are typical of those used in talking to children.

Many of the highly structured programs are based on order of acquisition. If the program is teaching concepts, those that are learned first are presented first. The same statement holds for the order of teaching phonemes, morphology, syntax, and semantics.

SPECIFIC LANGUAGE PROGRAMS

All language programs have the same general goal—utilization of adequate linguistic skills. The organized programs stress one or two of the major aspects of language. Some deal with the sound system, others are concerned with grammatical structures, and others are oriented to vocabulary. Some have been designed specifically to be used on a daily basis in classrooms, with the teacher presenting the lessons. Others were planned for clinicians who are working with language-impaired children. When teachers use programs designed for a one-to-one or small group relationship, they must modify the programs to meet the needs of classroom activity. When clinicians utilize programs designed for classroom participation, they tend to select techniques and ideas that will help them with children with various language problems. Programs designed for the classroom or the clinic tend to utilize the procedures which we have described above. The programs either have been developed and field tested or they have been designed as a part of specific research. Many of them require materials like pictures, toys, and furnishings in addition to the descriptive manual. Since new language programs are being marketed every year, we have chosen to present only a few examples.

Most of the programs that are based on the structure of the language are organized on the basis of developmental norms. Since there is some evidence that certain inflections are likely to be used correctly by children earlier than others, the programs take this into account. We also know that when children are learning to talk, they leave out the functors such as the prepositions, the articles, and the conjunctions.

Programs that teach structures that are learned easily may not contribute a great deal to intelligibility. Two that are easy to teach are the prepositions and the verb form *will* or its contractions *I'll* to designate future time. If more basic structures need to be taught then start with those. Selection of a program for children should be guided by two questions: What does the child or the group need most? and What will contribute most to their skills in communication?

Regardless of what program is utilized, there are specific requirements for the child and corresponding set for the clinician or teacher. The child must attend to whatever is being taught. For instance, the child who is learning ten new vocabulary words usually needs to look and listen. The clinician or the classroom teacher may be utilizing pictures, toys, or objects as stimulus materials. The child's task is made easier if the right materials are selected.

Just as children practice their writing and their reading skills, so they must work on the linguistic unit they are learning. Practice may be of two types: oral or rehearsal to oneself. Oral practice includes the direct imitation of the model and responses to structured activities such as sentence completion or answering questions.

To show whether there is carry-over of the new structure, the child must use it in many situations. As he learns the plural noun inflections, he must begin to select the correct inflection for the various nouns he is using and use all of them easily and spontaneously in his speech.

THE JOHNSON-MYKLEBUST PROGRAM

The Johnson-Myklebust Program (1967) is based on the assumption that children with delays in language learning have auditory or expressive language deficiencies. These interfere with all kinds of academic learning. They spill over into arithmetic, reading, and other school subject matter. As a result, the authors recommend that this group of children be identified and carefully evaluated so that the classroom teacher can begin a program at the level of the child's performance.

The authors identify disordered language as encompassing (1) generalized deficits in auditory learning, (2) deficits in auditory verbal comprehension, and (3) disorders of auditory expressive language. The programs that they recommend are directly tied in with the individual's major problem and the level at which he is functioning. They consider the child with a generalized deficit in auditory learning as one who hears, but is unable to interpret. He understands neither spoken words nor the sounds of the environment and therefore is unable to structure his auditory world. All the activities which they suggest involve the development of meaningful auditory experiences. They include materials and exercises designed to increase the auditory awareness of the child, the ability to determine where sounds or an order comes from. The child may require selective discrimination training, work on auditory memory, auditory reflection, and rhythm patterns. In their text Johnson and Myklebust provide direction for establishing some competency in each of these particular areas.

Those who have auditory verbal comprehension deficits are unable to relate the spoken language to an experience. As a result, simultaneous presentation of the experience with its related linguistic unit is the major technique of this approach. The program includes some repetition of modeled utterances, selective teaching of the understanding of all the parts of speech. Every word or utterance that is taught is associated with an experience. It may be the experience of feeling the objects as they are presented or looking at the pictures as they are being described. The children are expected to comprehend longer and longer sentences.

Many of the suggested activities can be tape-recorded. Then the child can turn on his tape to find out what he is to do. In this way he can practice listening and immediately carry out the exercise whether it be in a sequence of one, two, or ten parts.

The authors assume that generalized auditory skills and auditory verbal comprehension will precede expressive language. Within the group of expressive language deficits they identify three types: (1) difficulty in remembering or retrieving words and word units for spontaneous use, (2) difficulty in execution of the motor patterns necessary for speaking, and (3) inability to organize words to express ideas in complete sentences. Morphologic and syntactic errors are present in the expressive language of this group long after normally developing children have acquired them. To facilitate recall they recommend activities such as usage of words in context, word associations, words in series or categories, use of visual cues, rapid naming, self-monitoring, and continued use. For those children who are unable to program the movements for expressive language, the approach is motoric. They are taught to feel the muscles involved in speech production, to observe those movements visually, and to move from single sound production to the blending of sounds into words.

Those children with sequencing and morphologic problems must learn the structure of language. This is done through sentence patterns associated with experience. Many of the activities dealing with plurality, verb tenses, and other specific morphologic inflections from Distar (Engelmann, Osborn, and Engelmann, 1972) and other programs could be utilized in this program as long as they were restructured not for drill but in line with specific experiences.

A GUIDE FOR LANGUAGE AND LISTENING DEVELOPMENT

The program, a Guide For Language and Listening Development, was used and field tested in the Hartford, Connecticut, public schools (Graber, 1971). It cuts across the morphologic, syntactic, and semantic aspects of language. The authors utilize the units in the kindergarten curriculum, including subject matter such as safety, seasons, family, transportation, people of the community. For the most part the authors use an experiential approach. One unit, called "Myself and My Family" is divided into eight parts. Each part has a set of purposes and the materials to be used in that part are identified for the classroom teacher. For example, activities described in the first part of the unit are designed to have each child say his own name, encourage each one to listen to the other children and learn the names of the others, have the children listen to a story and recall a specific detail. The children begin their school day by saying "hi" or "good morning" to Mr. Bear, a large, cuddly teddy bear. Each one introduces himself to Mr. Bear. Then, in order to help the children to listen for one another's names and for their own, a jumping game is introduced. The teacher says, "John, will you jump?" and "Joe, will you jump?" Each child has an opportunity to jump individually and then in partnership with someone else in response to commands such as "Will Cathy and Helen jump?" or "John, will you tell someone to jump with you?" The third activity involves the children's listening to a story of the teacher's choice and being able to recall at least one detail from the story. There is a great deal of stress on language use for naming, conceptualization, and for problem solving. Teachers who do not have the time to develop their own activities may be able to use materials from this syllabus. Not every unit is comparable in either completeness or in the explicitness of the goals. However, it is sufficiently well organized that teachers of kindergarten and first-grade children and those in special classes can utilize the materials with the specified goals in mind.

DISTAR

Distar (Engelmann, Osborn, and Engelmann, 1971), a two-year program planned originally for preschool culturally different children, is appropriate for both preschool and older handicapped children. The program is designed to teach the language of instruction which children need to understand and use. Each of the two parts of the program, Distar I and Distar II, has 180 lessons that are presented at a fast pace. The daily lessons take about half an hour. In Distar I, 22 language concepts are taught (Table 7–1). The language learned in Distar I is further expanded and generalized in Distar II. The latter focuses on qualities and relationships in the child's world and provides practice of the skills learned in Distar I.

Before the teacher begins Distar I, she administers the placement test individually to each member of the class. It evaluates the child's ability to understand identity statements such as "This is a car," "That's a book," action statements such as "The girl is running," "Can the girl run?" and "Is the girl running?" polars such as *long-short*, *big-little*, and prepositions such as *in*, *on*, *under*. In addition to comprehending these forms, the child's ability to use them in complete statements is also evaluated.

On the basis of the children's responses to the placement test, they are grouped for the Distar program. Those who have minimal or no language probably will need the preprogram. Others will start at points that take into account what they know and what they do not know.

Tests are administered at the end of the series of lessons on each concept. In that way the teacher can determine whether or not the children have learned the concept.

Table 7–1. Concepts Taught in Distar I

Concepts	Examples
Identity statements	This is a _______ . This _______ is _______ .
Polars	long-short, loud-soft
Prepositions	in, on, under
Pronouns	I, you, we
Multiple attributes	tall and full
Comparatives-superlatives	longer, longest
Locations	grocery store, park
Same-different	boy-boy, girl-boy
Only	only hamburger
Action statements	What is she doing? Hiding under the table
Categories	vehicles
Plurals	regular plural inflection: cats, dogs
Why	Why is the girl smiling?
Verbs of the senses	I see, I hear
Verb tense	Regular and irregular inflections for past tense; future tense
If-then	If he flies, he'll get home faster.
Before-after	After he ate the hamburger, he ate the pie.
Parts	Parts of a train, of a body
Or	She gives him the book or the paper.
All	All are smiling.
One	One boy will dive.
Some, all, none	Some matches are burning, all are burning, none are burning.

Source: S. Engelmann, J. Osborn, and T. Engelmann. *Distar.* Chicago: Science Research Associates, 1972.

Those who fail a test repeat the lessons on that concept and are retested. Engelmann indicates that most instances of failure to learn are a reflection of inaccurate placement in a group, rather than failure of the individual. If the teacher has grouped pupils on the basis of the placement test and any other information available about them, they should learn at a similar rate and therefore be able to pass the tests at the same time.

The program itself is organized into tracks, formats, and tasks. A *track* is a subject or a concept that is presented for several days in the lessons. Examples are the identity statements, which are used in lessons 1 through 23, or the action statements, in lessons 1 through 78. A *format* is the way the exercises are presented. For instance, the teacher points to each item and says to the group, "This is a book, this is a car, this is a boy." Then, the teacher points to the items, and asks the pupils, "What is this?" The first level of response is the single word, "car." Then the teacher adds the instruction, "Say the whole thing," when he asks the question. At this point a complete sentence, "This is a car," is the expected response. This format is used a great deal in the lessons. As the pupils progress, the format becomes more complex.

Tasks are group and individual activities in a lesson, and each has several exercises. Each exercise requires a response from the children.

In summary, then, the track is the concept to be taught over time, the format is the way or the how the concept is taught, and the task is an exercise selected to teach the concept.

In addition to the placement test, the tracks, and the tests for the concepts, there are review sections to ensure maintenance of the concept. If the class has not generalized what they have been taught, they will fail the reviews. At that point, the teacher returns to the appropriate sections of the program.

The Take Homes are a child's "reward" to show his parents what he has been doing. He gets a Take Home when he has successfully completed a unit.

Because this instructional system is based on the assumption that failure on a task by one individual is an indication of the group's lack of understanding or correct use, there is little time spent in individual teaching. Engelmann suggests that the teacher spend no more than five seconds in helping an individual child on an exercise.

Teachers who have been utilizing this program have modified it to some extent. They use the contraction *it's* rather than *it is*. Also they have slowed down the pace of presentation of items because the pace has not given some children sufficient time to think about and rehearse their answers. The research on this program has indicated that it helps the rote reading of the children, but not necessarily reading comprehension (Spicker, 1971). What specific effects Distar has on the spontaneous expressive language of children has not been evaluated. Teachers report that it is effective in developing communication skills, but we need more measures to support or negate the teachers' clinical hunches.

PEABODY LANGUAGE DEVELOPMENT KITS

The series, Peabody Language Development Kits (Dunn, Smith, and Horton, 1965), was designed to stimulate language use of educable retarded and culturally different children. There are four sections: (1) level p (mental ages 3–5); (2) level 1 (mental ages 4½–6½); (3) level 2 (mental ages 6–8); (4) level 3 (mental ages 7½–9½). For each of the four levels a manual has been developed which describes 180 lessons. The list of materials for each lesson is included in the manual. Each level has pictures, puppets, posters, and plastic color chips. Level 2 includes a Teletalk. The Teletalk set can be used as a telephone, a two-way radio, or any other communication system that the teacher selects. The materials are attractive and the children enjoy utilizing them. Although the authors indicate that the programs can be presented to classes of 30 children, there are more opportunities for individual recitations if the lessons are presented to smaller groups. There is sufficient material in the four levels for language development programming for children over a four-year period.

This language development program provides still another approach to the stimulation of language comprehension and use. It stresses an overall oral language development program. A great deal of stress is placed on conceptualization and cognitive processing. Children who have not been exposed to programs like "Sesame Street" or who have had little exposure to storybooks can be introduced to a world of words associated with pictures and be given opportunities to develop their imaginations through the story pictures. The program was not designed to correct specific linguistic structures. There are no tests designed as a part of the approach and therefore no direct means of measuring the effectiveness of the program. It is an enrichment program and should be viewed as such by the classroom teacher.

Clinicians use many of the materials in these kits for purposes for which they were not originally designed. When the clinician is teaching categories, she may withdraw those picture cards dealing with different categories from the kits for her clinical language program. She also may utilize many of the pictures to teach vocabulary to individual or small groups of children. The large posters are resources for teaching and measuring sequencing ability of children.

The authors of this program have directed research studies which indicate that verbal intelligence, psycholinguistic achievement, and school achievement were raised significantly as a result of these lessons.

THE CHILD SPEAKS

The speech improvement program described in *The Child Speaks* (Byrne, 1965) is based on research in two midwestern school systems. The research showed that children improved in many facets of language arts when their teachers presented this program daily. Individual children and entire classes of children at both the kindergarten and first-grade levels made spectacular gains in the use of correct articulation. Some of their reading skills also improved more than those of children who did not receive the program.

The plan includes one unit which emphasizes the development of adequate listening patterns and identification of the speech mechanism. The rest of the units stress specific sounds. The [p] sound, which is used correctly by almost all children at age 5, is reviewed during the second week. At least one week is spent on each of the 13 consonant sounds which Templin (1957) and others have identified as those that are learned last by children. The central theme for each unit and the object used to identify each of the sounds are listed in Table 7–2.

The order in which the units are taught is flexible. In the program as listed in Table 7–2 the units were arranged to coincide with children's interest in holidays such as Thanksgiving and Valentine's Day, but they can be arranged to suit the purposes of each teacher or clinician. For example, the sounds might be introduced at the first-grade level in line with the reading program.

The approach to teaching each sound involves the following steps.

1. Identification of the sound
2. Listening for the sound
3. Discrimination between the sound and those with which children tend to confuse it
4. Production of the new sound
5. Carry-over of the new sound in key phrases

The five steps and the types of activities recommended to attain each one are outlined in Table 7–3.

The materials used with the syllabus include animals, objects, pictures, filmstrips, records, hand mirrors, and a class scrapbook. The animal, Mr. Frog, introduces all the sounds, and the Sound Box is his "home." He "lives" there with the listening ears

Table 7–2. Order of Presentation of Sounds in The Child Speaks Speech Improvement Program

Unit	Central Theme	Identifying Object
1	sounds around us	
2	*p* sound	pig
3	*k* sound	Captain Kangaroo
4	*s* sound	Timmy Teakettle
5	*z* sound	buzzing bee
6	Review of *p, k, s, z*	
7	*g* sound	gray goose
8	*sh* sound	seashell
9	*l* sound	telephone
10	*f* sound	funny face
11	Review of *g, sh, l, f*	
12	*v* sound	valentine
13	*ch* sound	choo-choo-train
14	*j* sound	jack-in-the-box
15	*r* sound	rooster
16	Review of *v, ch, j, r*	
17	voiced *th* sound	airplane
18	unvoiced *th* sound	thumper
19	review of entire program	

Source: M. C. Byrne. *The child speaks—A speech improvement program for kindergarten and first grade children.* New York: Harper & Row, 1965.

Table 7–3. Outline of Daily Goals and General Activities for Each Sound in The Child Speaks Speech Improvement Program

Day	Goals and Activities
First day	I. Introducing the sound of the week[a] A. Association of the sound with the name of an animal or a familiar object B. Words in which the sound is found 1. Identification of children whose names contain the sound 2. Objects or animals that make the sound 3. Names of colors, objects in the room, or numbers which contain the sound
Second day	II. Listening for the sound A. A story which stresses vocabulary that requires the sound B. Questions based on the story or other activities that require answers which utilize the sound
Third day	III. Discriminating between the new sound and other sounds Picture materials which require children to determine whether or not the sound of the week is present in the names of the pictures
Fourth day	IV. Producing the correct sound in isolation and in words A. Action games B. Stories C. Activities
Fifth day	V. Sharing time—carry-over of correct sound production in show and tell time Utilization by the children of a key phrase which includes the sound

Source: M. C. Byrne. *The child speaks—A speech improvement program for kindergarten and first grade children.* New York: Harper & Row, 1965.

[a] More than one week can be spent on each sound, depending upon the speech needs of the children and the number of activities utilized.

and all the other animals that symbolize special sounds. The only pictures available at the time this program was developed were small. However, they are colorful, and if the children were in a circle, they had no trouble seeing them. Large pictures are now on the market.

If an instructor feels that a different set of words might be more effective with the class, there is no reason why they cannot be substituted for those in the book for any of the phonemes, as long as the words provide the appropriate practice for a sound. For instance, in the unit on the phoneme [s] the children are to listen for differences between the [s] and its typical substitutions. The program suggests pictures for words with [s], such as *sailor*, *sled*, *swing*, *school*, and *house*, and for the words without [s], such as *thumb*, *telephone*, *shoe*, *shirt*, and *radish*. If the children don't know about sleds or radishes, more familiar words should be substituted. Also, the stories suggested for story time were based on the recommended books for children just prior to the publication of the program in 1965. Since that time other stories have appeared that can replace the suggested ones.

Teachers spend 15 to 40 minutes daily on the lessons. They are encouraged to incorporate the work on the speech sound in as many other activities as possible. Many kindergarten teachers have used the syllabus as a core curriculum, with the week's sound determining their activities for art, music, story telling, physical education, and arithmetic.

Teachers can carry out these activities with minimal in-service training. The original research on the effectiveness of the program indicated that the number of children requiring a special speech program after its use was reduced by one-third (Byrne, 1966). Follow-up questionnaires directed to the original teachers who participated in the research project indicated that they were still using this approach to speech sound learning ten years after the program was initiated. They introduced new materials, but utilized the basic outline of the program.

GRAY-RYAN PROGRAM FOR THE NON-LANGUAGE CHILD

The Gray-Ryan Program for the Non-Language Child (1973) is a highly organized approach to teaching grammatical forms. It should be used under the supervision of the clinician. Teachers and specially trained aides can administer it. The authors have developed 40 units to teach a group of nouns and the basic grammatical structures (Table 7–4). The order of presentation of the 40 units is based on their teaching value. When unit 1 is learned, those responses are combined with the next unit. In other words, the language learning is cumulative.

Most of the steps in each unit utilize some form of imitation or prompting. The initial steps require that the model presents a stimulus, the child imitates the stimulus, and the child receives a token. Each child response that is being trained is conditioned, and it is then coordinated with the next response he must learn. He is given no trial examples before the unit begins, but is expected to catch on to the procedure quickly. If the child's first 10 responses in a step are wrong, he can be given some short instructions. If his next 10 responses are also wrong, the instructor uses a branching index to return the child to an earlier step where he had success. If he continues to fail the task, the instructor can try anything that might work. No attention is given to comprehension of the modeled stimulus presented to the child.

Table 7–4. Program Units in the Gray-Ryan Program for the Non-language Child

A. Core programs
   1. Identification of nouns
   2. Naming nouns
   3. *In/on*
   4. *Is* (copula)
   5. *Is* + present progressive form of the verb
   6. *Is* interrogative
   7. What is
   8. *He/she/it*
   9. *I am*
   10. Singular form of the noun + present tense of the verb
   11. Plural form of the noun + present tense of the verb
   12. Cumulative plural and singular forms of the noun + present tense
   13. Article *the*

B. Secondary programs
   14. Plural form of the noun + *are*
   15. *Are* interrogative
   16. *What are*
   17. *You/they/we*
   18. Cumulative pronouns
   19. Cumulative *is/are/am*
   20. Cumulative *is/are/am* interrogative
   21. Cumulative *what is/are/am*
   22. Cumulative noun/pronoun/verb/verbing
   23. Singular and plural + past tense

Source: B. Gray and B. Ryan. *A language program for the non-language child.* Champaign, Ill.: Research Press, 1973.

Before the program is begun a screening test, Programmed Conditioning for Language Test, is administered to determine what linguistic structures the child does not have. A criterion test is then given for the first of the structures on the list that the child appears to lack. If his score on the criterion test is less than 80 percent, the instructor begins with that unit. There is a criterion test for each of the 40 units.

Let us say that the instructor has selected unit 4 as the place to begin with a child. Unit 4 teaches the copula *is* in 22 steps. The goal for the child is that, when all the steps in the unit have been completed, he will routinely use the following combinations correctly.

1. Noun Phrase + *is* + a noun
   Example: The baby is a girl.
2. Noun Phrase + *is* + an adjective
   Example: The boy is little.
3. Noun Phrase + *is* + a prepositional phrase
   Example: The book is on the table.

The unit employs pictures or objects and tokens. If the child is in a group of three or more, the criterion for advancing from step to step is 10 consecutive correct responses. If the child is working alone or with one other pupil, the criterion for moving is 20 consecutive correct responses. The number of modeled utterances for each step will vary depending upon the accuracy of the child's responses.

In order to prepare the child to utilize *is* correctly in spontaneous speech, the models are gradually modified to require more fill-in by the child. An example of the procedure is given in Table 7–5. The first model type is called immediate complete (IC). The instructor presents the complete model as he expects the child to say it and the child is to respond immediately. The second model type is called delayed complete (DC). The child is given the structure, but no additional cue. He must remember it briefly before he responds. In the third type, called an immediate truncated (IT), the instructor models only a portion of what the child is to say and he must complete the utterance. Delayed truncated (DT), like delayed complete, requires a brief lapse of time before the child responds. In the final model type no model is given (N).

Just as fewer and fewer clues about his response are given, so the ratio of reinforcement decreases. At first every correct response is reinforced by the presentation of a token, then every other correct response, and finally only one in ten.

When the pupil has completed a unit, a home carry-over program is initiated. The parents are asked to obtain child responses for five to ten minutes a day for eight days in a two-week period. Parents are to keep track of the child's use of the correct form and praise him when he does well. Parents report the carry-over to the teacher.

During the period of the home carry-over program, the child takes a post-criterion test. If he passes it, he takes a criterion test for the next unit and the process begins all over again.

This approach to teaching language is being used in many schools. The authors report that the field data from users indicate that it is successful. It leaves nothing to chance. The modeler, whether it is a teacher, clinician, parent, or aide, knows what to do and what to expect. However, its structure is monotonous and we wonder about the need for so much rigidity.

INTERACTIVE LANGUAGE DEVELOPMENT TEACHING

One detailed program that clinicians utilize is called Interactive Language Development Teaching (Lee, 1975). It is based on a set of stories built around grammatical structures children need to learn. The stories utilize experiences and materials that are familiar to children. By analyzing a spontaneous speech sample of the child, the clinician determines which grammatical structures are either missing or misused, which are below average developmentally for his age, and which should be the target for her teaching. She then develops a set of stories to help her to teach the target structure or uses the ones provided in the program.

Since many of the children in language therapy programs have minimal vocabulary and since it is necessary to build upon the language the child is already comprehending and using, the clinician may have to develop the first story on only 30 or 40 words. For instance, the clinician could build several stories around the vocabulary of the child we discussed in Chapter 3 who had only 40 words. Since the child tended to use these as single-word responses or occasionally in two-word combinations, the clinician's story would be told in short, simple sentences. The target response might be the use of the present progressive inflection [ing], since that is one of the first inflections a child normally uses correctly. The clinician might introduce a toy dog and a mother doll

Table 7–5. *Is* Program in the Gray-Ryan Program for the Non-language Child

	Model Says	Model Type	Child Response	Reinforcement
Series A				
Step 1.	The girl is big, Tom.			
	is	IC	is	1:1
Step 2.	The dog is black, Tom.			
	is black	IC	is black	1:1
Step 3.	The car is blue, Tom.			
	The car is blue.	IC	the car is blue	1:1
Step 4.	The girl is happy, Tom.	DC	the girl is happy	1:2
Step 5.	The cat is black, Tom.			
	cat	IT	the cat is black	1:2
Step 6.	The book is big, Tom.			
	book	DT	the book is big	1:2
Step 7.	The boy is captain, Tom.	N	the boy is captain	1:10
Series B				
Step 8.	The book is on the table, Tom.			
	is on	IC	is on	1:1
Step 9.	The boy is in the house, Tom.			
	is in the house	IC	is in the house	1:1
Step 10.	The dog is in the house, Tom.			
	The dog is in the house.	IC	the dog is in the house	1:1
Step 11.	The cup is on the floor, Tom.			
	cup is on	IT	the cup is on the floor	1:2
Step 12.	The dish is on the table, Tom.			
	the dish	IT	the dish is on the table	1:2
Step 13.	The pencil is on the chair, Tom.			
	the pencil	DT	the pencil is on the chair	1:2
Step 14.	The man is in the car, Tom.	N	the man is in the car	1:10
Series C (In each step the combinations *is* + noun, *is* + adjective, *is* + prepositional phrase are used.)				
Step 15.	The lady is big, Tom.			
	The lady is big.	IC	the lady is big	1:1
Step 16.	The glass is on the table, Tom.			
	the glass	IT	the glass is on the table	1:2
Step 17.	The car is red, Tom.	N	the car is red	1:10
Series D (Model asks questions about pictures.)				
Step 18.	Where is the boy, Tom?			
	The boy is in the car.	IC	the boy is in the car	1:1
Step 19.	What color is the car, Tom?			
	car	IT	the car is blue	1:2
Step 20.	Is the girl pretty or ugly?	N	the girl is pretty	1:10
Series E				
Step 21.	(Model tells a story, then asks questions to elicit *is* responses.)	N	girl is at the table her dress is blue	1:10
Series F				
Step 22.	(Model engages in conversation and asks questions to elicit *is* responses.)	N	car is in the garage daddy is big	1:10

Source: B. Gray and B. Ryan. *A language program for the non-language child.* Champaign, Ill.: Research Press, 1973.

and tell a story that would require the child to use a present progressive inflection, in his response. The first story might go something like this.

CLINICIAN	CHILD
1. This is a dog.	
2. This is mommy.	
3. Mommy is looking at the dog.	
4. What is mommy doing?	Target response: Mommy is look*ing* or Mommy look*ing*

Similar sections can be built around other verbs the child uses in the noninflected form—*cut* (mommy is cutting), *sit* (mommy is sitting), or *go* (mommy is going).

A set of stories might involve the dog and a bone, the target being the use of the third person singular form of the verb.

CLINICIAN	CHILD
1. Here is the dog.	
2. Here is his bone.	
3. The dog wants his bone.	
4. What does the dog want?	Target response: The dog *wants* his bone or He *wants* his bone.

The clinician would present stories that require the desired target structure until the child demonstrates to the satisfaction of the clinician that she knows it. The criterion is usually 9 out of 10 correct responses. Of course, if it is obvious that the child cannot handle the target, the clinician must return to one that is also necessary for continued language development but perhaps easier to master.

Lee suggests several ways to obtain the desired response if a child gives the incorrect one. The clinician can give him the correct model following his incorrect response (expansion) and ask him to imitate her. She can also give him a reduced model, in which she presents only the word he has omitted. For example, in working on the copula *is* in sentences like *it is hot*, if the child says, "it hot," the clinician gives the reduced model *is* and the child is then expected to respond, "it is hot" or "it's hot." Another way is to request the child to "say all of it" or "tell me some more." If the clinician wants the child to figure out his own error, she can ask, "What did you say?" or repeat the child's response with a questioning voice. For example, if the child continues to say, "He hitted the ball," the clinician might reply, "Hitted?" until the child learns that the correct response is *hit*. Asking the child if his reply is correct is a technique which works only when the child is fairly well along in his number of correct responses.

This type of approach is based on the child's grammatical status and as such is especially suited to his needs. It can be utilized in small group therapy as well, even if the clinician is trying to elicit several different grammatical structures from different children. Lee's book provides many stories that can be adapted to the needs of the children and is especially useful for clinicians who are beginners. More experienced ones will create their own within the format of this approach.

IDEAS AND MATERIALS FOR DEVELOPING SPECIAL UNITS BASED ON PARTS OF SPEECH

Since we use so many visual stimuli in teaching, we are always looking for new materials that are attractive and serve many functions. Much of the work on accurate phoneme production of both elementary and junior high school students has been dependent on pictures that have labels with a specific phoneme. Pictures provide a stimulus for the response we want to obtain. As a result of this interest quantities of pictures are now available commercially for the teacher or clinician who does not choose to develop his own materials.

Before a child can build his own sequences of words, he must have something to say and a vocabulary to express himself. The instructor can help him to acquire a functional vocabulary with objects he can feel and manipulate and with pictures. After all, both stand for the words the child wants for communicating an idea.

Pictures for teaching a vocabulary should depict names of things, actions, spatial relations, and descriptive adjectives (Brown, 1974). Some school children will need to learn basic words that most children have at 2 or 2½ years. These include *doll*, *car*, *here*, *there*, *this*, *that*, *dog*, a word for *mother*, and one for *father*. If they do not add to this set, then they have difficulty expressing themselves. Gestures help, but we have a limited number of those.

The Peabody Articulation Cards (Smith, 1973) are a set of over 300 large picture stimulus cards organized for practice on 27 consonant sounds including blends. With these cards either a classroom teacher or a clinician can plan improvement or clinical training activities. They are arranged according to initial, medial, and final positions of phonemes within words. The name of the picture is printed on the back of each card to provide identification for the teacher or clinician. The cards have multiple purposes. For instance, the picture of the *valentine* can be used for the initial [v], the medial [l], the medial [n], and the final [n]. In order to make it easy to locate the pictures and to rearrange them for practice for a specific phoneme, the cards are color-coded and a sorting rod is included as part of the kit.

For children who have very limited language, the instructor might consider using a series of action pictures (Ideal, 1974). This is a series of twelve pictures (7½″ × 8″) in full color that illustrate action verbs such as *play*, *ride*, *go*, *walk*, and *jump*. They can be used for teaching the present tense of the verb and then the present progressive. The pictures are particularly applicable for children who come to school with almost no expressive language. They are designed also so that the children can begin to put a few words together in sequence as they describe the very simple pictures. For instance, there is a picture of a girl sitting at the table with a spoon in her hand and a bowl of cereal in front of her. It is an illustration for the verb *eat*. While the instructor is teaching the verb *eat*, he can model short sentences for the children and ask them what is happening in the picture. These pictures are large enough so that they can be placed on a stand or in the chalk trough.

When the class or group has problems with verb tenses, a series called the Language Making Cards (Lippke, 1974) can be utilized. These pictures can also be arranged for teaching sequencing of words in sentences. The cards are considerably smaller (4½″ × 2¾″) than those in the Peabody kits. They are in color and are varnished for longer wear. Since they can be used for many purposes, they have been numbered for easy filing and indexing.

Many children leave out prepositions. There are a limited number of them and they have been taught easily to average children who are learning English as a second language. It is easy to demonstrate prepositions such as *in*, *on*, *under*, *beside*, *inside*, and *over*. In addition, there are sets of materials specifically designed for teaching prepositions, such as the Spatial Relations Picture Cards (Rogan and Larson, 1974).

There are five other categories of words that we utilize a great deal—adjectives, adverbs, pronouns, conjunctions, and articles. However, children with severely delayed language may know very few of these or use them incorrectly. Adjectives enhance the language, but they are not a necessity for the person who has a meager linguistic repertoire or limited control of speech.

Materials for teaching adjectives, except for colors, are more difficult to find. There are some in the Language Making Cards (Lippke, 1974), but they are small. It is just as easy to use objects and people to demonstrate the words to be learned.

Most teachers and clinicians use contrast as a technique. For instance, adjectives like *big* and *little*, *light* and *heavy*, *smooth* and *rough*, can be demonstrated with objects of different sizes, weights, and textures. Children can identify the *tall* and *short* members of the class. They can be asked to show they are *sad*, *happy*, *sleepy*, or *angry*. They can select the *short* and *long* lines drawn on the chalkboard.

When they have learned these words, the instructor can introduce the comparative and superlative forms of the same adjectives. Everyone can draw a *big* tree, a *bigger* tree, and the *biggest*. We can show them a *little* crayon, a *littler* one, and the *littlest*.

Adverbs, like the adjectives, can be demonstrated readily. As we have said, average children are using *here* and *there* before they are 2 years of age. Children with minimal language may have only a few, such as *here*, *there*, *up*, and *down*. These are the first adverbs which should be taught if they are missing from a child's vocabulary.

The adverbs utilized in obtaining information—*why*, *how*, and *when*—should also be taught. So frequently we ask the question, "Why did you do that?" Children ask *why* long before they learn to listen for your answer. *When* questions are related to the time concept, which is important for young children.

Picture material that portrays action is helpful for teaching these adverbs. After describing a scene or telling a story, the instructor can ask, "Why did he do that?" "When will he come?" or "How did it happen?" These words are part of the academic language and children must understand their use. They must also learn how much information they can obtain by using them.

Personal and indefinite pronouns should be a part of language use before children enter kindergarten. Reports indicate that the personal pronoun *I* is used by most children before they are 2 years of age. Other forms, such as *me* and *my*, may be misused initially and then maintained in their incorrect forms until the children get to school. Like the adverbs and adjectives, pronouns can be taught without specially prepared materials. The instructor needs only to point to people and objects in the room and in pictures and ask questions designed to elicit pronoun use, for example, "Who are you?" is answered "I am Mary"; "Whose pencil is this?" elicits the response "That's her pencil."

Coordination is a stage of language development that requires the use of conjunctions. The conjunctions heard most frequently in children's speech are *and*, *but*, and *or*. These too can be taught without special visual aids. The instructor can model directions: ("John and Joe, get the cookies and milk.") and ask pupils to give two or more directions to their peers ("John, go to the window and then to the chalkboard."). The instructor provides a model when he says, "Pour your milk in the glass, but don't spill it." A pupil might respond to a question about what he likes and dislikes saying, "I like to swim, but I don't like to get water in my eyes" or "I want to play soft ball or ride a horse." Action pictures and questions about them may also be used. After the pupils have had several seconds to look at a picture of a woman walking toward a bus, they might be asked "What is she doing?" or "Why do you think she has both an umbrella and her sunglasses?"

The articles, *the*, *a*, and *an*, are a part of a noun phrase. They never stand alone. Some programs for the retarded are based on the premise that the memory span of the child is so limited that he should be given only the content words at first. Instead of saying *the boy jumps*, the program begins with the two-word utterance *boy jumps*. There are rationales for doing it either way. Some clinicians have indicated that the phrase *the boy* becomes one word and the children are not able to separate *the* from *boy*. On the other hand, the rhythm of our language is broken when we present materials such as *boy jumps* without articles. Since our concern is to expose the children to the natural flow of language and at the same time to give them opportunities to use it, we prefer to attach the articles to whatever noun we are teaching. Therefore, we suggest the model of *the boy* or *a girl* or *an apple* be presented; and encourage the pupils to respond with the same model.

SUMMARY

The material in this section has dealt with the many facets of expressive language. Whether the units or the programs are taught by teachers or clinicians, the two groups should coordinate their activities. The most effective team in a school that is concerned with speech and language development will be a combination of the two.

LISTENING PROGRAMS

The child first learns about his world through sensorimotor explorations, through the experiences and the activity in which he engages. As adults, however, the two major modes of learning are reading and listening. We spend much more time listening, however, than we do in reading. Many of us listen to TV for the news, for music, and for entertainment of all kinds. We spend much less time reading the paper, the novels, or even the magazines. Listening skills are required for interpersonal exchanges. Since we use listening as a primary mode, we should be concerned about the development of listening skills of children.

Listening is generally taught as a skill through the presentation of stories and instructions of increasing length and complexity. The instructor expects the child to be able to attend to, retell, and answer questions about a story. He provides instructions for activities and expects the child to be able to carry them out. The child's listening skill and comprehension can be evaluated on the basis of his responses to questions about the story and his performance of the activity.

Conditions for high-level listening differ somewhat from individual to individual. Some individuals require a quiet environment with no distracting sounds. Others can tune out distractions or even listen better in a noisy environment because of the concentration required to focus on what they are listening to. Some listen best when they are sitting quietly, while others pace around the room or engage in all kinds of physical gyrations. We know some children who listen more carefully when they are sitting under the table than when they are in their assigned chairs. In university classrooms students listen and write simultaneously. They transfer what they are hearing to a piece of paper. When we pick up a telephone, we listen to the party at the other end while we doodle on the telephone pad.

Some parents report that their children "listen" to television for hours. Actually the children may be sitting in front of the television, but not listening in the sense of comprehending what is on the tube. Programs such as "Sesame Street" have been designed to encourage true listening through active participation in the activities presented. As a result of this type of involvement, many children have learned basic concepts and some problem-solving techniques even before they are enrolled in preschool. The characters, activities, and presentations are of sufficiently high interest that some children watch the program twice a day and demonstrate they have learned something from each viewing.

AUDITORY DISCRIMINATION

One aspect of listening is auditory discrimination. Only a few facts have been established about auditory discrimination. We know that it improves with age and levels off at about 8 years of age. Also, children from low socioeconomic environments seem to demonstrate less precise discrimination than children from high socioeconomic environments.

There is no evidence that the auditory skill involved in discrimination of nonspeech sounds of various kinds transfers to discrimination of phonemes. There seems to be some relationship between a child's discrimination ability and his misuse of phonemes, if he has multiple errors. In addition, the literature provides little support for the assumption that training on auditory discrimination should precede direct therapy to modify the production of the phonemes.

About half of the studies of pupils with reading problems indicate that these children also have difficulty in auditory discrimination. Whether there is a cause-effect relationship between these skills is not known. It may be that the two deficits spring from a common cause. One skill uses the visual and the other the auditory mode for learning. Perhaps both modes and skills need to be approached in other than the usual ways.

One study (Flynn and Byrne, 1970) considered the relationship between the auditory abilities and the reading abilities of children at the third-grade level in both high and low socioeconomic environments. The study was conducted in schools that had been previously identified as representative of the highest and lowest socioeconomic groups in the town. All the students were at least one year ahead or behind grade level in reading achievement as measured by the Iowa Test of Primary Reading Abilities. The IQ range was 85 to 131.

The results indicated that as a whole superior readers were significantly different from the retarded readers on most of the auditory tasks. The two tests on which the retarded readers did as well as their advanced peers were those in which the child mimicked the examiner. The results relative to the socioeconomic levels are not so clear-cut. The advanced readers in the high socioeconomic subsample had significantly higher scores than their retarded reader counterparts on the Templin, Pitch, and Schiefelbusch Discrimination Tests, and the examiner-designed blending test. The advanced readers from the low socioeconomic groups had significantly higher scores than their retarded reader counterparts on the Wepman, Templin, Schiefelbusch, and two blending tests. Thus, regardless of socioeconomic level the superior readers performed at a superior level on the Templin and Schiefelbusch Discrimination Tests and examiner-designed blending test.

If tests and observations of the students show diminished auditory discrimination, then programs to improve this skill will need to be developed. Some may require practice in identifying gross or precise sounds. Others may need work on specific sound discriminations, such as [s] and [ʃ].

As with so many other parts of language programs, the creative clinician and teacher with time can develop their own materials for the needed discriminations. For teachers who have little time, the Auditory Discrimination In-Depth Program (Lindamood and Lindamood, 1974) has been utilized in many school systems for kindergarten and later grades, depending on what the students need. The first section of the program introduces the concept of listening selectively to sounds. The ear is identified as the monitor for analyzing what goes in through it.

The second section on the oral-aural level enables students to determine tactual as well as auditory relationships among the phonemes of the language. Some speech pathologists do not like the labels which the designers of the program have used for sounds like [p] and [b] (lip poppers) and [f] and [v] (lip coolers), but the program can, of course, be used without the labels or with different ones.

The third section provides a series of problem-solving auditory discrimination exercises that utilize colored wooden blocks for individual sounds. At this stage the child learns to associate a colored block with a particular phoneme. He then can "spell out" nonsense syllables and eventually words. The designers hypothesize that this intermediate step is useful particularly in the prereading stage prior to the association of the visual symbol in the alphabet with the auditory unit.

The fourth and final level is concerned with the association of the phoneme with the written symbol. Exercises and games with playing cards and lotto cards are utilized for the development of association of the oral sound with the written symbol. This system is carried further in the area of spelling and reading.

SUMMARY

In a society that rewards those with excellent oral communication skills, we expect everyone to master at least the rudiments of a language system. Whether or not parents are conscious of their linguistic interactions with a child, they and their substitutes have the first chance to influence the child's language acquisition. At a later point teachers further the development of communication.

When there is a lack of acquisition or inadequate development, the speech and language clinician is the professional person who evaluates the nature and extent of the problem and plans programs of intervention. Whether the problem is one of dysfluency, voice, aspects of comprehension, or use of oral language, the clinician is trained to provide direction for those children and adults who need help.

Sample programs have been reviewed for clinician and teacher use. Each has its strengths and weaknesses, and none of them may be what is necessary for a particular classroom or group of children. Careful record-keeping of the progress of individuals can supply the information necessary to modify the programs to meet special needs.

REFERENCES

Bankson, N. W., and Byrne, M. C. The effect of a timed correct sound production task on carry-over. *Journal of Speech and Hearing Research, 15,* 160–168 (1972).

Brown, E. *Picture Cards.* Boston, Mass.: Teaching Resources Corporation, 1974.

Byrne, M. C. *The child speaks—A speech improvement program for kindergarten and first grade children.* New York: Harper & Row, 1965.

Byrne, M. C. A speech improvement program for kindergarten and first grade. *The Instructor, 75,* 75–82 (1966).

Dunn, L. M., Smith, J., and Horton, K. *Peabody language development kits.* Circle Pines, Minn.: American Guidance Service, 1965.

Engelmann, S., Osborn, J., and Engelmann, T. *Distar.* Chicago: Science Research Associates, 1972.

Farquhar, M. S. Prognostic value of imitative and auditory discrimination tests. *Journal of Speech and Hearing Disorders, 26,* 342–347 (1961).

Flynn, P., and Byrne, M. C. Relationship between reading and selected auditory abilities of third grade children. *Journal of Speech and Hearing Research, 13,* 731–740 (1970).

Guess, D., Sailor, W., and Baer, D. To teach language to retarded children. In Schiefelbusch, R. L. and Lloyd, L. L. Editors. *Language perspectives—acquisition, retardation, and intervention.* Baltimore, Md.: University Park Press, 1974.

Graber, K., and Gunier, K. *A guide for language and listening development.* Waterloo, Iowa: Black Hawk–Buchanan County Board of Education, 1971.

Gray, B., and Ryan, B. *A language program for the non-language child.* Champaign, Ill.: Research Press, 1973.

Ideal School Supply Company. *Action pictures.* Oaklawn, Ill.: Ideal School Supply Company, 1974.

Johnson, D. J., and Myklebust, M. *Learning disabilities.* New York: Grune & Stratton, 1967.

Kirk, S. *Illinois test of psycholinguistic abilities, Revised edition.* Champaign, Ill.: University of Illinois Press, 1968.

Lee, L. *Interactive language development teaching.* Evanston, Ill.: Northwestern University Press, 1975.

Lindamood, C. H., and Lindamood, P. C. *Auditory discrimination in depth.* Boylston, Mass.: Teaching Resources Corporation, 1974.

Ling, D., and Ling, A. H. Communication development in the first three years of life. *Journal of Speech and Hearing Research, 17,* 146–159 (1974).

Lippke, B. A. *Language making cards.* Salt Lake City, Utah: Word Making Productions, 1974.

Loban, W. Oral language and learning. In Walden, J. Editor. *Oral language and reading*. Champaign, Ill.: National Council of Teachers of English, 1969.

MacDonald, J. D., et al. An experimental parent-assisted treatment program for preschool language delayed children. *Journal of Speech and Hearing Disorders, 39*, 395–415 (1974).

National Society for Crippled Children and Adults. *Search*. Distributed by the National Society for Crippled Children and Adults, Chicago, Ill. No date.

Rogan, L. H., and Larson, C. F. *Spatial relations picture cards*. Niles, Ill.: Developmental Learning Materials, 1974.

Smith, J. O. *Peabody articulation cards*. Circle Pines, Minn.: American Guidance Service, 1973.

Spicker, H. H. Intellectual development through early childhood education. *Journal of Exceptional Children, 37*, 629–641 (1971).

Templin, M. *Certain language skills in children*. Minneapolis: University of Minnesota Press, 1957.

Winitz, H., and Reeds, J. A. Rapid acquisition of a foreign language by the avoidance of speaking. *International Review of Applied Linguistics in Language Teaching, 11*, 295–317 (1973).

SPEECH PROGRAMS IN THE SCHOOL Chapter 8

Schools have always faced major challenges in providing quality education for everyone. Growth and population shifts require different solutions. When neighborhoods change, there is a need to modify the educational pattern to suit the new population.

In addition, all those social forces that shape other institutions impinge on the schools, too. As a result school clinicians must be able to adapt to the shifts in emphasis and provide professional leadership. Within that framework we shall now present some information about the organization of the school's speech and language program.

ORGANIZATIONAL ARRANGEMENTS

In most school districts the speech and hearing personnel are responsible to a director of special education. Depending upon its size and its commitment to special education, the district may employ in addition to audiologists, clinicians with special interests in language, speech, and dysfluency. In small districts one or two clinicians handle a wide variety of communication deficits and delays and may also direct the hearing screening program.

Some clinicians are responsible for the program in only one school, but others may be responsible for the programs in several. Because of distances between schools some clinicians may be located in a central school and those who need her services are brought to her clinic office.

Even though the school board determines overall school policy, the implementation is left to the superintendent and his administrative staff. That staff includes the school principals. They really set policy for their own buildings, so long as it does not conflict with overall school guidelines.

School clinicians and principals work together to facilitate the work of the clinician. If principals understand and agree with the clinicians' goals, they can smooth the path for their acceptance by teachers and aides. Principals can also be the buffer between the clinician and the irate parent who does not want his child in a clinical speech program.

Early in the school year the clinician, with the assistance of the principal, explains her responsibilities to the teachers. She may have an intensive in-service program for them at that time or may spread out her in-service over the year.

Since teachers make referrals of all those pupils who are not screened on a regular basis, they need to know several things. First of all, what is a communication deficit? How can they determine whether any of their students have deficits? What kinds of deficits are there? What criteria will the clinician use in determining which pupils are to be enrolled in a remediation program? In order to provide some answers to these questions, the clinician must explain and demonstrate types of deficits—all those that have been described in Chapters 3 and 4. Her skill in explaining these will determine what kind of referrals she gets.

Surveys in the schools have shown that the incidence of serious voice disorders among the school population is considerably higher (3 to 10 percent) than the referrals made by teachers. However, teachers rarely refer a student for evaluation of voice production and use probably because they have not been given the guidelines to enable them to identify vocal deviations.

CASE SELECTION

In some communities the school speech clinician can enroll all children with even minor deviations. The clinician, if he is well-prepared and has an ideal environment in which to work, will not need to train teachers to carry out speech and language development programs. Rather, he will work with teachers only on identification of communication problems and ways of achieving permanent carry-over for those in the clinical program.

In most communities, however, there are not enough clinicians to provide services for all the children who need them. Therefore, the clinician must select those who he considers have the highest priorities. He may use severity of the problem as his primary criterion for enrolling pupils. Sometimes he will consider the prognosis for improvement if therapy is initiated. He may consider the relationship between the chronological age and the language age or the suitability of a student for an already existing remedial speech group. Some clinicians try to include some pupils from each of these categories. Then he must plan with the teachers how best to handle the others.

School speech clinicians face a serious professional dilemma with regard to management of children with articulatory deviations. The problem has arisen because there are too few clinicians for the number of children who are referred for clinical speech assistance and clinicians lack adequate evaluative tools to differentiate those children who will attain normal speech as a result of the developmental process from children whose speech patterns will not change without clinical services. In spite of the dilemma the clinician must cope with parents, teachers, and other community pressures to enroll children who may improve without a therapy program. The group who have articulatory deviations without any motor aberrations probably cause the most concern.

Studies indicate that many kindergarten, first-, and second-grade children have phonetic errors. The percentages vary from 3 to 50 percent depending on the criteria used by the clinician for the various age groups. Almost all of the kindergarten children in the low socioeconomic classes in a speech improvement project (Byrne, 1966) had some errors on the 13 consonants that were tested prior to the beginning of the program. Many parents want the speech sound errors to be eliminated before their children begin reading programs and they insist that the children have special instruction to prevent additional reinforcement of the errors.

In order to deal with the problems of selection of children and effective utilization of time, some clinicians advise ignoring phonetic errors until the children reach the third grade. At that point all who are going to change will have reached normal phonetic competency (Templin, 1957). Other clinicians, however, do not like the postponement. They feel that by the third grade the errors are sufficiently stabilized so that they are unable to bring about the changes as efficiently as might have been possible at an earlier age.

There are alternatives. Rather than ignoring the problem of articulatory deviancy, clinicians can provide speech improvement programs for the classroom which either they or the teachers can conduct. A review of the literature indicates that speech improvement programs have been conducted for many years in several school districts. Sometimes they are part of the language arts program, and the children engage in creative dramatics, choral reading, and oral presentations of all kinds. In other instances the speech improvement has been organized and maintained as a part of the clinical speech program.

SPEECH IMPROVEMENT PROGRAMS

In recent years there has been some interest in special speech improvement programs that focus on specific sounds for children in kindergarten, first, and second grades. The research indicates that these approaches to articulatory learning are effective in reducing the number of phonetic errors (Wilson, 1954; Sommers et al. 1961) and also in decreasing the number of children who need a clinical speech program (Byrne, 1966).

If the clinician decides that the best way to manage his clinical time is to supplement his services through a speech development program, what role does he play in such a program? The clinician should be the resource person for the program and in some instances its director. The speech clinician should evaluate the children who are engaged in the speech program, if the teacher recommends an evaluation, and he should train the classroom teachers to carry out the speech work.

Although several rationales have been expressed both for and against speech improvement programs, the most frequent one on the positive side is prevention of speech defects and enrichment of one aspect of the language arts program. Teachers report its effectiveness in fostering effective listening patterns. Some administrators feel that the program also improves reading skills, and some studies support this viewpoint (Sommers et al., 1961). Those who favor speech improvement assume that normal articulation per se is a desirable skill for all children and that the classroom environment can be structured to foster and accelerate accurate learning of speech.

Some administrators and teachers oppose speech improvement programs. We shall present some of their reasons, and some answers which we feel override the objections. They emphasize that many articulatory problems disappear as a function of age and the school environment. Most children with errors "outgrow" their deviations and the others will need speech therapy regardless of early attempts through a classroom speech program. There is sufficient evidence that control of correct phonetic production as measured on tests improves with age (Templin, 1957). However, as we have indicated, the process of learning to utilize sounds correctly can be accelerated. Studies by Sommers (1961) in Pennsylvania, by Byrne (1966) in Kansas, and by Wilson (1954) in Indiana have demonstrated the effectiveness of speech improvement work in reducing articulatory errors in kindergarten and first-grade children. Templin and Byrne have shown that children from high socioeconomic environments learn correct sound patterns at an earlier age than children from low socioeconomic families. If acceleration of the learning process can be accomplished by one segment of the population, should we not provide additional opportunities for all children to learn correct speech sound patterns as rapidly as possible?

Another objection is that such programs penalize the children who do not need speech help, that the use of 15 to 30 minutes of each day to help only 10 to 25 percent of the class deprives the good speakers of other types of learning experiences. The answer to this objection is that a good speech improvement program provides ample opportunity for the good speakers to further develop their oral skills. In addition, these children also need to develop better listening habits—skills that are fostered by the speech improvement work.

Some clinicians feel that they should not be in the classroom with children who have minor articulatory errors when their time is needed for those children who cannot

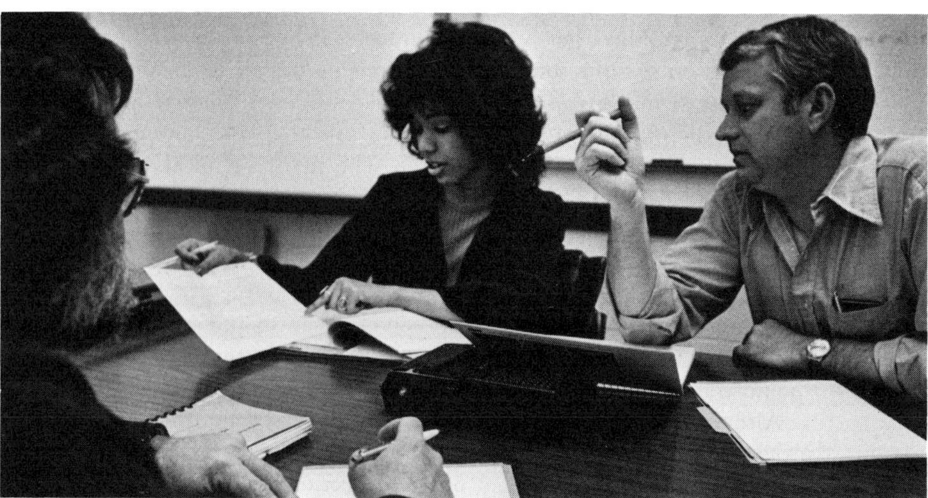

function adequately without lengthy, time-consuming therapy. With this point of view, we agree. The classroom teachers in one three-year speech improvement study (Byrne, 1966) were given one day of demonstration as a part of their in-service training and met once a month with the clinical director. They did not need a speech clinician to carry out the program in the classroom.

Some speech clinicians feel they are not qualified to provide in-service training and supervision to teachers who are engaged in speech improvement work. The young clinician may need some time to develop his professional role before he undertakes such a program. He must feel comfortable in his relationships with teachers and must be confident of his own ability in changing speech patterns. If he is willing and takes the opportunity to learn about the goals of a speech development program and how it can be carried out, he will find the experience most rewarding. His large case load of children with articulation errors can be reduced, and he can spend his time with the complex language and speech problems that require intensive therapy.

The role of the clinician in effective language planning for children who are mentally retarded, learning disabled, emotionally disturbed, or physically handicapped is still being clarified. In our experience these children who have concomitant language deficits require a concentrated all-day approach that should be teacher- rather than clinician-oriented. The communication breakdown of these pupils requires more help than clinicians can usually provide. Classroom procedures and the language goals for each student, however, can be delineated by the clinician with the teacher as his partner and co-worker.

IN-SERVICE TRAINING IN SPEECH AND LANGUAGE DEVELOPMENT

If classroom teachers are to modify the speech and language behavior of large number children within the classroom, they must be given an in-service program. There are several general principles that the clinician must keep in mind if his in-service work is to be successful. First of all, training must be planned carefully. Administrators, such as the superintendent and his curriculum advisors and the principals in the elementary schools, must understand the nature of this work. They must be willing to accept the philosophy of utilization of the classroom teacher for this aspect of the program. All of them should be enthusiastic about such a venture. If they indicate enthusiasm and support, then the teachers will volunteer to enroll in in-service training. The clinician, however, should not encourage the principals to force teachers who are not interested to enroll. A few enthusiastic volunteers can change the negative or neutral attitude to a positive and highly desirable one.

Wherever possible the in-service training should begin with kindergarten and first-grade teachers. Children's behavior can be modified at an earlier age more readily than at a later age. Therefore, their teachers should begin the speech and language programming as early as possible. In addition, it seems easier to modify the curriculum at the primary level than it is later on. Also, there is some evidence that some aspects of reading skills are improved as a result of these programs and that the children who learn to listen and develop discrimination patterns have tools which are essential for later learning.

The clinician and the teachers must decide together what is to be gained by the speech program. The clinician must select concrete materials to achieve the goals and demonstrate their uses to the teachers for whatever maturational group the program is geared. Most teachers feel that they understand the principles of such programs if the principles are not only discussed, but also demonstrated with a small group of children.

The clinician can instruct teachers so that they can evaluate and record the progress of the children with regard to the language behavior they are teaching. For instance, if the goal for the week is to increase correct use of plural inflections, the teacher can chart how often each child uses the inflection correctly and incorrectly in a three-minute spontaneous speech sample. The teacher may elect to chart the performance of 8 children per day, if she has forty in her class, or a smaller number depending on class size. It would take less than a half an hour a day. Teachers need to know how to chart, what to chart, and how to use the information in their weekly plans. Figure 8–1 is an example of such a chart.

Teachers receive many routine structured responses from their students during the course of a day. The clinician can show teachers how to use these responses for speech improvement practice. For instance, if students are required to ask for things, such as paint, their milk, or a piece of paper, teachers can suggest a simple question form to be used, such as "May I have ______?" If each child is required to introduce himself before he participates in sharing or talk time, they can encourage the use of the simple sentence "I'm Joe." In the reading program, they can ask, "Whose turn is it?" and request that the answer be given in a sentence form, "It's my turn."

In-service training cannot be a one-lecture or even a one-term program. It must be continued for many years until the philosophy has been well developed within a school system. In addition, teachers at different grade levels experience different kinds of problems. They must have an opportunity to discuss their special problems with the clinician. The clever clinician can suggest many ways in which the teacher can be

Name of student ____________________
Dates ____________________
Target behavior to be modified ____________________

	Total number used	Correct use	Incorrect use
Monday			
Tuesday			
Wednesday			
Thursday			
Friday			
Monday			
Tuesday			
Wednesday			
Thursday			
Friday			

Figure 8–1. Form for recording information about speech and language behaviors.

freed for 20 to 30 minutes once a month during the regular school day. For instance, the PTA can arrange to supervise the children on the playground so that the teachers can meet to discuss aspects of the program. Some mothers or teacher aides can be invited to supervise the children for a film scheduled so that the teachers can be freed from classroom responsibilities.

Clinicians can encourage teachers to take courses in speech and language development and can encourage local colleges and universities to teach the courses both in the summer and in after-school hours for classroom teachers. Clinicians can also encourage their superintendents to obtain state funds for consultants to help them with the in-service training and can encourage state departments to arrange for additional workshops. The clinician can disseminate information at many levels—to the superintendent, principals, teachers, PTA groups, board of education members.

COORDINATION OF THERAPEUTIC AND CLASSROOM PROGRAMS

Once the clinician has determined which students should be enrolled in therapy schedules must be arranged with the teachers. It is often difficult to find a time for therapy which does not interfere with classwork or other activities. Sometimes, the teacher and the clinician must compromise because some students need extra help in everything. In such cases, they must consider priorities—what is needed most, next, and so on.

Some clinicians schedule pupils two or three times a week; others work with them four or five times a week. The amount of time is related to the amount of time the clinician has in the building, the severity of the problem, and the need for intensive work.

Both group and individual sessions are utilized. In some instances the clinician does individual, concentrated work until a particular skill is partially acquired and then places the pupil in a group for more peer activities to reinforce the newly acquired skill. However the schedules are arranged, they must be flexible to allow for change within the school year.

When the schedule for the children in one room has been settled, the clinician can then provide the teacher with a calendar, indicating when the students will have speech therapy.

At the same time the clinician can work with teachers in setting up supportive classroom programs. The teachers should be provided with information about the target structures for each student, how to help the students achieve the specific goals, how to assist in carry-over, and how to keep records of the students' progress. The clinician can provide materials and methods for eliciting the target structures. In addition procedures for recording the correct and incorrect responses can be reviewed and the reinforcement to be utilized can be identified.

In many school districts there is a manual for the clinicians. It may be one prepared by the state coordinator of speech and hearing or by the local clinical group. The *Manual for School Speech, Hearing, and Language Programs* (American Speech and Hearing Association, 1973) can be utilized as a guide for those districts that want to develop their own or can be adopted in its present form.

REPORTING RESULTS OF PROGRAMS

When there is a shortage of funds, programs must be reduced or eliminated. The programs most likely to be cut are those with which the public is unfamiliar and those which have not demonstrated the benefits they have provided. For this reason clinicians should try to document their work as thoroughly as possible with accurate statistics on enrollment, descriptions of tasks, records of results, and reports on follow-ups. Sometimes only limited data about the tasks, the results, and the relationship of the program to total education have been given to the superintendent, the principal, and teachers. Reporting how many students received therapy during the year is a meager bit of information for the person who must defend the existence of the program.

The federal government has ruled that every school district must have an approved plan for educating all students, including the exceptional. That principle is important, but its application to the implementation of speech programs depends on public knowledge of such programs. How committed are the tax payers to providing speech and language services to all? If the community does not know what the speech specialist does, there is no reason to expect support for more than a minimal program.

AN INTEGRATED PROGRAM

The ideal program in language and speech is one that is concerned with all its facets—listening, speaking, reading, and writing. The facets cannot be divided and assigned to one or another specialist. There must be overlapping responsibilities for the various pieces, and the entire staff must be involved in developing and modifying a philosophy of language teaching and learning. All must be willing to cooperate and work together toward a common goal. We know that the average adult spends about 90 percent of his time listening and speaking and less than 10 percent reading and writing. We cannot afford to slight any of the four facets, however. Parents particularly will not permit us to ignore reading skills, so essential for later information-gathering.

Both improvement and remedial aspects of the program must be identified and designed to fit the special needs of each school's students. They must contribute to and support one another. A multidisciplinary approach to the school's curriculum is needed and should have a high priority in the list of *musts* of the school district.

SUMMARY

Clinicians in the school have a unique opportunity to work on a daily basis with different members of the educational staff. We have provided some guides to assist them and school personnel to develop a greater degree of mutual understanding about a speech and language program. It must be coordinated with the rest of the scholastic program, so that all students who need our assistance will have a well-integrated approach to learning.

REFERENCES

American Speech and Hearing Association. *A manual for school speech, hearing, and language programs*. Washington, D.C.: American Speech and Hearing Association, 1973.

Byrne, M. C. *The child speaks–A speech improvement program for kindergarten and first grade children*. New York: Harper & Row, 1965.

Byrne, M. C. A speech improvement program for kindergarten and first grade children. *The Instructor*, *75*, 75–82 (1966).

Templin, M. *Certain language skills in children*. Minneapolis: University of Minnesota Press, 1957.

Sommers, R. K., et al. Effects of speech therapy and speech improvement on articulation and reading. *Journal of Speech and Hearing Disorders*, *26*, 27–38 (1961).

Wilson, B. A. The development and evaluation of a speech improvement program for kindergarten children. *Journal of Speech and Hearing Disorders*, *19*, 4–13 (1954).

EPILOGUE

The ability to communicate is one of the prized possessions of our society. When we lose even a part of our communication skills, we feel its effects in our relationships with other human beings. Those who do not develop normal or close to normal communication experience frustrations that are difficult to handle.

In this book we have described the language system which most of us use in communication. It is complex and requires many years for most of us to master. Speech, which uses the language symbols as well as a paralanguage for communication, requires facile control of the speech mechanism. Both speech and language utilize the cognitive abilities of the individual.

When something goes wrong in this total process, we hope we can find out why and how it happened. If we remember that speech and language are multiply determined, it will help us to explain to an anxious parent or a concerned teacher why we cannot pinpoint causes of failure.

There is much we can do, however, to assist those who are delayed or deficient. Until we have more answers to our queries than we have at present, we must strive to deal as effectively as we can with those whose communication skills are faltering.

We wish we could promise immediate and permanent results with our approaches, but we cannot. We have no magic, we have no pills. As a profession we do have compassion for those who have communication disorders, and we hope that we can help them to develop and improve their abilities to the limit of their capacities. Each of us is an individual with human rights as well as obligations. We must use our talents as a profession to learn more about these disorders and how we can assist in preventing them or reducing their impact.

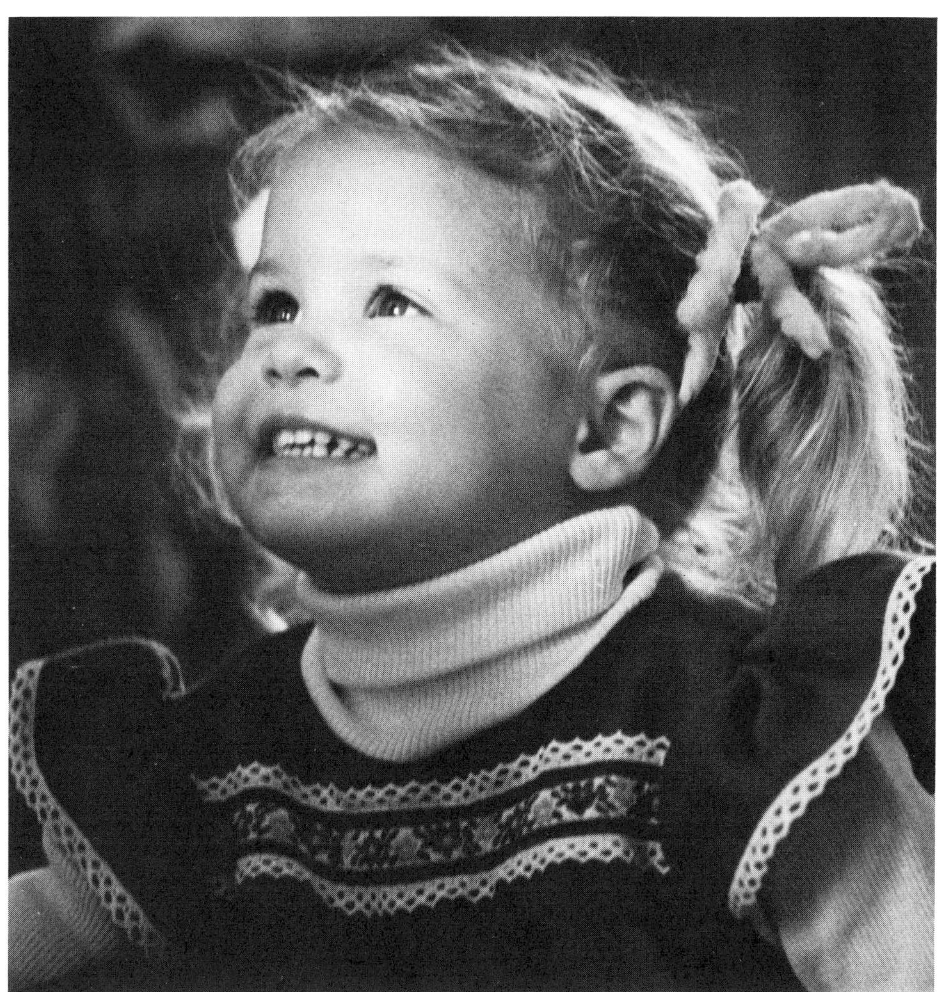

APPENDIXES

Selected Tests for Children

Name	Measures	Suitable for Age Groups	Time Required
Illinois Test of Psycholinguistic Abilities, Revised Edition	Specific communication abilities	2 to 10 years	60 minutes
Peabody Picture Vocabulary Test	Receptive vocabulary	21 months to 18 years	10–15 minutes
Northwestern Syntax Screening Test	Comprehension and production of grammatical forms	3 years to 7 years 11 months	15 minutes
Auditory Test for Language Comprehension, 1973 Edition	Comprehension of oral language units—form classes, function words, syntax	3 years to 6 years 11 months	20–30 minutes
Templin-Darley Screening and Diagnostic Tests of Articulation, 2nd Edition	141-item test—vowels, diphthongs, consonants, blends	3 to 8 years	30–45 minutes
McDonald Screening Deep Test	9 phonemes in 10 contexts	4 to 8 years	10 minutes
Photo Articulation Test	All phonemes	3 to 8 years	5 minutes
Goldman-Fristoe Articulation Test	Phonemes in words, sentences, syllables	3 to 8 years	30 minutes
Preschool Achievement Record	Ambulation, manipulation, rapport, communication, responsibility, information, ideation, creativity	1 month to 7 years	30–60 minutes
Denver Developmental Screening test	Gross motor, language, personal-social, fine-motor adaptive	1 month to 6 years	10–30 minutes

Distinctive Features of Consonants

Phonemes	r	l	p	b	f	v	m	t	d	θ	ð	n	s	z	tʃ	dʒ	ʃ	ʒ	k	g	ŋ	h
Vocalic	+	+	−	−	−	−	−	−	−	−	−	−	−	−	−	−	−	−	−	−	−	−
Consonant	+	+	+	+	+	+	+	+	+	+	+	+	+	+	+	+	+	+	+	+	+	−
High	−	−	−	−	−	−	−	−	−	−	−	−	−	−	+	+	+	+	+	+	+	−
Back	−	−	−	−	−	−	−	−	−	−	−	−	−	−	−	−	−	−	+	+	+	−
Low	−	−	−	−	−	−	−	−	−	−	−	−	−	−	−	−	−	−	−	−	−	+
Anterior	−	+	+	+	+	+	+	+	+	+	+	+	+	+	−	−	−	−	−	−	−	−
Coronal	+	+	−	−	−	−	−	+	+	+	+	+	+	+	+	+	+	+	−	−	−	−
Round																						
Tense																						
Voice	+	+	−	+	−	+	+	−	+	−	+	+	−	+	−	+	−	+	−	+	+	−
Continuant	+	+	−	−	+	+	−	−	−	+	+	−	+	+	−	−	+	+	−	−	−	+
Nasal	−	−	−	−	−	−	+	−	−	−	−	+	−	−	−	−	−	−	−	−	+	−
Strident	−	−	−	−	+	+	−	−	−	−	−	−	+	+	+	+	+	+	−	−	−	−

+ = present

− = absent

Modified from McReynolds, L. and Engmann, D. L. *Distinctive feature analysis of misarticulations.* Baltimore, Maryland. Univ. Park Press, 1975.

PUBLISHERS OF MATERIALS FOR SPEECH PROGRAMS

American Guidance Service, Inc.
Publishers Building
Circle Pines, Minnesota 55014

Bowmar Publishing Corporation
P.O. Box 3623
622 Rodier Drive
Glendale, California 91201

Curriculum Associates, Inc.
94 Bridge Street
Chapel Bridge Park
Newton, Massachusetts 02158

Developmental Learning Materials
7440 N. Natchez Avenue
Niles, Illinois 60648

Ideal School Supply Company
Oak Lawn, Illinois 60452

Learning Business Inc.
Dept. L B 2
Westlake Executive Center
790 Hampshire Road
Suite C
Westlake Village, California 91360

Learning Concepts Inc.
2501 N. Lamar
Austin, Texas 78705

Modern Education Corporation
P.O. Box 721
Tulsa, Oklahoma 74101

Science Research Associates, Inc.
259 East Erie Street
Chicago, Illinois 60611

Teaching Resources Corporation
100 Boylston Street
Boston, Massachusetts 02116

Word Making Productions
60 W. 400 South Street
Salt Lake City, Utah 84101

A BRIEF GUIDE FOR CHECKING SPEECH

The physician or parent should be concerned about a child's communication when any one or more of the fillowing conditions exist.

1. The child is not talking at all by age 2.
2. The child is using mostly the vowel sounds when he talks after age 2.
3. Speech is largely unintelligible after age 3.
4. Sounds are more than a year late in appearing, according to the developmental sequence.
5. There are many omissions of initial sounds in words after age 3.
6. There are no sentences by age 4.
7. There are many substitutions of easy sounds for difficult ones at age 5.
8. Word endings are consistently dropped after age 4.
9. Sentence structure is noticeably faulty at age 5.
10. There are unusual confusions, reversals, or telescoping in connected speech at age 5.
11. The child is noticeably nonfluent after age 5.
12. There is abnormal rhythm, rate, and inflection after age 5.
13. The child is distorting, omitting, or substituting any sounds after age 8.
14. The child is embarrassed and disturbed by his speech at any age.
15. The voice is monotonous, extremely loud, largely inaudible, or of poor quality at any age.
16. The pitch is not appropriate for the child's age and sex.
17. There is noticeable hypernasality or lack of nasal resonance at any age.

Modified from Herold Lillywhite. Doctor's manual of speech disorders. *Journal of the American Medical Association*, *167*, 850–858, 1958.

SUGGESTIONS TO HELP THE HEARING IMPAIRED FUNCTION MORE EFFECTIVELY

1. Get the attention of the person before you begin to talk.
2. Speak naturally, do not mumble, and do not overemphasize.
3. Look at the person as you talk to him.
4. Keep your hands and other interfering objects (like books) away from your face.
5. Make sure the person can see your face. Focus light on you, not on him.
6. Let the person select the seat that will optimize his ability to hear and see you.
7. With young children, check their batteries and their hearing aids for proper amplification.
8. If you are not understood, rephrase your idea rather than repeat the same words.

ORGANIZATIONS TO WHICH TO WRITE FOR INFORMATION ABOUT COMMUNICATION PROBLEMS OF SELECTED GROUPS OF CHILDREN AND ADULTS

Alexander Graham Bell Association
for the Deaf
3417 Volta Place, N.W.
Washington, D.C. 20007

American Association on Mental Deficiency
5201 Connecticut Avenue, N.W.
Washington, D.C. 20015

American Speech and Hearing Association
9030 Old Georgetown Road
Washington, D.C. 20014

Council for Exceptional Children
1920 Association Drive
Reston, Virginia 22091

American Cleft Palate Educational Foundation, Inc.
University of Pittsburgh
331 Salk Hall
Pittsburgh, Pennsylvania 15261

State coordinator of speech and hearing programs
Division of Special Education
State Department of Education

State and county health departments

SOME PAMPHLETS FOR PARENTS AND TEACHERS

Aphasia and the Family
Available from American Heart Association
44 East 23 Street
New York, New York 10010

For Parents of New Born Babies with Cleft Lip/Palate, 1975.
Available from American Cleft Palate Educational Foundation, Inc.
University of Pittsburgh
331 Salk Hall
Pittsburgh, Pennsylvania 15261

From "I" to "We" (DHEW Publication No. (OCD) 74-1033), prepared by Lois Murphy and Ethel Leeper for the Office of Child Development, 1974.
Available from Superintendent of Documents
U.S. Government Printing Office
Washington, D.C. 20402 (60¢)

Learning to Talk: Speech, Hearing, and Language Problems in the Preschool Age Child, 1969.
Available from Superintendent of Documents
U.S. Government Printing Office
Washington, D.C. 20402 (40¢)

Please Listen to Me, 1972.
Available from Maryland State Department of Education
Baltimore, Maryland

Project Headstart Speech, Language, and Hearing Program (DHEW Publication No. (OCD) 75-1025), 1975.
Available from Office of Child Development
Office of Human Development
U.S. Department of Health, Education, and Welfare
Washington, D.C. 20201

Statements on Deafness
Can Your Baby Hear?
Doctor, Is My Baby Deaf?
Hearing Alert
Available from Alexander Graham Bell Association for the Deaf
3417 Volta Place, N.W.
Washington, D.C. 20007

GLOSSARY

The words that are defined in this glossary are technical terms used in the text in discussing communicative disorders. The definitions express the most relevant and appropriate meanings for these words as used in the text.

Acoustic trauma—a sudden injury to any part of the hearing mechanism. It may destroy the hearing or cause a temporary hearing loss.

Adaptation—the adjustments an individual makes to meet the needs of the changing environment.

Affixes—prefixes, infixes, and suffixes added to a basic word to indicate a change, as in fud, fud*z*; frequent, *in*frequent*ly*.

Affricate—a combination of two sounds produced in such a way that they are perceived as one. A plosive sound precedes a fricative; and the explosive stage of the plosive is not heard. An example is the [tʃ] sound in the word *chew*.

Agnosia—the lack of ability to recognize the parts of one's environment. Visual agnosia is the inability to recognize the form or the nature of things. Auditory agnosia is the inability to understand the sounds of the environment or the words people use. There is no blindness or hearing loss. The problem is one of recognition and comprehension.

Air conduction—the transmission of sounds to the inner ear through the air that fills the outer and middle ear. When the sound is blocked somewhere in the outer or middle ear, it may be transmitted by the bones of the skull (*see* Bone conduction).

Air flow—the exhalation of air from the lungs through the larynx, nose, and mouth. Air flow is necessary if sounds are to be produced and understood.

Allomorphs—a variant of a morpheme that occurs in a specific environment. For example, the suffixes [z], [s], and [əz] are added to singular nouns with certain final sounds to show plurality, as in car—cars; book—books; dress—dresses.

Allophone—a speech sound that is produced in varying ways but is still recognizable as the same sound.

Anal stage—the second stage in the psychoanalytic theory of psychosexual development. According to the theory, pleasure and conflict center on the holding and letting go of feces.

Anxiety—an emotional state in which there is a generalized fear without a specific recognized source.

Aphasia—the weakening or loss of the ability to understand or to express ideas with language. It is a symbolic disorder, not the result of motor problems. This text is concerned primarily with its effects on speaking (expressive aphasia) or comprehension (receptive aphasia). Other aspects are related to reading (dyslexia) and writing (dysgraphia).

Aphonia—weakness of voice or loss of voice. Those affected may not be able to be heard because their voices lack sufficient volume to be carried to the listener; or they may not be able to produce any sound.

Apraxia of speech—a disorder involving the voluntary movements of the speech mechanism needed to produce speech, even though muscle power, sensitivity, and coordination in general are intact. The person has no difficulty chewing or swallowing yet cannot program those same muscles to produce speech voluntarily.

Articulation assessment—an analysis of the way a person produces the phonemes of English. It may include all the sounds or only those that are most likely to be wrong. The person who is testing may evaluate sounds in isolation, syllables, words, phrases, or sentences.

Articulation disorders—disorders that are associated with faulty production of the speech sounds, failure to produce speech sounds, or incorrect use of the sounds in words.

Assimilation—a person's incorporation of new elements into his or her current structure or view of the world.

Audiogram—a graphic record of the results of a hearing test. Special symbols are used to indicate hearing by air and by bone and for the right ear and left ear. Information about other hearing tests may also be on the form.

Audiologist—a professional person who provides appropriate clinical hearing tests and intervention and/or engages in research on hearing problems.

Audition—the sense of hearing, which enables us to listen to the speech of others and to monitor our own.

Auditory discrimination—the ability of an individual to determine whether two sounds are the same or different. Usually the sounds (nonsense syllables or words) are presented in isolation, and the listener must judge whether the tester is saying the same sounds or different ones.

Aversive conditioning—a type of conditioning in which punishment is used to extinguish or eliminate undesirable behavior. For example, when a child is being trained to sit on a chair for his lesson, he may be given a mild shock if he gets out of the chair.

Base line—performance of an activity or a task that is measured prior to the initiation of a program of remediation. For example, if we want to know how often a person substitutes [θ] for [s], we listen and record the frequency of the [θ] during a specific time period, perhaps ten minutes a day for each of three days.

Bone conduction—transmission of sound to the inner ear by way of the mechanical vibrations of the skull. The amount can be measured with an audiometer. *See* Air conduction.

Breathiness—a voice quality that results from a combination of incomplete lax vocal fold approximation and initiation of phonation after the air flow has begun. We can perceive breathiness in the voices of others, and we can create it ourselves by talking and exhaling simultaneously.

Carryover—the automation or spontaneous use of a newly learned sound, word, or grammatical rule. The clinician, whether measuring carryover in the classroom or at home, should keep track of carryover throughout each step of the therapy program. The clinician should look for carryover of the [s] phoneme, for example, in a few words he or she has taught, as the person uses them, then in untaught words, and finally in general conversation.

Case grammar—a set of rules governing the semantic roles of nouns in relation to verbs, in contrast to transformational or phrase structure grammar.

Central auditory disorders—disorders related to damage to the auditory nerve pathways, in the brain stem, in the relay pathways, or in the hearing centers in the cerebral cortex. Those with central auditory disorders neither hear nor understand sounds or language.

Cerebral palsy—the result of an intracranial lesion, this condition, which is usually present at birth, involves paralysis or muscular incoordination.

Cleft palate—a defect in the hard and/or soft palate caused by the failure of the structures of the palate to develop adequately to form the roof of the mouth.

Cleft palate and lip—(*see* Cleft palate); additionally, there is a defect in the alveolar ridge and/or upper-lip structures caused by the failure of these structures to develop adequately and join in midline.

Cochlea—a snail-shaped cavity in the inner ear that contains the essential end organs for hearing. When the cochlea does not function for any reason, hearing is impaired.

Cognition—a psychological process that we associate with knowledge. It has many levels, including awareness, perception, conceptualization, differentiation, and reasoning.

Communication—a process that includes: the expression of an idea; its transmission or conveyance to another person or group; its comprehension by the receiver(s) of the message; and the social and psychological impact of the exchange of ideas.

Competence—absolute and complete knowledge of the linguistic structures of a specific language. It can only be inferred, since it is not feasible to test such complete knowledge.

Comprehension—the ability of an individual to understand and give appropriate meaning to what he or she hears.

Connotative meaning—the emotional implication of a word or phrase that overlaps or supplants the concrete meaning. Certain words have special emotional meaning to people, as the word *baby* to new parents.

Consonant—a sound produced with partial or complete blocking of the air stream as it moves from the larynx through the mouth.

Constituents—the morpheme or group of morphemes in an utterance. In the sentence, *John goes, John* and *goes* are constituents, as is the complete utterance, *John goes.*

Contentives—the parts of speech that a child tends to use to convey meaning in his or her early language development. They carry the major part of the meaning and include nouns, pronouns, verbs, adjectives, and adverbs.

Conversion neurosis—a form of neurosis in which the underlying conflict is changed into a sensory or motor symptom, such as functional deafness or aphonia or paralysis of some kind.

Critical period—the optimal period of readiness for learning certain behaviors. The critical period for learning the basic structure of a first language is between two and five years of age.

Curriculum guide—a syllabus followed by the teacher at a particular grade level for the various subjects that he or she teaches.

Deaf mute—a person who is without any usable hearing and also without speech. Those who are deaf and can only communicate with signs fall into this category.

Decibel (dB)—a unit of measurement that indicates the ratio between two sound pressures; a measure of the loudness of a sound. A "15 dB loss in the right ear by air and bone" means a sound has to be that loud before the person can hear it.

Deep structure—underlying semantic relationships we identify in the sentence. *Visiting firefighters can be a nuisance* might mean that *firefighters* are a nuisance or that *visiting* is a nuisance.

Denotative meaning—the exact meaning of a word as it is defined or described in a dictionary.

Determinants—the causes or the explanations for both normal and abnormal communication. There are physical, psychological, and social determinants.

Deviant language—some or all aspects of an individual's language that are different or inappropriate in terms of complexity, correctness, and variety, in view of his or her age.

Diadokokinesis—a term used to indicate the speed with which a person can produce a series of speech sounds. For instance, when a person whose speech mechanism has been damaged tries to say *kʌkʌkʌ* or *pʌtʌkʌ* as fast as he or she can for a period of five seconds, there may be a slow rate of movement. This rate will interfere with the rapid flow of speech associated with normal speech production.

Dialect—the systematic variations in the speech or language of a group of persons. These variations are associated with a geographic or an ethnic community.

Diaphragm—a dome-shaped muscle that separates the thoracic from the abdominal cavity. It expands and contracts when air is taken into the lungs and then expelled.

Diphthong—a speech sound that glides continuously from one vowel to another; for example, *ou,* as in *bou.*

Discrimination—recognition of similarities and differences in stimuli. Auditory discrimination means we are able to hear when two sounds or words are the same or different.

Distinctive features—the bundle of relevant contrastive characteristics of a phoneme that distinguishes the sound from others. Only 13 have been identified by Chomsky and Halle in the laboratory.

Distortion—production of a sound that is perceived by the listener as either visually or acoustically different from standard but that still has the basic characteristics of the phoneme.

Down's Syndrome—a congenital defect having specific mental and physical characteristics; mongolism. Children born with this syndrome are retarded mentally, physically, and socially to varying degrees—from very low-level trainable to educable.

Dysarthria—an articulation disorder resulting from damage to that part of the central nervous system that controls the muscles of articulation. There may be a paralysis or weakening of the muscles; speech will be affected.

Dysfluency—abnormal disturbances in the rhythm or flow of speech; *stuttering*. Persons who are dysfluent may repeat or prolong sounds or words or block completely on them. Their speech may be accompanied by facial grimaces.

Echo—repetition of part or all of an utterance that a person has heard. Parents use this procedure when they have understood only part of what a child has said or when they want to make sure that they have heard correctly.

Ego—a psychological structure that maintains contact with the external world in the interest of the total personality and its needs. Freud described it in detail.

Egocentric speech—the monologues of the child as he talks to himself. According to Piaget, this type of speaking is characteristic of children between the ages of four and six years.

Elaborated code—the use of a language system that encourages rational thinking on the part of the listener. For example, by explaining the choices available to their children, parents encourage their children to problem-solve, instead of giving them a directive.

Embedded clauses—subordinate clauses within the sentence. In *The boy who ran away is now at home*, *who ran away* is an embedded clause.

Emphysema—a condition in which the air spaces in the lungs are enlarged. As a result, breathing is difficult and the voice may sound weak and breathy.

Eustachian tube—the tube that connects the middle ear with the nasopharynx. There are two of them. The end that opens into the nasopharynx may be blocked by overgrown adenoids, causing the middle ear to become filled with fluid. Many people have conductive hearing losses as a result of the blockage of these tubes.

Expansion—a type of response in which a parent or another adult repeats a child's remark immediately after it has been said but changes it to include any grammatical or semantic corrections that are needed.

Extinction—the gradual decrease in the frequency of a response that results from the withholding of a reward. Someone who has received immediate attention whenever he yelled will stop when yelling no longer gains the attention of others. The reward of "attention" is gone.

Farquhar Discrimination Test—a measure of the *same* and *different* aspects of a sound within the framework of a distinctive feature analysis. The specific sound to be identified by the child is randomly placed with others that have no similar features and, finally, with those with only one feature difference.

Fixation—according to psychoanalytic theory, a defensive adaptation of a person to his or her environment. Development at one of the early psychosexual stages is arrested, and the person does not progress to a higher or more mature level.

Fricative—a speech sound that is produced by forcing the air stream through a narrow opening. For example [s] is produced by forcing air through the spaces between the central teeth.

Functors—the parts of speech (prepositions, conjunctions, and articles) that children tend to omit during early language acquisition. Children seem to be able to convey their ideas without them.

General American dialect—the principal dialect spoken by those who live in the geographic area west of the 13 original American colonies.

Generalization—recognition of the commonality of characteristics among a group of things, occurrences, or problems. In speech therapy we "discover" that *book*, *baby*, and ten other words all begin with the consonant sound, [b].

Geneticist—a professional person with training in hereditary diseases and conditions. He or she may be a member of a team concerned with conditions such as cleft palate or with diseases such as multiple sclerosis.

Glottis—the space between the vocal folds when they are at rest. Air enters and leaves the lungs through the glottis.

Grammar—a description of a language; the sum total of the rules governing the use of a particular language.

Habitual pitch—the fundamental frequency used most often when a person talks; a person's characteristic pitch.

Harshness—an unpleasant vocal quality that results from a combination of many factors; sometimes described as strident or grating.

Hearing impairment—acuity that is below normal, ranging from mild to complete hearing loss. It requires some adjustment of the person's communication, since his reception is faulty.

Hertz (Hz)—a unit of frequency of vibration; formerly called cycles per second. Pure tones ranging from 125 Hz to 8000 Hz are used in hearing tests.

Hierarchical structure—the arrangement of the parts of a sentence that shows the relationship of each word and each group of words to the total sentence.

High-risk baby—one who shows physical and/or neurological abnormalities at birth. Symptoms such as being "blue" or jaundiced, having difficulty breathing, or being premature will alert the attending physician to possible difficulties in development, including speech and language.

Hoarseness—a vocal quality with the characteristics of breathiness and harshness. There is no vocal fold adduction. A sore throat or laryngitis may cause us to sound hoarse because of the failure of the vocal folds to come together appropriately.

Holophrase—a key word that a child uses to convey an idea. Usually the word has a specific meaning, but the meaning is different in the context in which the child uses it. The person to whom the child is talking may or may not understand what is meant by the single word—thus the person "guesses" until he finds out the child's meaning.

Human communication—the interpersonal situation in which a person creates and sends a message to another person who receives it, understands it, and initiates a reply.

Id—according to the psychoanalysts, the original animistic aspect of the individual, governed only by the pleasure principle.

Illinois Test of Psycholinguistic Abilities, Revised Edition—a measure with 12 subtests, each of which measures a specific psycholinguistic ability. The authors have organized the subtests to separate out various modalities (visual, auditory, gestural, verbal) at two levels: automatic and representational. The results are used by speech pathologists, educators, and psychologists to plan remedial language programs for children.

Imitation—a procedure that involves copying the behavior of another, whether it is speech or a motor activity. Sometimes a child must be taught to imitate gestures and other motor acts before he can imitate speech. Imitation does not imply that the individual understands what he is repeating.

Impedance audiometry—a diagnostic procedure that permits the audiologist to measure the effect of any blockage in the middle ear on a person's hearing.

Incidental learning—the result of internalizing what a person hears and sees and, through cognitive processing, learning many things that have not been taught. A person "figures something out for himself."

Induction of rules—the formulation of grammatical rules and the utilization of those rules in speaking or comprehending a language. After hearing several examples of past-tense verbs, an individual "induces" the rules that enable him to form the past tense to talk about past events.

Inner ear—the portion of the hearing mechanism that is located in the bones of the skull. It has two principal parts: the cochlea (*see* Cochlea) and the vestibular mechanism, which controls our sense of balance.

Intensity—a term used to indicate the degree of loudness of the voice or of other sounds. There may be voice problems associated with intensity, or hearing problems related to the degree of loudness of the sound or speech necessary for the listener to hear.

Internalization—the incorporation of attitudes, standards, and opinions within the individual. According to psychoanalysts, the superego is derived from the internalization of parental attitudes.

Language—a set of verbal symbols whose meanings the people in our community or our society have agreed upon. The meanings are attached to both individual words and groupings of words.

Language acquisition—the learning of the linguistic structure of a language. It occurs over time; complete mastery of the grammar of English, with all of its irregularities, is probably not completed until age 12, with the semantic aspect never being completed.

Language deficit—may be defined variously as below the norm of a particular test or what a specific society expects linguistically or how an individual feels about his language. Criteria are set by schools, homes, and other units of our society.

Language disorder—a disorder associated with the deviant, delayed, or missing structure or with the functions of language. The structure includes the phonological, morphological, syntactic, and semantic aspects. The functions are various purposes for which we use language.

Laryngectomy—a surgical procedure that involves the removal of the larynx because of disease (cancer) or injury. Without a voice box or vocal tract, the person must then learn a different way of talking.

Laryngologist—a physician with special training who diagnoses and treats problems of the larynx.

Latency period—an interval of time between the reception of a stimulus and a response. We hear a noise, and there is a pause prior to our response.

Learning—the acquisition of any relatively permanent behavior or knowledge as a result of experience and practice.

Learning disability—a condition of children with normal intelligence who have difficulty learning school subjects and do not function at their intellectual capacity in the regular classroom. Persons with learning disabilities may or may not have oral-language deficits. Their problem may be in any or all of the academic subjects.

Mainstreaming—the placement of exceptional children in the regular classrooms for most of their academic programs. Special service personnel supplement the work of the classroom teacher providing help in reading, speech, language, writing, or math.

Malocclusion—a condition in which the upper and lower teeth do not come together properly. The upper jaw may protrude over the lower one, or vice versa. There may be an open bite—the upper front teeth do not meet the lower front teeth when the person bites down on his molars.

Mean Morpheme Length of Utterance (MMLU)—the average number of morphemes in a set of utterances. The phrase *give me three books* has five morphemes. By averaging the number in a series of similar utterances, we can obtain a mean morpheme length of utterance.

Mental retardation—a group of conditions characterized by inadequate social adjustment, reduced learning capacity, and a slow rate of maturation due to below-average intellectual functioning. Most of the mentally retarded have some language deficiencies, ranging from minimal to severe.

Middle ear—an air-filled space containing three little bones: (1) the malleus is shaped like a club; (2) the incus, or anvil, is attached to the malleus; (3) the stapes, or stirrup, is attached at one end to the incus and the other end to the oval window, the entrance to the inner ear. Middle-ear problems occur when these bones cannot move freely to transmit sound to the inner ear.

Modelling—the name of the procedure that parents and others use when they talk to a child. They are "modelling" the language structure and at the same time providing a great deal of information about endless numbers of topics to the child.

Mongolism—*see* Down's Syndrome.

Monitoring—a listening situation in which the person who is talking evaluates what he is saying and how he says it; or someone listens and evaluates what someone else is saying.

Monomorpheme—two words that are not segmented but appear to be one word, as, *the man*, *a book*. As children talk, they run such units together not "knowing" that they have spoken two words rather than one.

Morphology—the branch of linguistics concerned with the smallest identifiable linguistic unit that is grammatically pertinent, as, *book*, or the [s] added to make the noun a plural form.

Negative reinforcement—the use of coercive stimuli to reduce or prevent the probability of reinforcement. An example is a mild electric shock used when a person stutters, to reduce the stuttering.

Neurosis—an emotional or a psychological disorder that manifests itself in varying symptoms and degrees of instability. The repeated failure to complete class assignments on time is a neurotic symptom.

Object permanence—a step in child development when the child recognizes that objects continue to exist even when they are not in sight. He "knows" that toys are in the toy chest even though he cannot see them.

Occupational therapist—a professional person who works with patients to improve their skills in using their hands and the other upper extremities.

Operant behavior—a voluntary act that can be strengthened or weakened as a result of its consequences (the stimuli it invokes).

Oral communicative disorders—speaking and listening behaviors that deviate from the accepted pattern of the society or that signal a negative evaluation to the speaker or listener.

Oral stage—according to psychoanalysts, the first period of development, when the infant derives pleasure from nursing, biting, chewing.

Organismics—all aspects of our physical appearance, including physique, that affect our communication.

Orthodontist—a dentist with special training in straightening teeth. This specialist places braces on teeth. Persons with these braces may or may not have speech sound problems that are related to the malocclusion.

Orthography—the art of writing or printing the letters of the alphabet to spell the words of the language. Some persons have deficits in writing that are not related to any motor problem involving the hands; rather, they cannot conceptualize how words should be spelled and they may write an indiscriminate arrangement of letters that do not make sense.

Orthopedist—a physician with special training in the diseases of the bones, joints, muscles, tendons, and cartilages.

Otitis media—any infection of the middle ear.

Otologist—a physician with special training in the diseases of the ear and their treatment.

Otosclerosis—a disease of the middle ear, in which new bone forms and interferes with the movement of the third bone, the stapes. It results in a hearing loss.

Overgeneralization—the inappropriate application of any rule of the language, as when a child says *foots* for *feet*, *hitted* for *hit*, *climbeded* for *climbed*.

Palate—the roof of the mouth. The anterior part, called the hard palate, is bony. The posterior part, called the soft palate, is made up of muscle and tissue.

Paralanguage—the vocal characteristics and vocalizations that are a part of the production of oral language; and the body movements.

Peabody Picture Vocabulary Test—a receptive vocabulary test that requires the individual to select from four pictures the one that identifies the word the tester gives him. Although educators use it as a measure of intelligence, speech and language clinicians recognize that it measures only one facet of intelligence. The test is useful to us as an indicator of what vocabulary the individual understands.

Perception—the awareness of an auditory signal that may be a noise, a pure tone, a word, or a phrase. It does not necessarily include understanding of the signal.

Performance—the concrete, measurable use of the linguistic rules of a language.

Personality—according to Freud, the integration of the id, the ego, and the superego; the organization of all those psychological and physical aspects that determine an individual's behavior and thought.

Pharynx—the muscular and membranous tube situated in the posterior part of the mouth between the nose, or nares, and the esophagus. It is a part of the vocal tract and is continuous with the larynx.

Phenylketonuria (PKU)—a metabolic disorder present at birth. If it is diagnosed and treated early, the child may not be mentally retarded.

Phobia—a strong irrational fear elicited by specific stimuli or situations. Examples are the fear some people have of falling from high places and the fear of darkness.

Phonation—the production of a voiced sound generated by the vibrations of the vocal folds.

Phoneme—a single speech sound that functions analogously in a language, for example, [s].

Phonetics—the description and classification of the speech sounds of a language.

Phonology—the branch of linguistics concerned with the sound system of a language, including the rules that govern the use of the sounds.

Phrase structure grammar—the rules that enable us to analyze the surface structure of a sentence in terms of noun phrase and verb phrase.

Physical therapist—a professional person who works with patients to improve their ambulation and other lower-extremity actions.

Pivot-open word arrangements—a combination of two words, one of which appears frequently as the first word, in combination with many different words, as in *that book, that car, that truck.*

Pleasure principle—the law that we are governed by the search for pleasure and the avoidance of pain.

Plosive—a speech sound produced by building up air pressure in the mouth and then suddenly releasing it, as with [p] or [b].

Positive reinforcer—one that increases the occurrence of a particular response when the reinforcer is presented as a consequence of that response.

Presbycusis—a term generally used to describe hearing losses associated with old age.

Presentence—a two- or three-word utterance that is not a sentence; it does not have a noun phrase and a verb phrase.

Primary process—according to psychoanalytic theory, the means used by the id to obtain direct satisfaction of instinctive wishes.

Processes—the relevant parts or operations required for an activity like *communication* to take place.

Prognosis—a prediction the clinician makes about the future performance of an individual, based on all the information available about the person and his speech and language. The clinician often recommends a specific therapy program and predicts how useful it will be for the individual's speech and language problem.

Projection—an ego defense mechanism by which the individual attributes his own undesirable feelings and traits to others in order to avoid recognizing them as his own.

Prosodic features—the characteristics that accompany the production of segmental phonemes, for example, length, loudness, quality, and juncture points.

Prosthodontist—a dentist with special training in making and placing dental appliances. The person with a cleft palate may require a special plate to serve as a roof in the mouth. The plate is fitted and evaluated regularly by the prosthodontist.

Proxemics—the use and arrangement of space as an aspect of our communication. It involves our closeness to and distance from people.

Psychoanalysis—a system of psychology that seeks the roots of human behavior in unconscious motivation and conflict.

Psychosomatic disorder—one that is caused by a combination of organic and psychological factors. A person having a cleft palate (an organic problem) can also have an abnormal psychological reaction to the cleft. He may be unwilling to make friends because he thinks the cleft draws negative attention to his speech or personal appearance.

Quality—the characteristic of the voice associated with vowel production. For example, we say that the voice has a "musical" quality or "nasal."

Reality principle—the awareness of the demands of the environment and the need to conform to those demands.

Referent—the object, event, experience, or abstraction to which the meaning of a word points.

Reinforcement—a term used in two ways: (1) Skinner describes *operant reinforcement* as the presentation of a reinforcing stimulus when a response occurs. When a child is being taught plural forms, the clinician may give him a chip, or say "Good" each time the child gives the correct response. (2) Pavlov said that reinforcement takes place when the conditioned stimulus is presented simultaneously or at an effective interval before the unconditional stimulus.

Reliability—the degree to which we can depend on test scores as a measure of some skill. Some tests have two forms that can be administered and compared. When clinicians look at their reliability as testers, they measure their percent of agreement with themselves when they score the same material twice, or they can compare their judgments with those of other clinicians.

Resonance—the response of the cavities of the mouth, nose, larynx, and pharynx to the sound produced by the vocal folds. These cavities act to amplify or depress the sound.

Restricted code—a type of oral communication that uses concrete, here-and-now references. It reflects the authority of the speaker, such as the father in the family.

Retrocochlear hearing loss—a loss associated with areas beyond the cochlea (*see* Cochlea). There may be damage in the auditory nerve or at the level of the temporal lobe.

Roots—words that cannot be divided into any smaller units and still be meaningful, as, *fud*.

Rubella—a term synonymous with German measles. When pregnant women are exposed to or contact rubella during the first three months of pregnancy, there is a danger that the newborns will have a hearing impairment and other physical problems.

Screening—a procedure that employs a short battery of tests and/or observations to determine whether speech, language, and hearing are within or below normal limits. It identifies with those individuals who need further testing to identify the nature of their problems.

Secondary sexual characteristics—characteristics not related to the genital organs but typical of one sex or another. For example, the pitch of male voices is lower than that of female voices.

Segmental phonemes—phonemes arranged in a linear sequence, as in *but*.

Semantics—the branch of linguistics concerned with the meanings of words or groups of words.

Sentence—an utterance that contains a noun phrase and a verb phrase.

Separation-individuation—the concept of the self and the recognition of the separateness of others. Children develop it during the early years.

Shaping—the conditioning of a response through successively rewarding gross approximations and then closer ones until the desired response is attained. We can reward the child's gross production of [r], at first, then upon closer approximations, and finally upon the correct production.

Signs—motions, gestures, finger spelling, or manual language used to convey a message by themselves or in combination with oral language.

Social classes—categories based on the educational, occupational, and financial status (low, middle, high) of individuals.

Socialization—the teaching of behaviors and patterns of thinking that enable a child to fit into his or her society.

Sociologist—a professional person who studies social institutions and social relationships.

Somatopsychology—the discipline that studies the relationships of physique to psychological situations and the reactions of individuals.

Sound spectrograph—an instrument that graphically records the changing intensity of the various frequencies in a sound wave.

Speech and hearing scientist—a professional person who studies the normal and abnormal aspects of hearing and speech.

Speech pathologist—a professional person who provides appropriate speech and language services and/or engages in research in speech and language.

Speech production—the making of individual and combinations of sounds or phonemes by the speech mechanism. We are concerned with speech production as one part of oral communication.

Speech Reception Threshold (SRT)—the degree of loudness of speech required for an individual to understand it.

Speech sound discrimination test—a measure of the ability of an individual to identify similar and dissimilar phonemes. It employs sounds in syllables and words.

Spontaneous recovery—according to behaviorists, the reappearance of a conditioned response following a period of rest after experimental extinction. Unless reinforcement is given, the response will extinguish again.

Stimulus generalization—the learning that takes place when a person who has been conditioned to make a response to a stimulus can make the same response to other similar stimuli.

Stroke—a cerebral vascular accident that can damage the brain. Persons who have had strokes may have a resulting speech or language problem. Some recover their communicative skills without therapy; others require therapy of either long or short duration. Some never fully recover their facility in talking.

Sublimination—according to psychoanalytic theory, an ego defense mechanism in which unacceptable drives are expressed by adopting indirect socially approved behavior.

Substitution—replacement of a sound or a word with another one that is inappropriate or does not follow the correct rule. The child who says θɪθtɝ for *sister* is substituting the phoneme [θ] for [s].

Superego—according to psychoanalytic theory, a personality structure representing the internalized values of society.

Surface structure—the grammatical rather than semantic relationships of the words in a sentence to one another. In *he has a book*, *he* is the subject; *has* is the verb; and *book* is the object.

Symbols—the words and combinations of words that have meaning to us and to those in our environment. The words represent or replace the actual objects or events.

Symptom complex—a group of functional or structural changes in the individual indicating the presence of a disease or disorder. The person may have signs of a cold, laryngitis, and sinus drainage.

Syntax—the order or arrangement of words in an utterance. In a simple affirmative declarative sentence the subject comes first and the predicate follows.

Telegraphic speech—a shortened form of speech used by children; it contains the most important or key words. A child may say *book*, *table*, meaning *the book is on the table*.

Test—any systematic procedure that permits comparison of an individual's performance with the norms of the test or his own performance over time. Tests are available to measure many aspects of speech and language problems. Some tests are more reliable than others.

Tinnitis—a condition that consists of ringing, hissing, or roaring noises in the ear.

Trachea—the tube that descends from the larynx to the bronchi; it is needed for the free passage of air from the lungs to the mouth.

Transformational grammar—a set of rules that permits us to rearrange, add, delete, and change the words in a sentence and still have a meaningful sentence.

Unconscious—according to psychoanalysts, the psychic process that cannot be brought to a level of awareness by ordinary means.

Utterance—a word or string of words that may or may not be grammatically and semantically correct, as, *a big girl*, *who that boy?*

Velopharyngeal closure—the seal that is accomplished when the muscles of the soft palate are raised and approximate the wall of the pharynx. Air is then prevented from entering the nasal passages.

Vocalics—vocal characteristics that affect the communication of an idea.

Vocal nodules—callouses or growths on the vocal folds that prevent the vocal folds from approximating one another.

Vocal disorders—those associated with faulty pitch, loudness, or quality or with the absence of vocalization.

Vowel—a voiced sound characterized by the unobstructed passage of the air stream from the larynx through the oral cavity.

INDEXES

AUTHOR INDEX

SUBJECT INDEX

81 82 83 5 4 3